Musculoskeletal Ultrasound for the Orthopaedic Surgeon

ER, OR AND CLINIC

Christopher M. Jobe, MD, RMSK. Dean W. Ziegler, MD

CONTENTS

Chapter 6 Knee Ultrasound

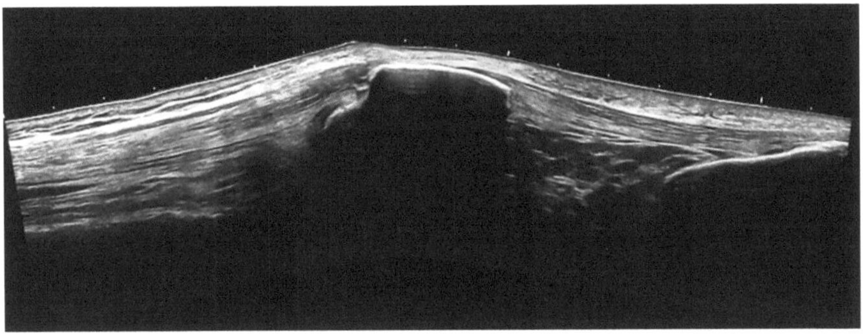

- Christopher M. Jobe, MD, RMSK

Introduction

Ultrasound is used more often at the knee for therapeutic purposes than for diagnosis. This is because the structures which are most frequently investigated, the menisci and the cruciate ligaments, are poorly visualized with ultrasound – if they are seen at all. On the other hand, ultrasound opens up other tissues and structures to investigation and at a lower cost than MRI. Many of the structures around the knee are close to the skin and parallel to the skin, which allows the sonographer to use positive and negative anisotropy to visualize them and differentiate them from adjacent tissues. Visualization of many of these structures will be superior to that obtained with MRI.

This chapter begins with the different ultrasound views and a brief review of the normal anatomy. We then cover some associated pathologies. Most of the chapter will be dedicated to ultrasound procedures in the office and operating room.

Normal Anatomy and Positions by Region

General notes on positioning

The structures we are examining are, in general, close to the skin and parallel to it. This will allow higher frequency and the use of anisotropy. The more anterior structures are usually better visualized in some degree of flexion and the more posterior in extension. The lateral side of the knee is more complicated, and in the posterior knee some degree of flexion is necessary to move arteries and nerves away from the joint and bones especially during procedures.

Distal Thigh Region/Quadriceps Mechanism

The anterior or quadriceps compartment of the thigh is made up of the four heads of the quadriceps as well as the adjacent nerves and arteries and skin. This area will usually be examined with a linear probe in smaller individuals and the curvilinear probe in larger individuals.

The pathology we are seeking in this area include: supra patellar effusions and infections; damage to the quadricep mechanism; and the adjacent nerves and arteries.

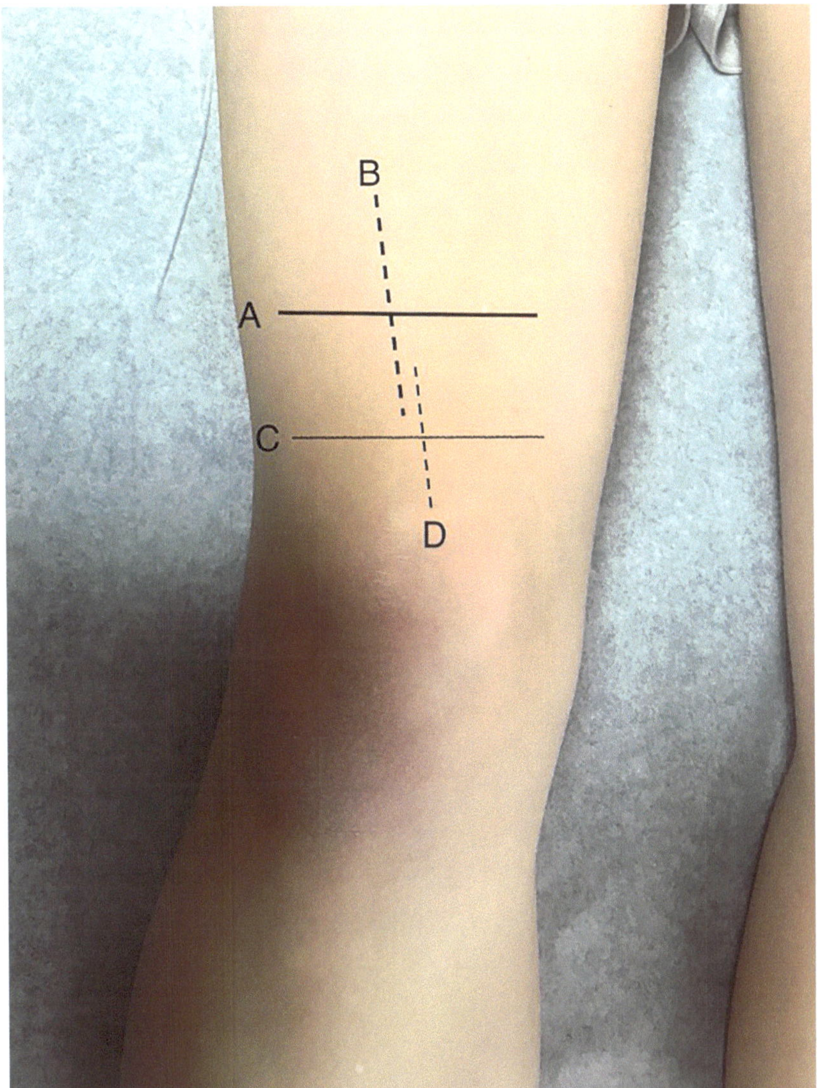

Figure 6-1a: probe contact lines A-D. A: short axis over the most distal muscle. B: Long axis over the tendon. C: Short axis over the most distal tendon just above the insertion into the patella. D: long axis of the insertion of the quadriceps insertion into the patella.

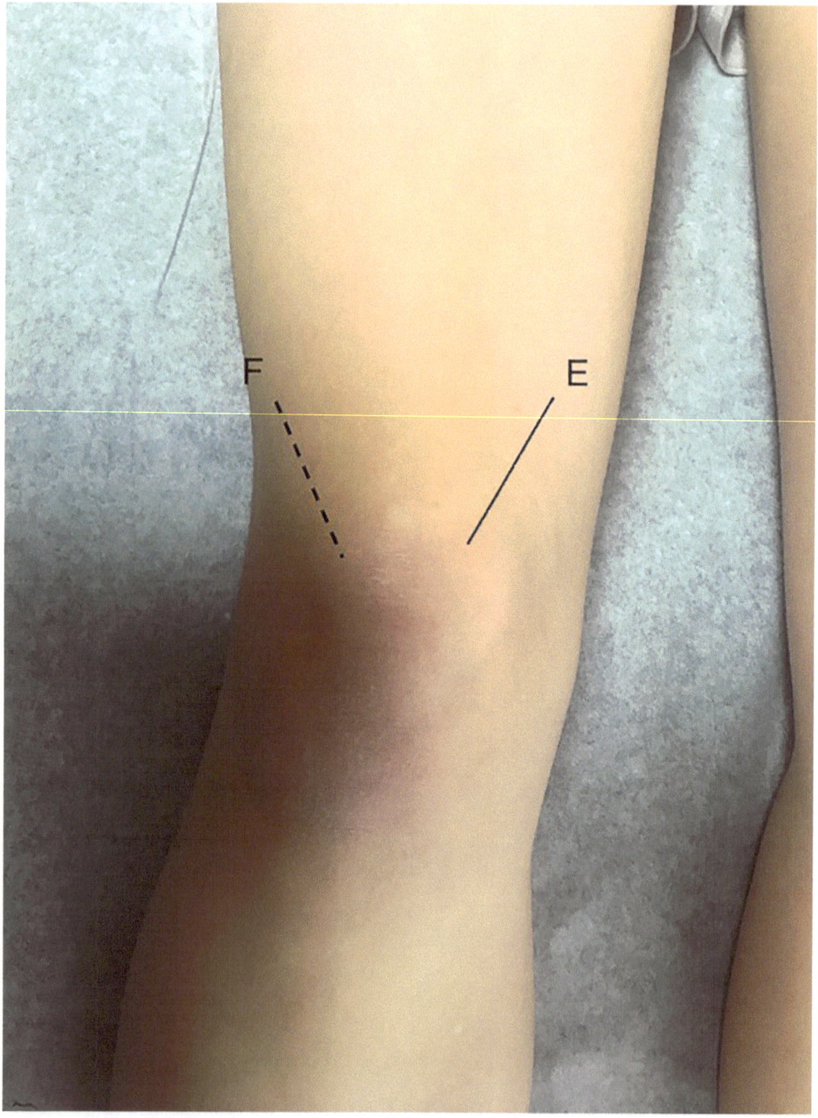

Figure 6-1b: additional probe sites: E: the long axis of vastus medialis. F: Long axis of vastus lateralis.

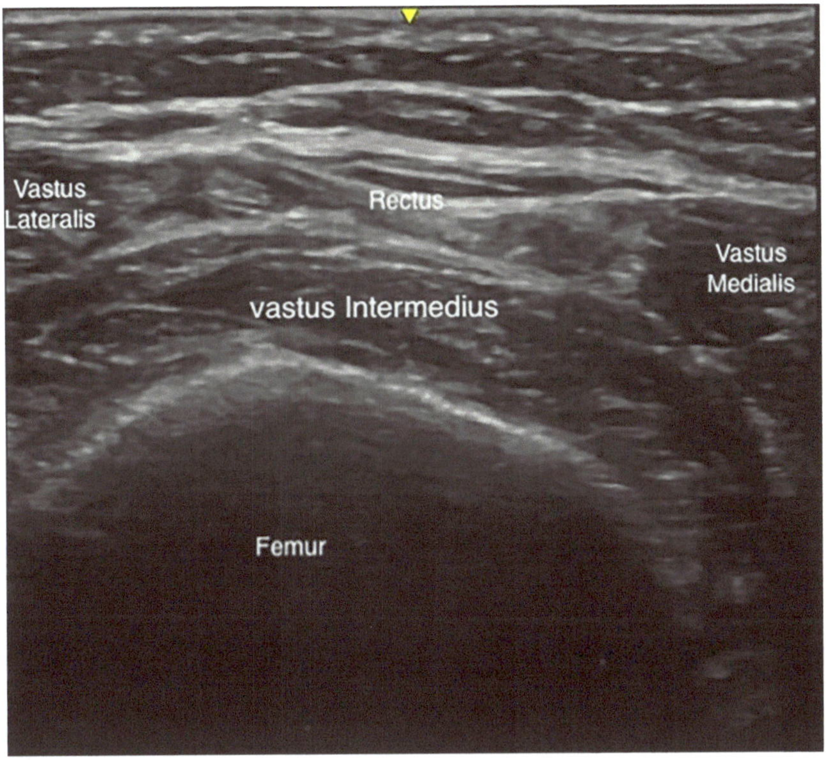

Figure 6-2a labeled.

All four heads of the quadriceps are represented at this level (Figure 1a: line A). The rectus at this point is just a tendon.

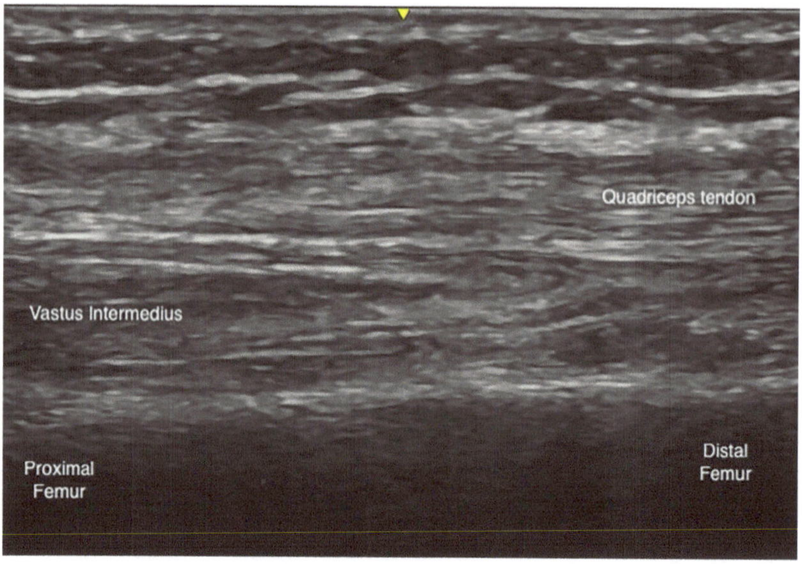

Figure 6-2b: Long axis view of quadriceps mechanism with the vastus intermedius rising to join the main tendon. (Figure 1a: Line B). The left is proximal, the right is distal.

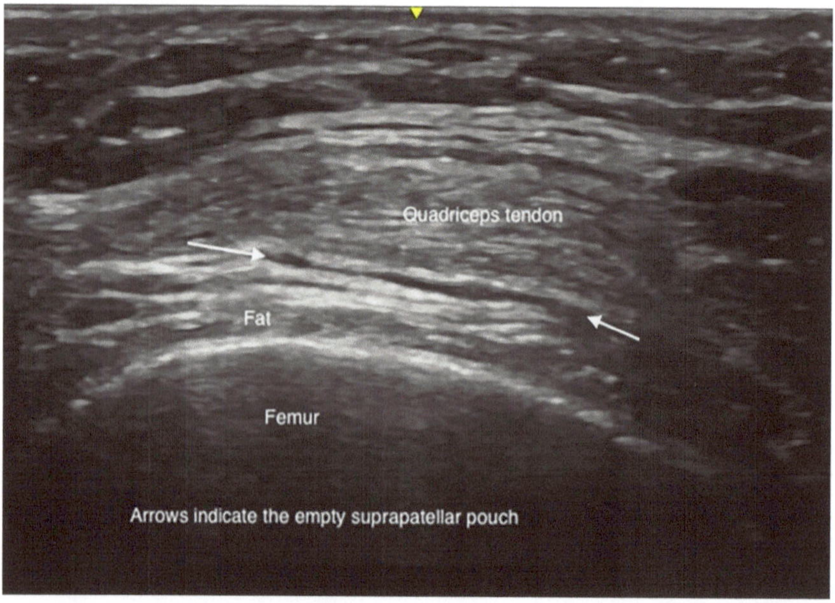

Figure 6-2c labeled: Arrows point to the empty recess of the suprapatellar pouch. (Figure 1a: Line C).

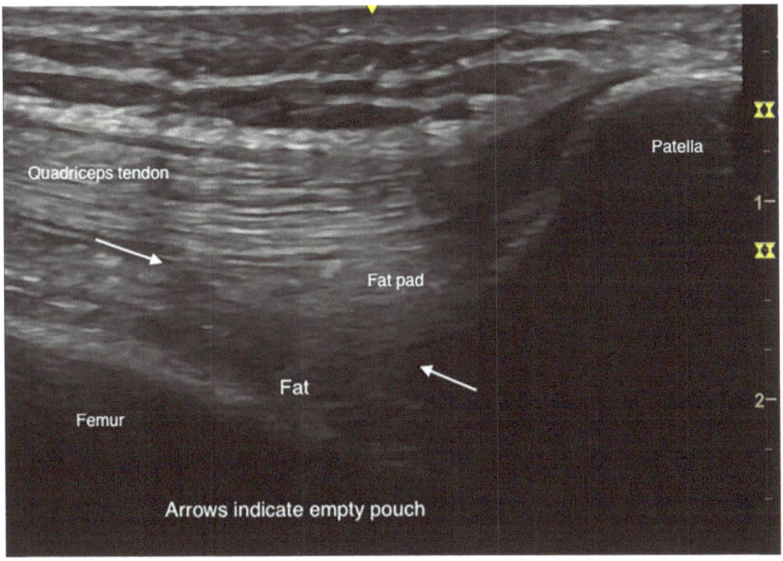

Figure 6-2d: Long axis pouch and insertion of quadriceps tendon onto the patella. The arrows point to the empty recess between the fat on the anterior femur and the fat pad at the superior pole of the patella (Figure 1a: Line D).

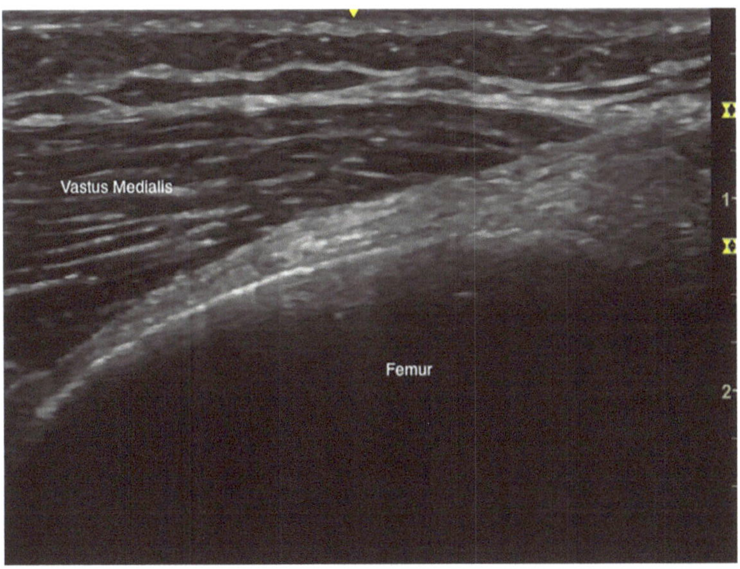

Figure 6-2e: Vastus Medialis as it approaches the patella. No fluid is seen between rectus and the femur (Figure 1b: Line E).

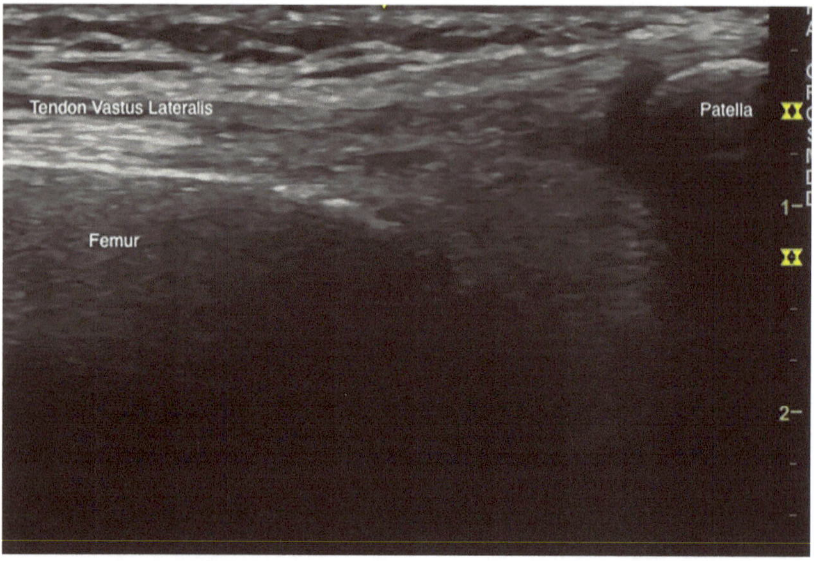

Figure 6-2f labeled: Vastus lateralis with its longer tendon but thinner structure approaching the patella. (Figure 1b: Line F)

Anterior Knee

The study of the anterior knee is essentially the study of the extensor mechanism. We can see the distal quadriceps tendon along with the retinacula and insertions onto the patella. Distally we can see the patellar tendon and its insertion onto the tibia and the fat pad behind the patellar tendon. And with Doppler we can see the blood vessels associated with the patellar mechanism.

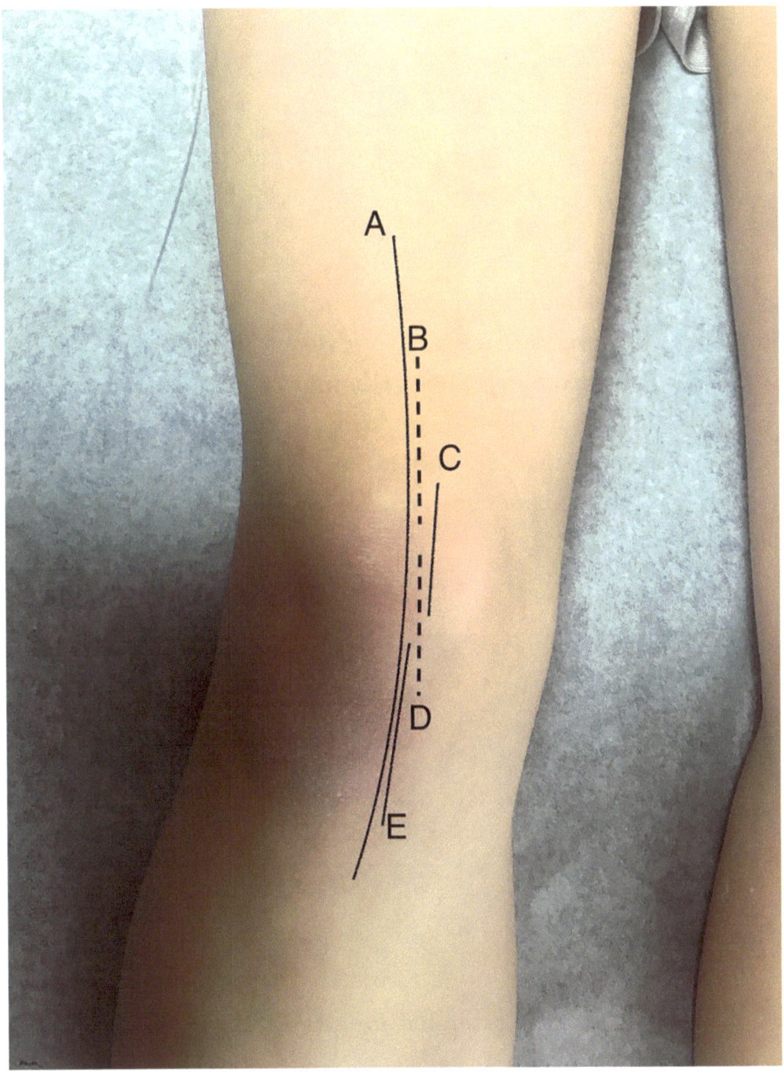

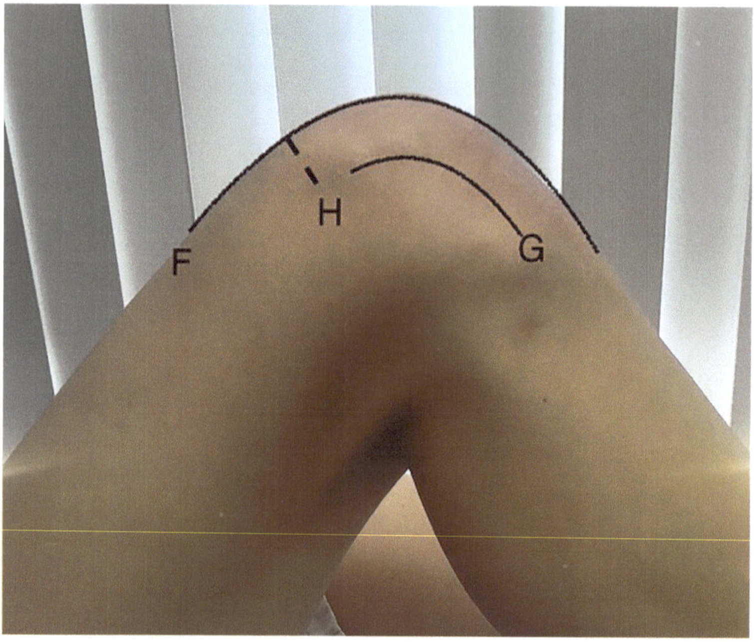

Figure 6-3: Photo of anterior knee with probe sites. A: extended long axis view of the mechanism; B: Quadriceps insertion. C: Long axis of Patella; D: Inferior pole of patella and origin of Patellar tendon; E: Long axis of patellar tendon and tibial insertion; F: Extended long axis of extensor mechanism in flexion with long axis view of upper trochlea; G: Long axis of condyle; and H: Short axis of the trochlear cartilage.

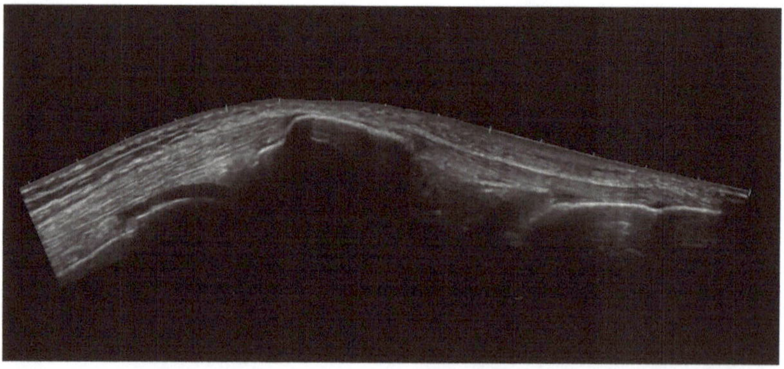

Figure 6-4: Ultrasound extended longitudinal view of tendons and patella.

Flexion puts tension on both the quadriceps and patellar tendons so that the observer can take advantage of anisotropy in viewing tendons and their insertions (Figure 3: Line A).

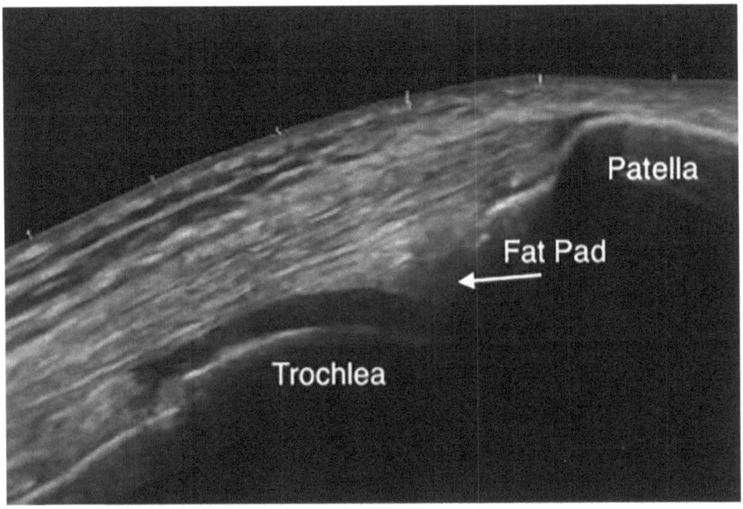

Figure 6-5: Ultrasound quad insertion with fat pad at the superior pole of the patella

(Figure 3: Line B). The hypoechoic area on the trochlea is articular cartilage.

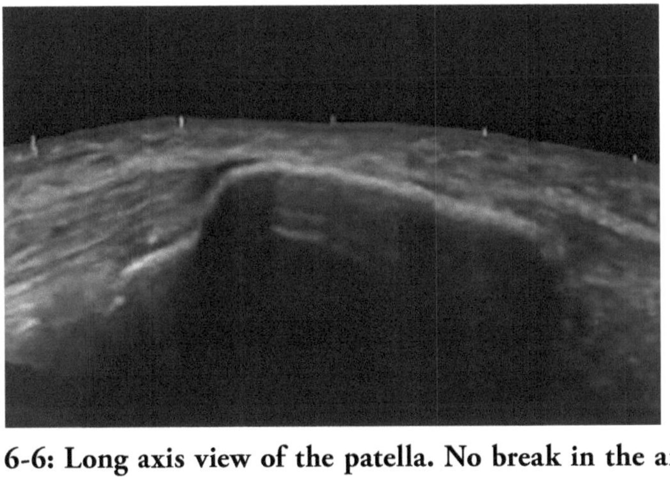

Figure 6-6: Long axis view of the patella. No break in the anterior cortex nor bursal fluid seen. Line 3 C

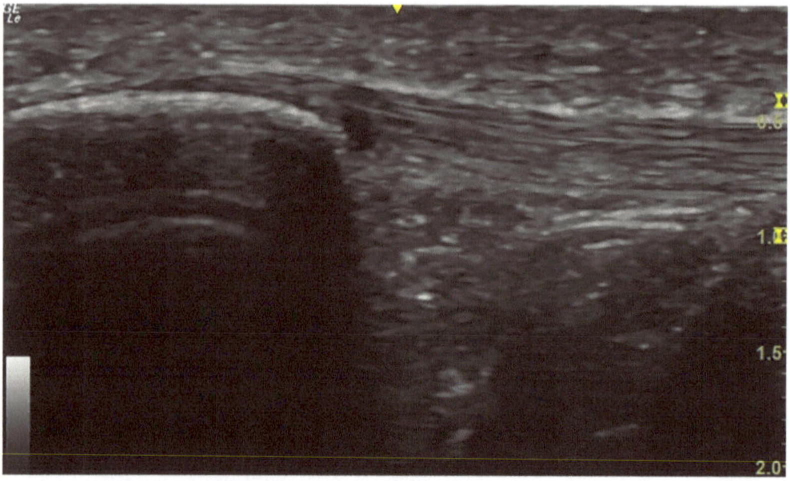

Figure 6-7: The patella tendon origin from the inferior pole has no change in echogenicity nor vessel invasion. Line 3 D

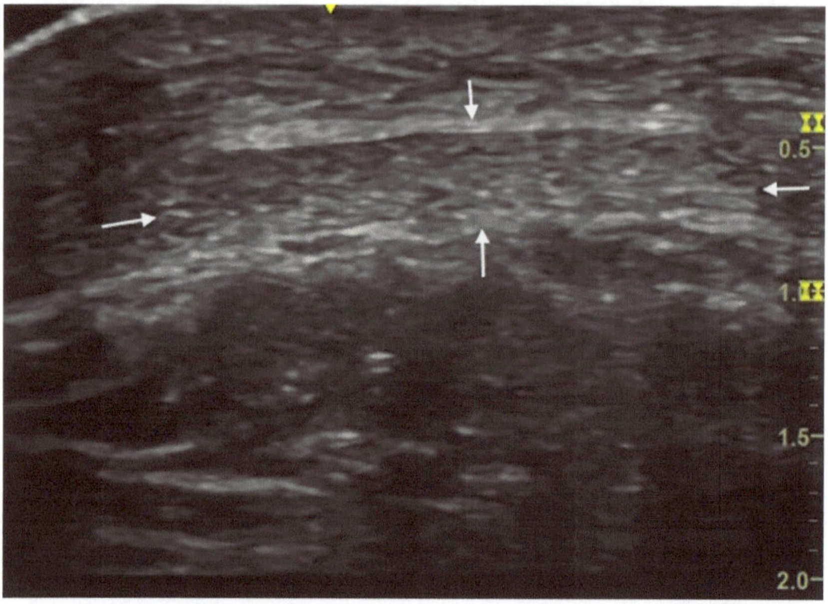

Figure 6-8a: Short axis view of patellar tendon with normal echogenicity.

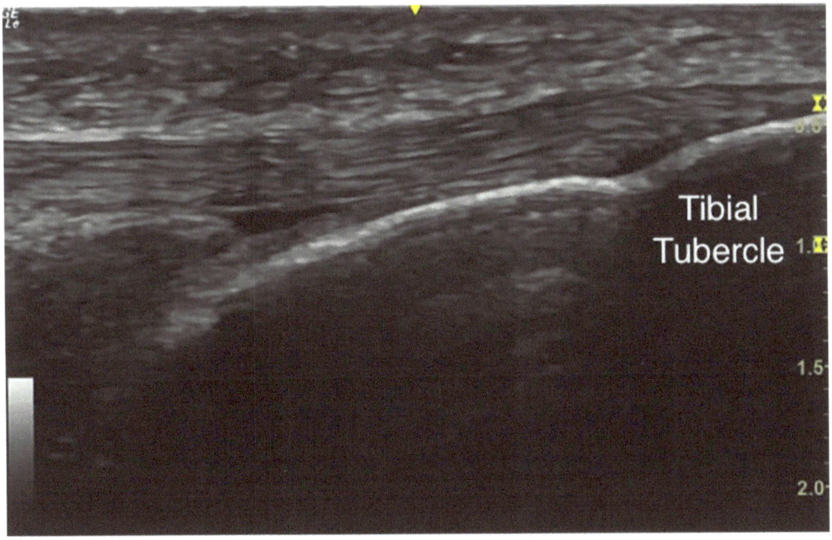

Figure 6-8b: Long axis view of the patellar tendon and its insertion (Fig 3 line E)

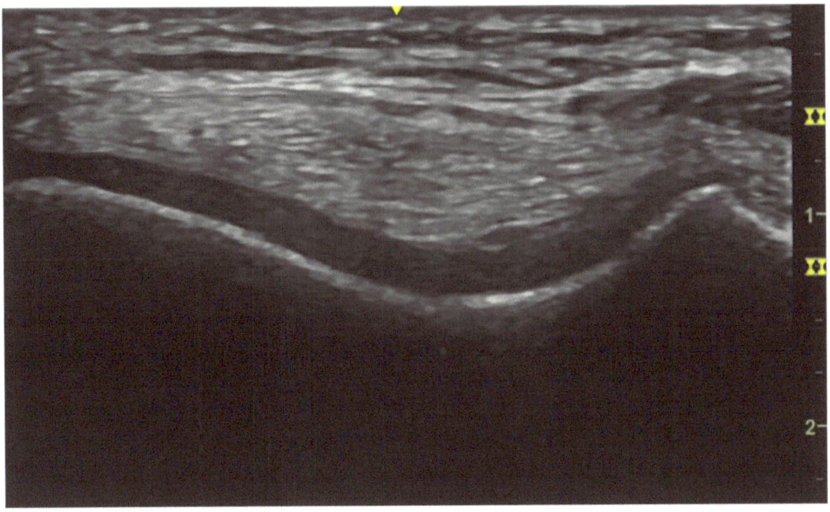

Figure 6-9: Short axis view of trochlea with the knee in flexion shows a normal trochlear cartilage and a short axis view of the quadriceps tendon (Figure 3: Line H).

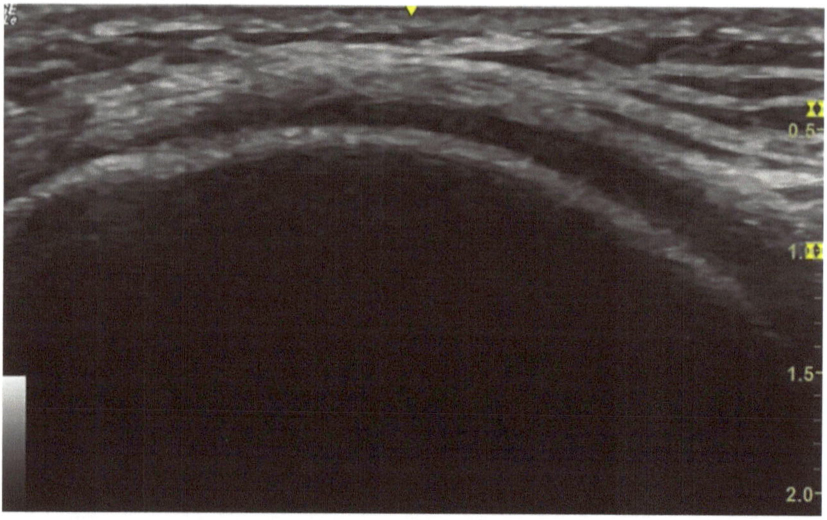

Figure 6-10: Moving to either side of the patellar mechanism with the knee in flexion we can look at the articular cartilage on the condyle. The cartilage is the dark hypoechoic area attached to the hyperechoic bone layer (Figure 3: Line G).

Medial knee

On the medial side of the knee there are two main long axis approaches, one overlying the medial collateral ligament, MCL, and the other over the posterior oblique ligament, POL. In the MCL view one can see, in addition to the MCL, the medial meniscus, the inferior medial geniculate artery and the pes anserine tendons. In the POL view one can see the semimembranosus in its groove in the tibia and some of the medial meniscus, when the knee is in partial flexion. In full extension the posterior medial muscles move anterior and obscure the posterior medial corner somewhat.

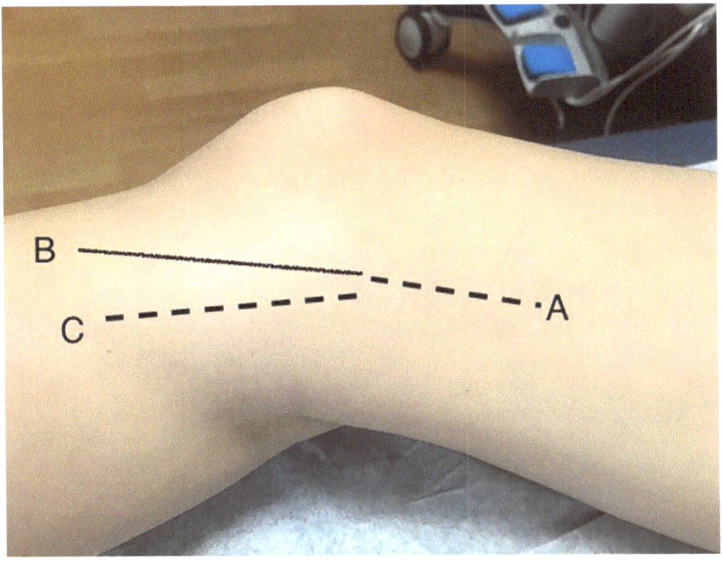

Figure 6-11a: Medial side in slight flexion. The thigh is to the right and the leg to the left. Line A: medial flair of the femur. Line B the lower MCL, medial meniscus and short axis of the pes insertion. Line C Posterior oblique ligament, semimembranosus insertion and more meniscus.

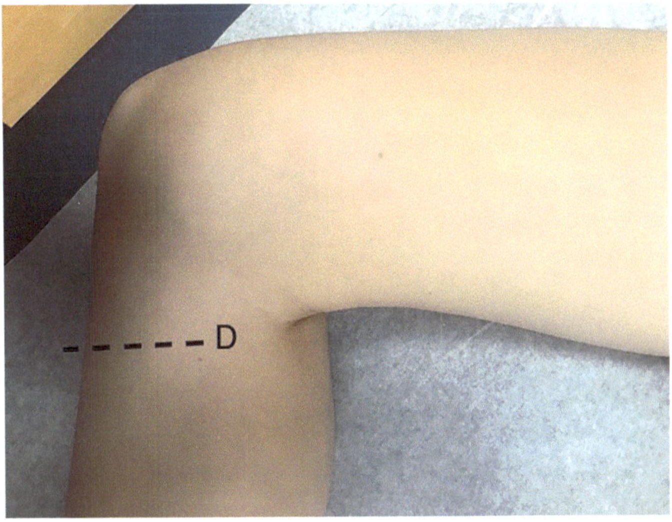

Figure 6-11b: Medial side of the knee in 90 degrees of flexion. Line D images short axis of upper tibia but long axis of pes insertion.

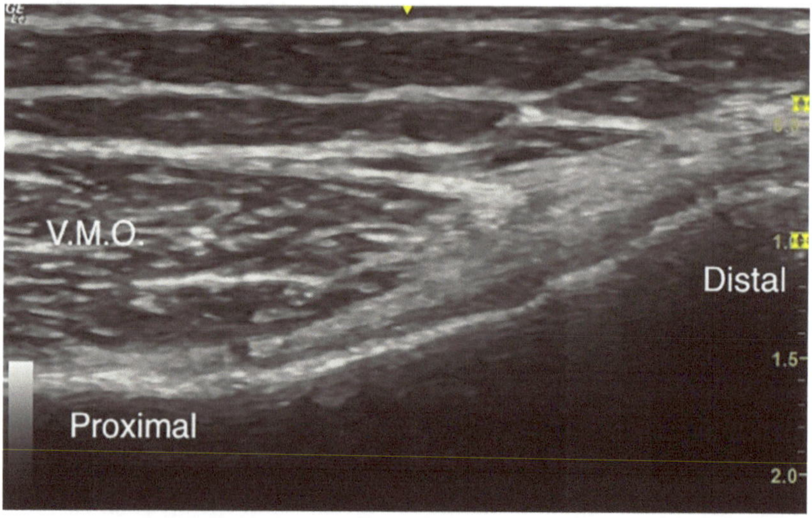

Figure 6-12a: Medial flair of the femur with the VMO on the left (Figure 11: Line A).

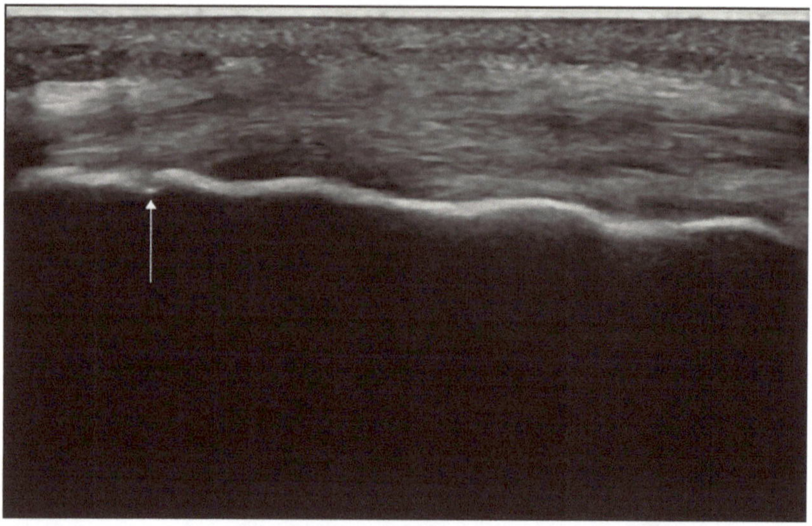

Fig. 6-12b: The proximal insertion of the MCL (arrow) (Figure 11 A line B).

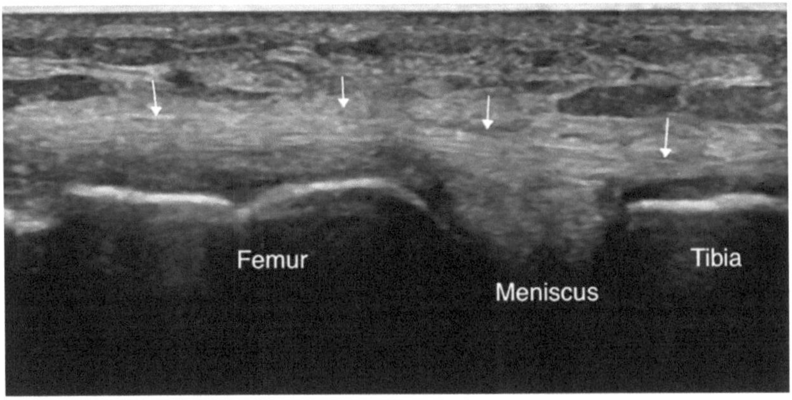

Figure 6-12c: The medial meniscus with the upper MCL lying against the medial femoral condyle (Figure 11a: Line B).

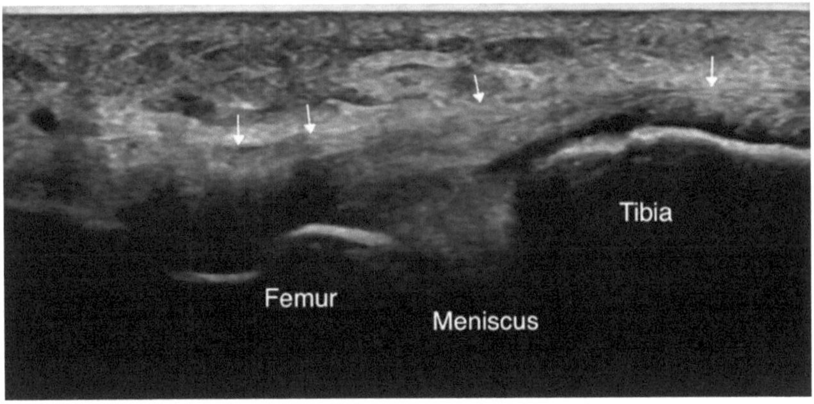

Figure 6-12d: Posterior MCL (arrows) in slight flexion. Note the slight laxity of the ligament.(Figure 11a: Line B).

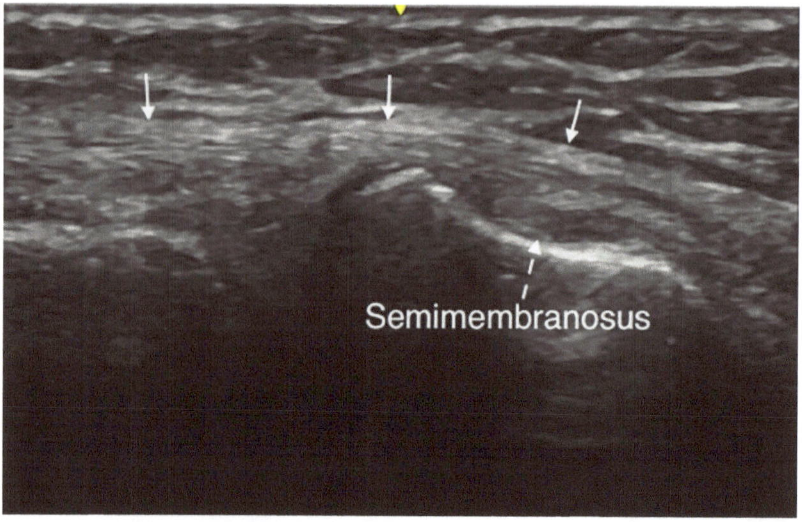

Figure 6-12e: Posterior portion of the MCL (arrows), arching over the anterior arm of the semimembranosus (Figure 11a: Line C).

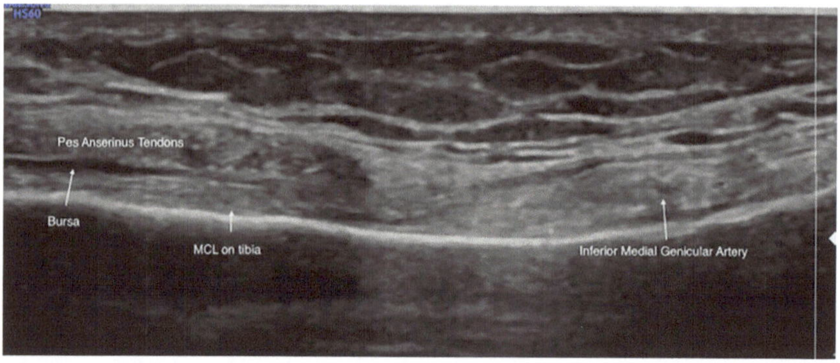

Figure 6-13a: The medial flare of the tibia, in the long axis of the tibia, shows the lower MCL in long axis and the tendons of the pes anserinus in short axis (Figure 11a: Line B).The proximal tibia is to the right and the distal to the left.

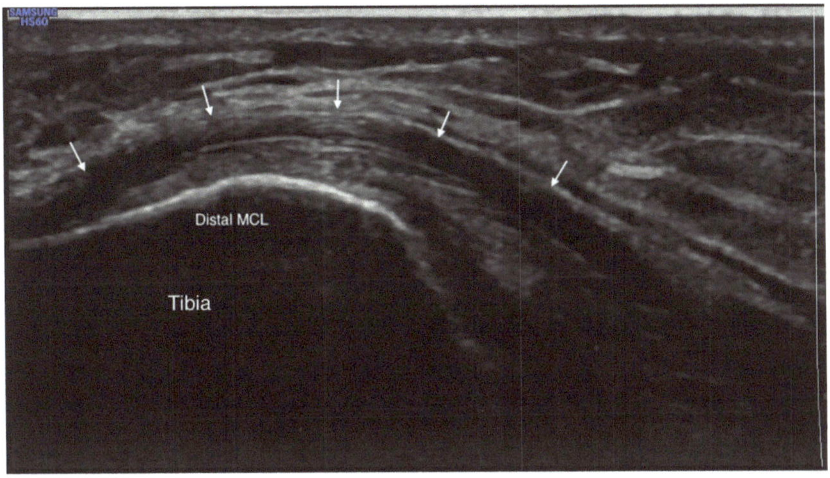

Figure 6-13b: The semitendinosus (arrows), which is dark with anisotropy, crosses the MCL which is lying on the tibia (Figure 11b: Line D).

Lateral Knee

Motion at the knee is a combination of spinning, rolling and sliding. The medial side is the site of tibial rotation and for the first 90% of flexion is essentially a spinning motion in the sagittal plane. The lateral side, as it is farther away from the axis of tibial rotation, has more rolling and sliding and therefore a more complex ligamentous arrangement.

One goal of the sonographer is to put the ligament or tendon being examined under tension so that the effects of anisotropy are more uniform. We therefore show the positions of the ligaments and their alignment, but we also need to list the position of the knee with respect to: flexion-extension, varus-valgus and tibial rotation.

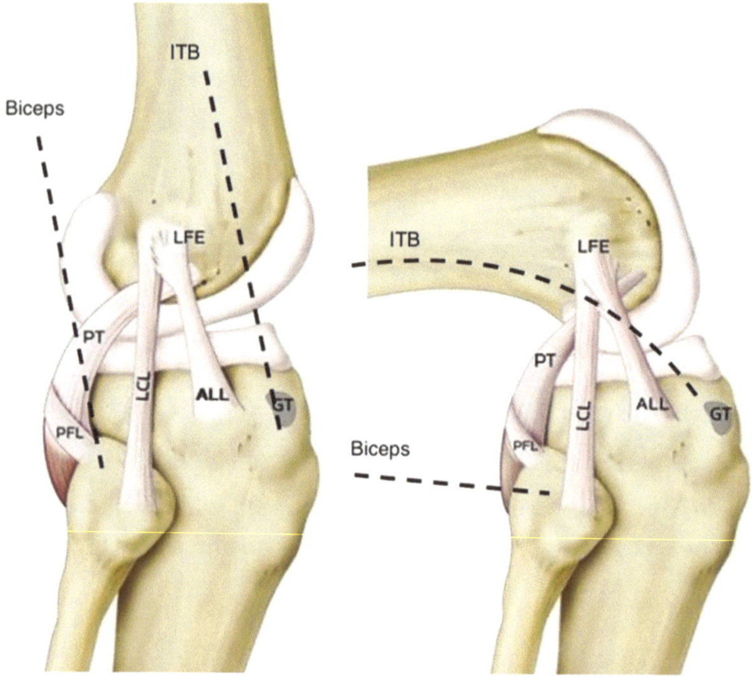

Figure 6-14: Positions of the ligaments and tendons in extension and flexion. Varus stress is helpful to greater and lesser degrees.

Table 1: Positions for tensioning ligaments/tendons.

Ligament/Tendon	Flexion/Extension	Varus/Valgus	Tibial Rotation
Popliteus	Flexion	Varus	Lateral
Popliteus-Fib. Lig.	Flexion	Varus	Lateral
Fibular Collateral	Extension	Varus	Lateral
Antero-Lateral	Flexion	Varus	Medial
ITB	-----	Varus	Medial

The positions of the tendons and ligaments vary more on the lateral side of the knee. For this reason there are not standard positions delineated as on the other three sides

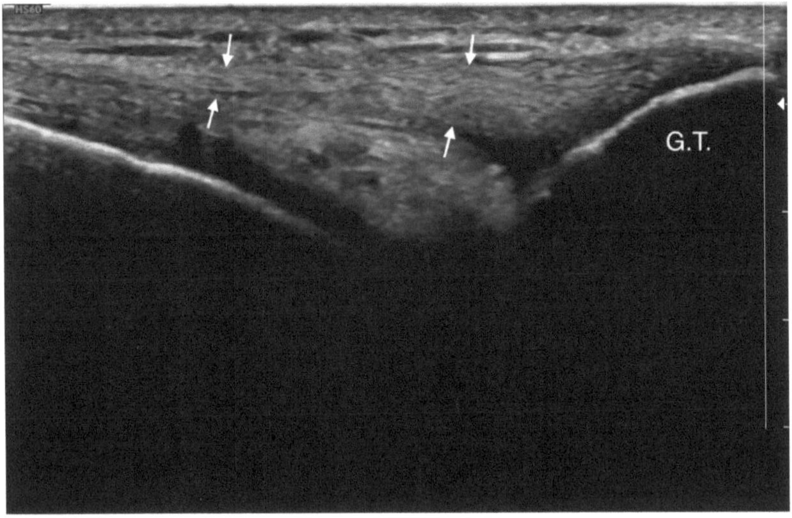

Figure 6-15: Iliotibial band (arrows) inserts on Gerdy's tubercle after passing over some fatty tissue with blood vessels.

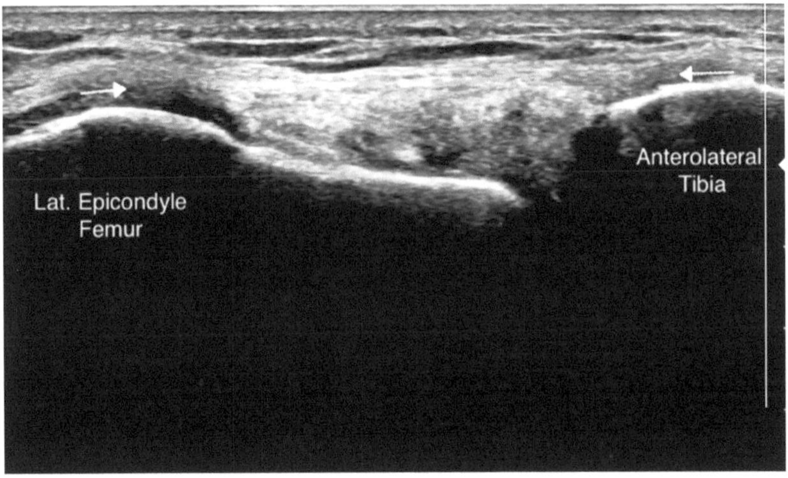

Figure 6-16: Anterolateral ligament (lateral capsular ligament) takes origin just in front of the origin of FCL (right pointing arrow) and inserts into the tibia behind Gerdy's tubercle (left pointing arrow).

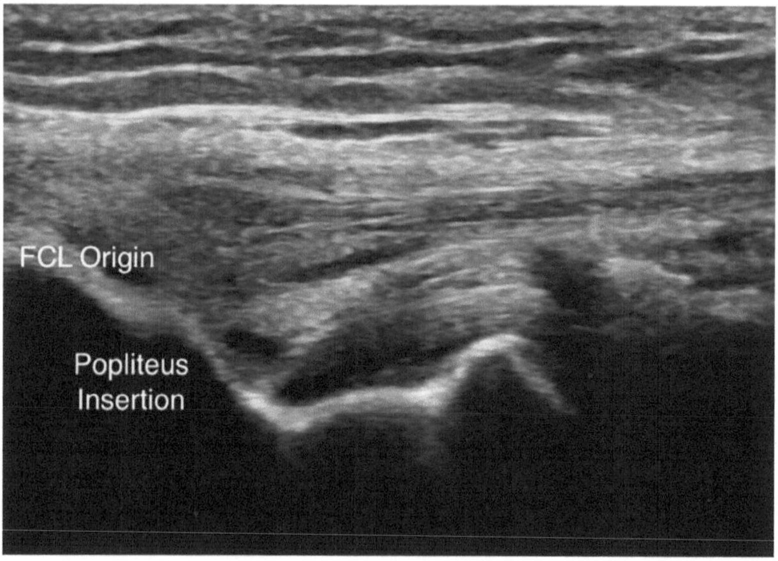

Figure 6-17a: The popliteus tendon inserts into the femur just deep and distal to the origin of the FCL. Because of its curved course one cannot observe the entire popliteus in one view. Because the popliteus is a weak extensor of the knee, flexion pulls a little bit more of the tendon into the knee. Flexion also makes these two structures more parallel. (See Fig. 14)

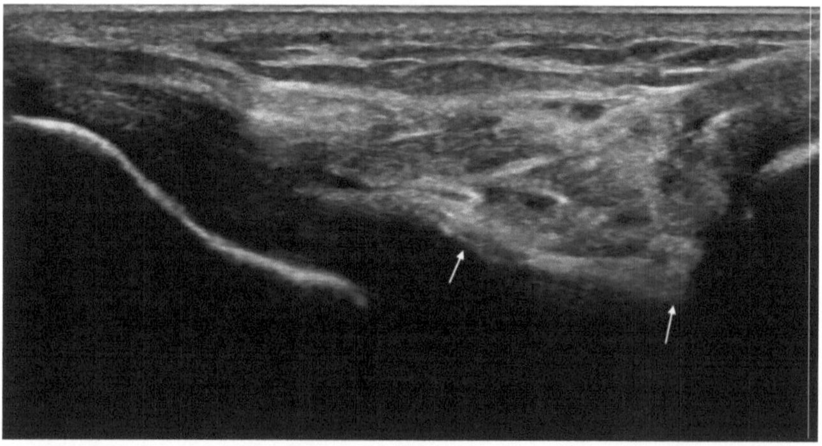

Figure 6-17b: Above, popliteal fibular ligament (curved arrow) is probably seen better, or at least easier, on MRI. It is difficult on ultrasound.

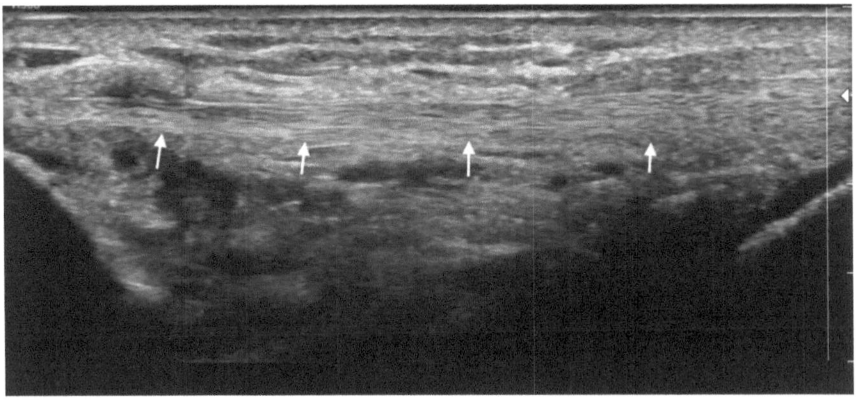

Figure 6-18a: Under varus stress the lateral collateral ligament is taut and more easily seen.

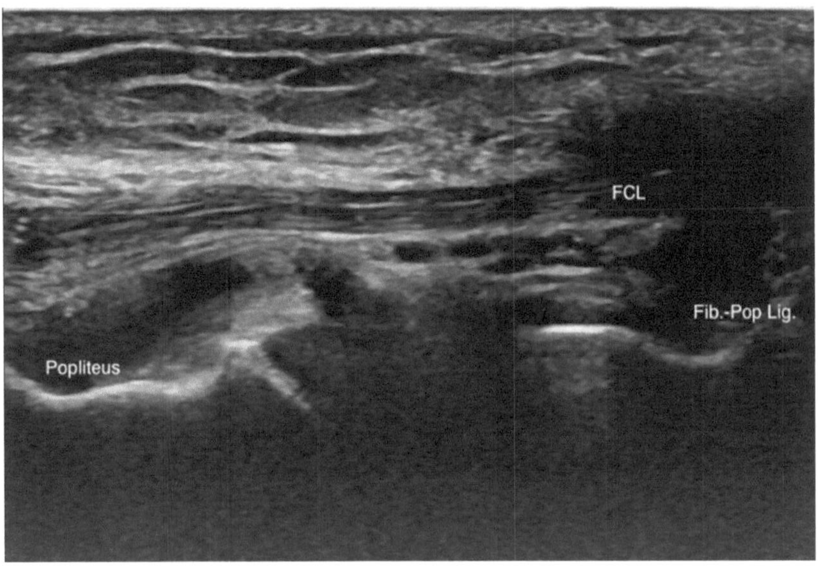

Figure 6-18b: This view shows the FCL origin just superior to the femoral attachment of the popliteus and in proximity on the fibula to the popliteal fibular ligament.

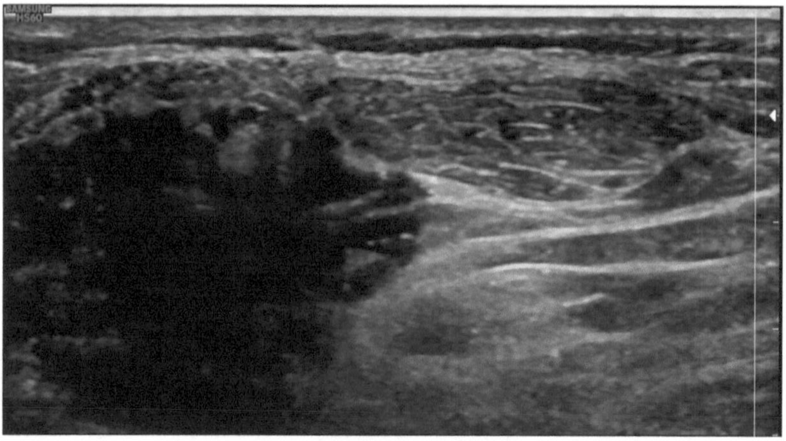

Figure 6-19a: A tendon develops along the posterior biceps muscle.

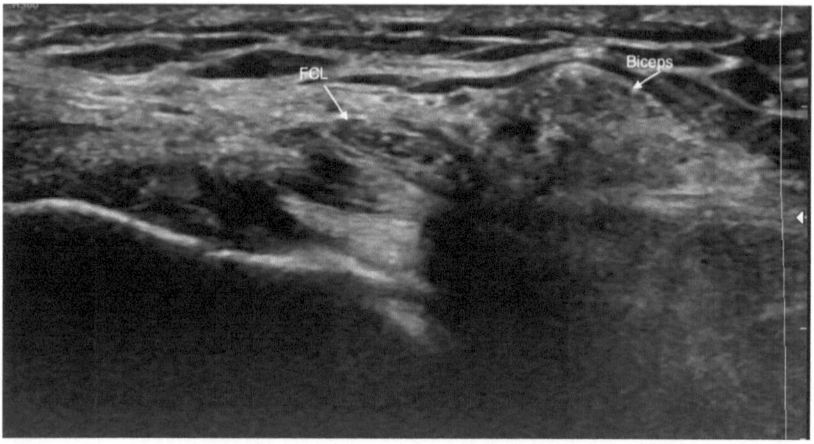

Figure 6-19b: Viewed in extension the biceps tendon and the FCL get closer to each other as they approach the fibula. The biceps splits as it inserts with a large portion going lateral.

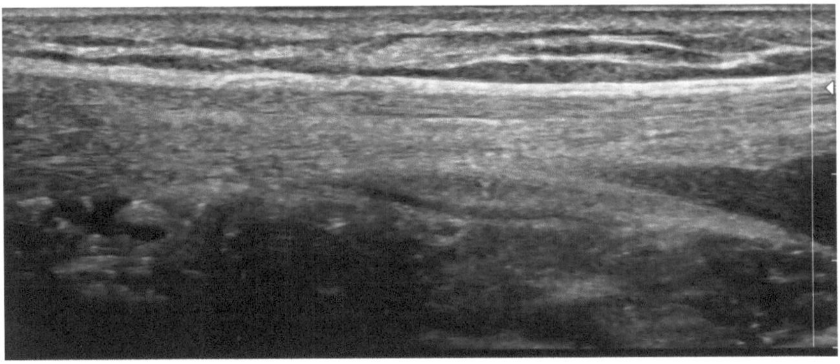

Figure 6-19c: A long view of the biceps tendon.

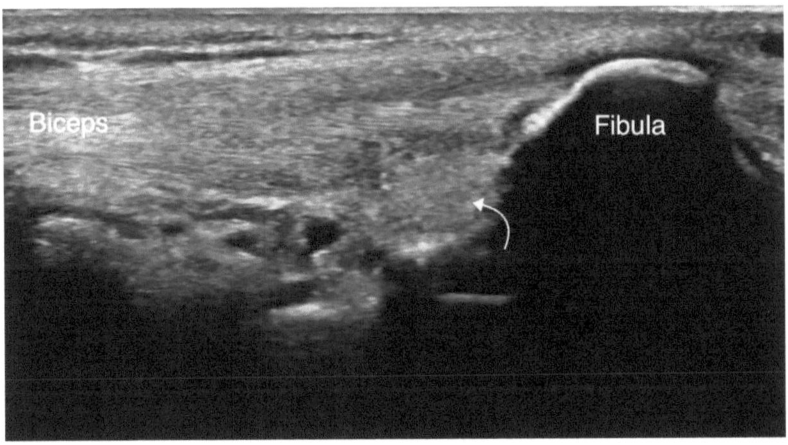

Figure 6-19d: Note how the biceps tendon divides as it inserts. It goes on either side of the FCL insertion (curved arrow), providing a dynamic tension to that ligament when biceps femoris is active.

A short axis view of the biceps femoris.

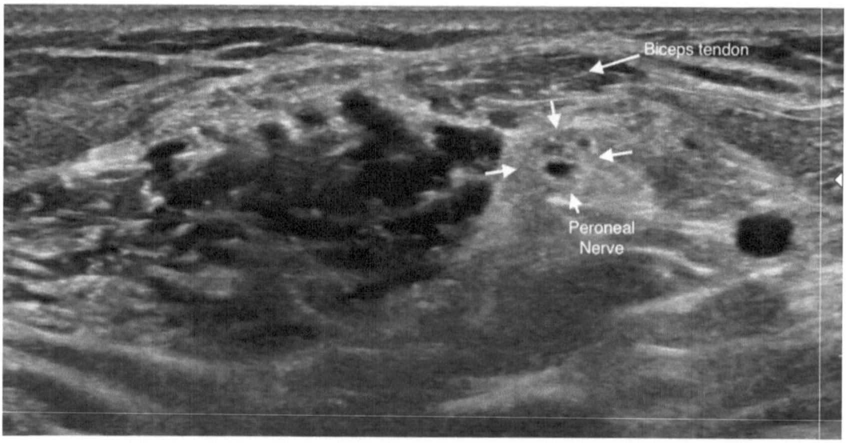

Figure 6-19e: The peroneal nerve travels posteriorly just medial to the biceps tendon. In this view the probe is on the lateral surface proximal to the knee.

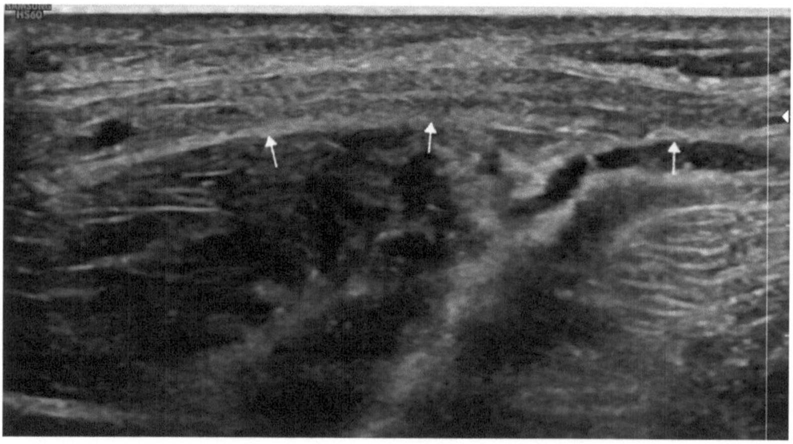

6-19f: Long axis view of the peroneal nerve as it passes into the anterolateral leg. Left is proximal and right is distal.

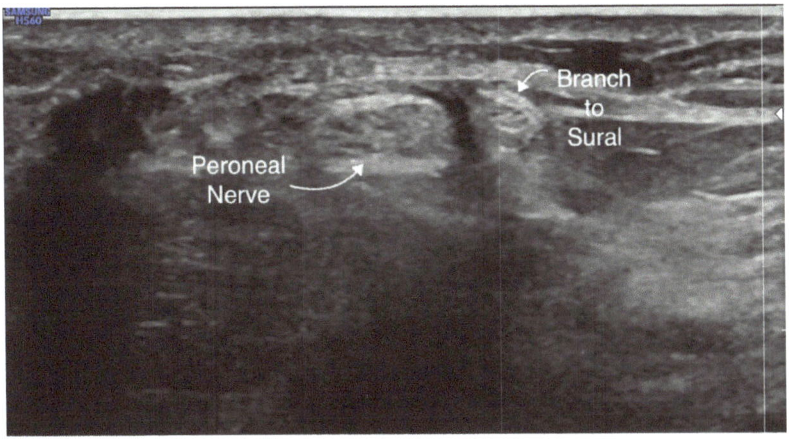

Fig 6-19g: The peroneal branch to the sural nerve separating from the parent nerve proximal to entering the leg.

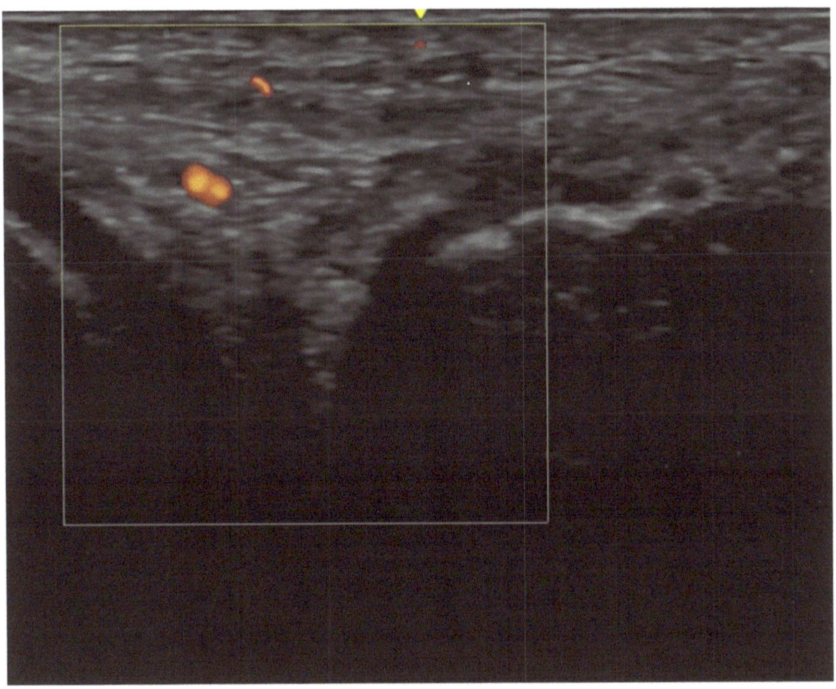

Figure 6-20: Lateral meniscus and lateral inferior genicular artery with Doppler. The lateral inferior genicular artery travels just at the outside periphery of the lateral meniscus.

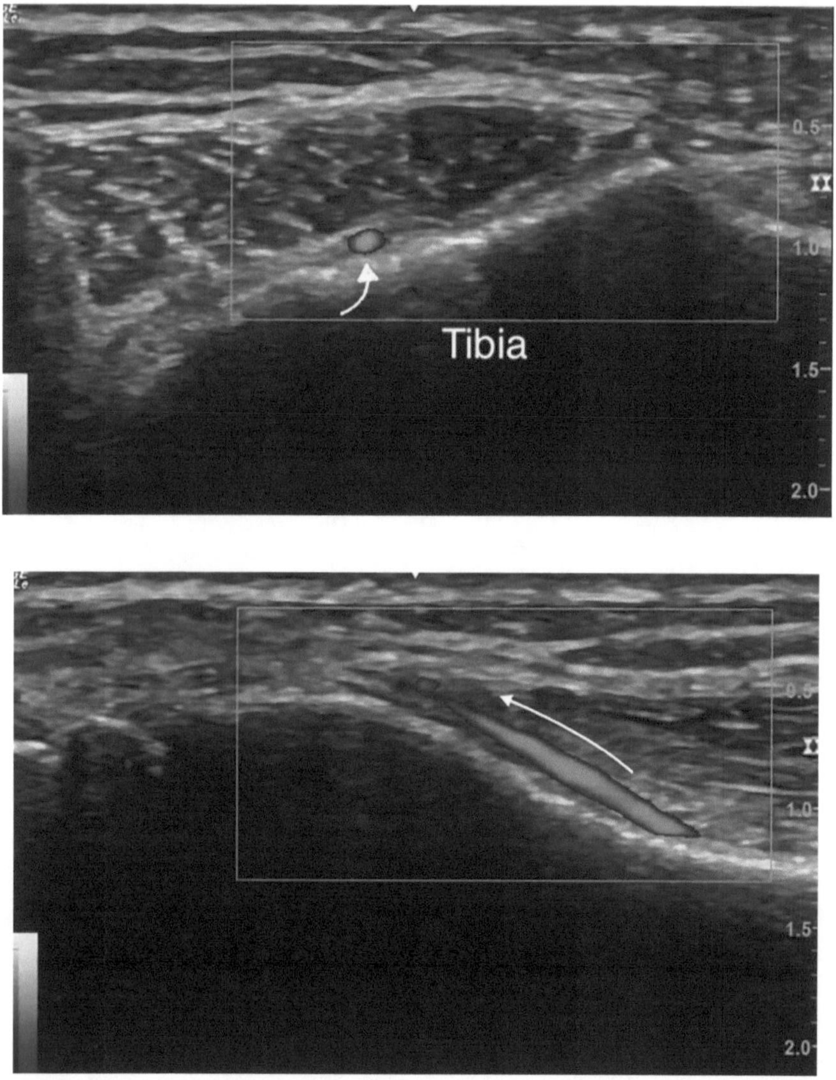

Figure 6-21a & b: Short and long axis views of the recurrent anterior tibial artery. The artery comes off of the anterior tibial artery and serves as part of the blood supply of the knee.

Posterior Knee Anatomy

The posterior knee contains proximally the muscles: semimembranosus, semitendinosus and biceps femoris. More distally we see both heads of the gastrocnemius and the origin of plantaris. The more visible nerves are the common peroneal and the tibial. In addition, we see the popliteal artery and vein system and its genicular branches.

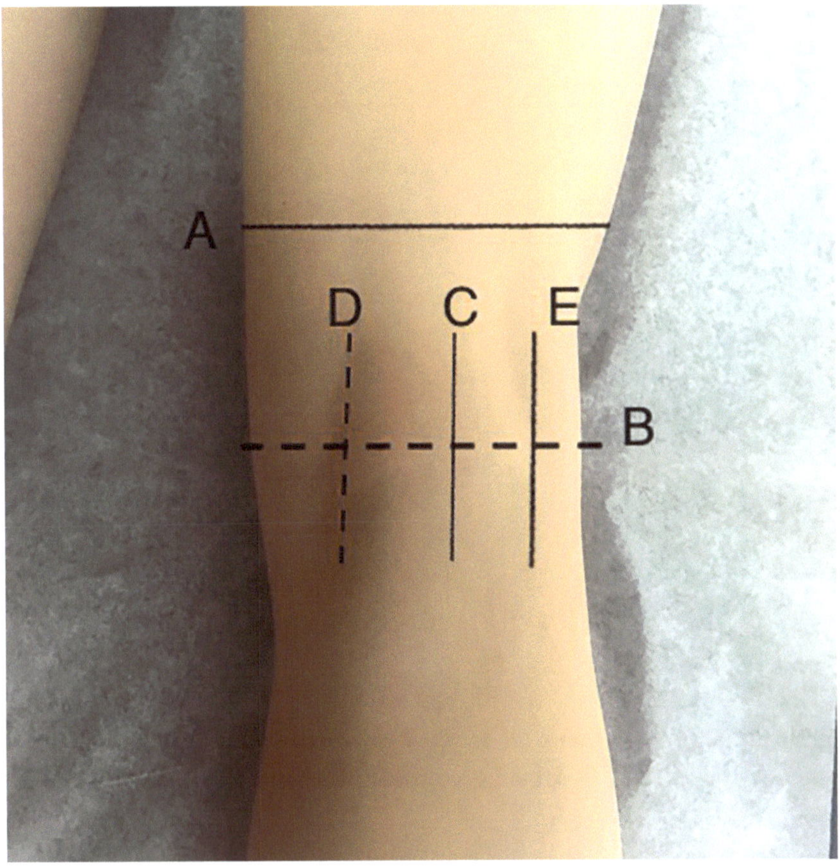

Figure 6-22: Photo of posterior knee with probe contacts A: short axis of the limb above the condyles; B: short axis at and below the condyles; C: long axis view in the mid-line of the knee; D: long axis over the medial compartment; and E: long axis view of the lateral compartment.

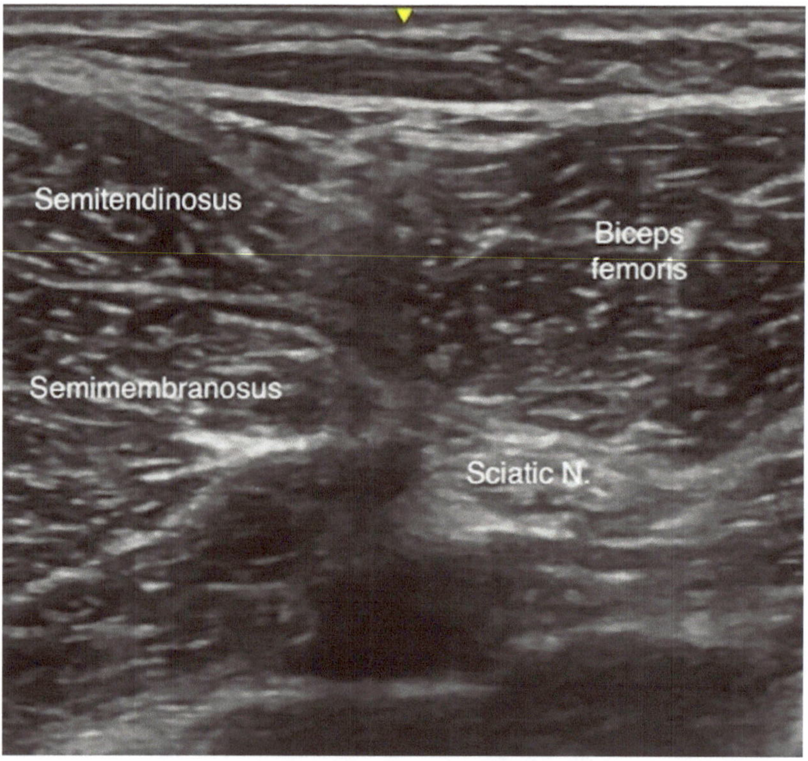

Figure 6-23a : Ultrasound transverse distal posterior thigh above the condyles. The lateral side is right and the medial left (Figure 22: Line A).

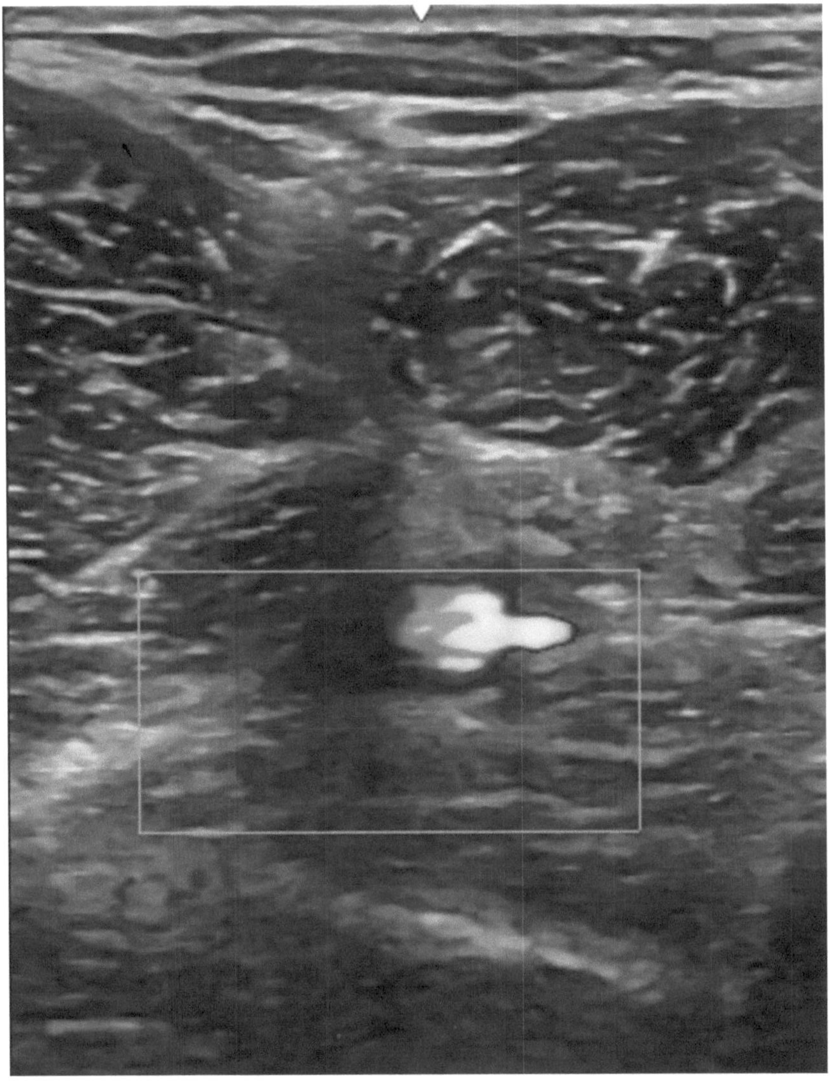

Figure 6-23b: This is a Doppler view of the popliteal artery at the same level as the previous figure. (Figure 22: Line A).

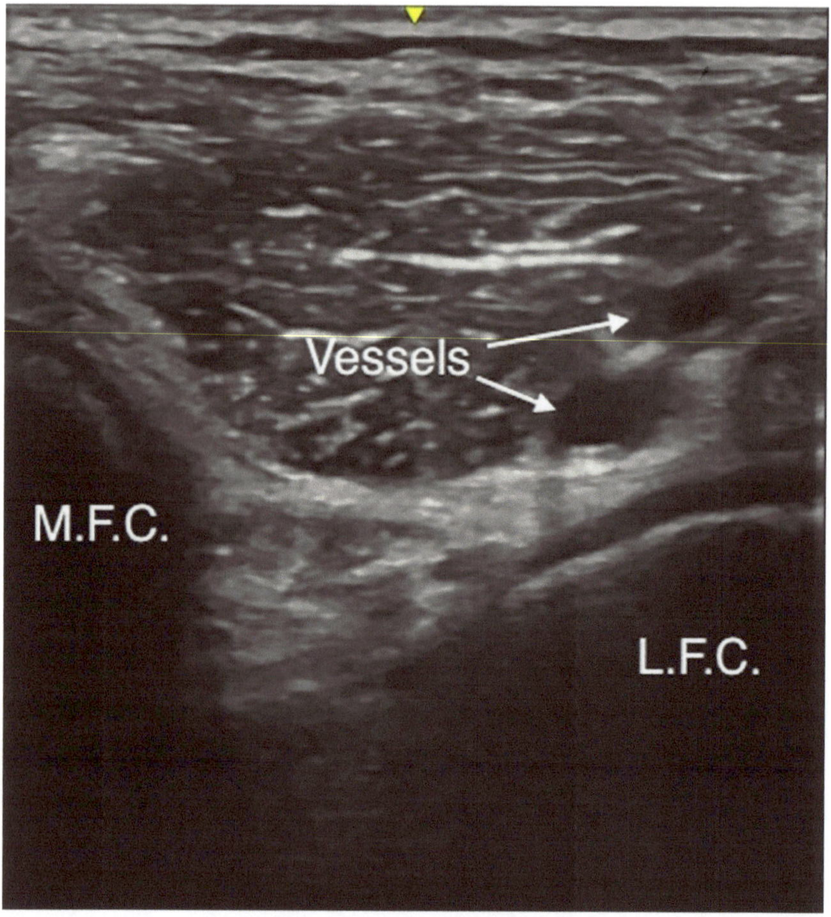

Figure 6-24: Ultrasound short axis at the condyle level. Note that the vessels are not exactly in the middle between the condyles. (Figure 22: Line B).

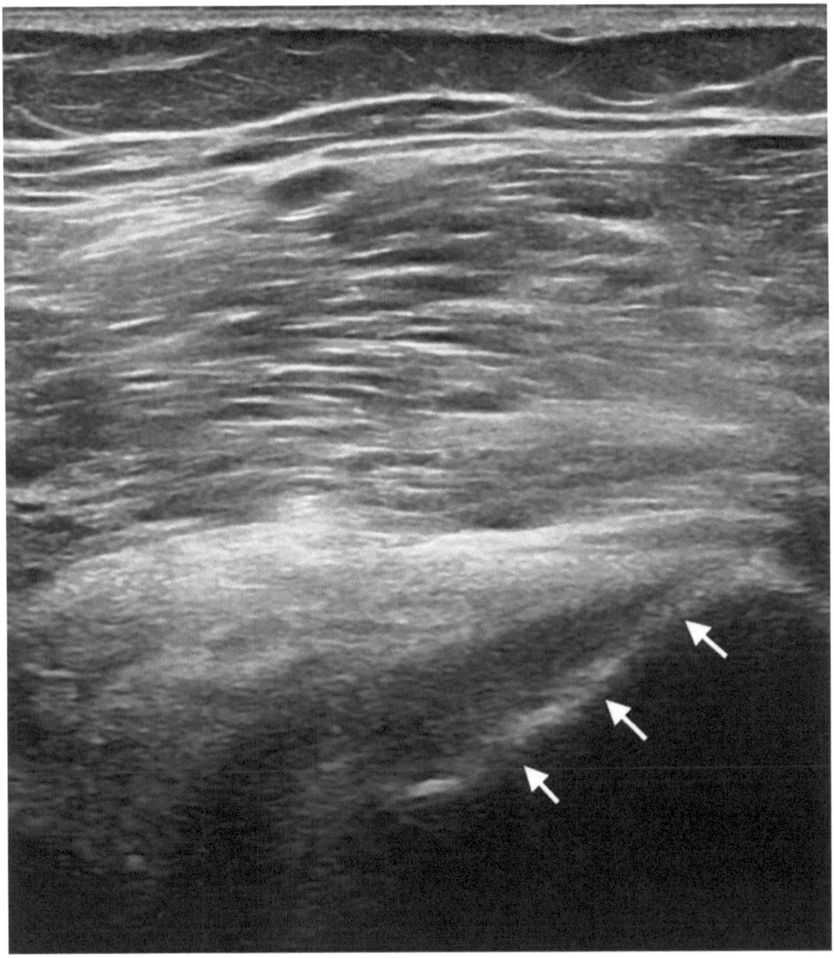

Figure 6-25a: Posterior long axis view of the knee in the midline. The knee is in mild flexion. Arrows indicate the insertion of the PCL onto the tibia. The PCL is hypoechoic because of anisotropy. The hyperechoic tissue just above the PCL is fat and then capsule with muscle occupying most of the upper half of the image. Note that the vessels do not directly overly the PCL. This is frequently the case. (Figure 22: Line C).

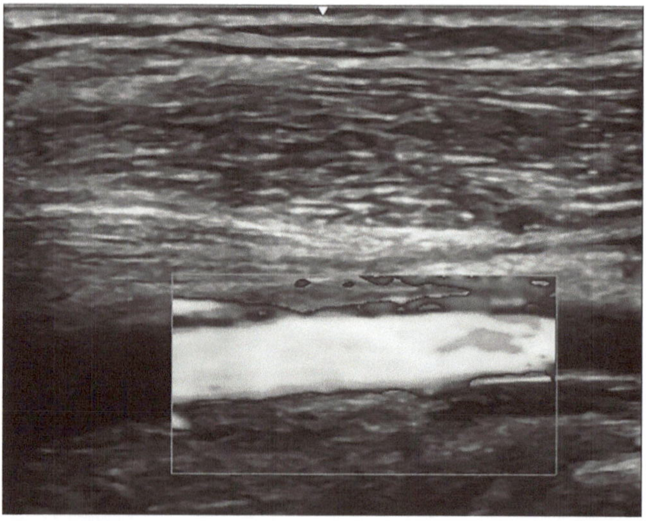

Figure 6-25b: The popliteal artery can also be seen on Doppler in the long axis view (Figure 22: Line C).

Medial condyle

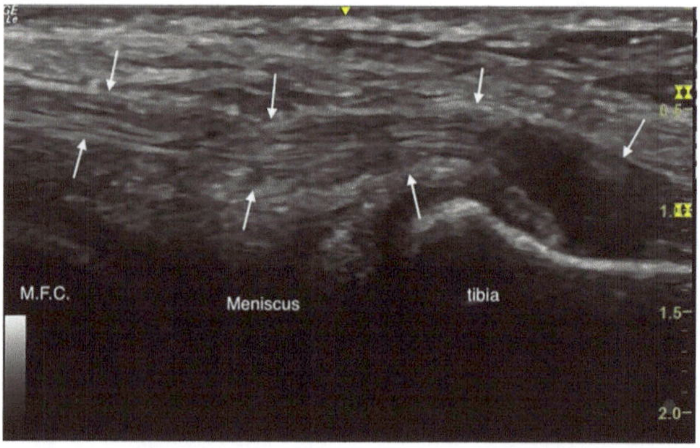

Figure 6-26a: On the medial side, we can see the tendon (arrows) of the semimembranosus, and the direct insertion. In this view the direct insertion is dark because of anisotropy. There are 5 insertions of the semimembranosus: the direct into the tibia, into the popliteal ligament, into the medial meniscus, into the fascia of popliteus, and finally the medial insertion into a groove into the proximal medial tibia. This last insertion is seen best in the posteromedial view (Figure 22: Line D).

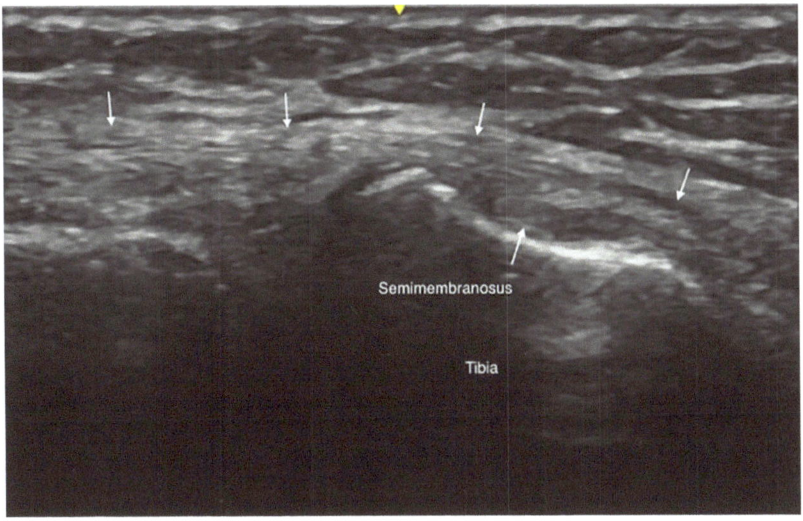

Figure 6-26b: The arrows point to the posterior portion of the retinaculum arching over the semimembranosus in the groove on the tibia (Figure 22: Line D but more medial and angled laterally perpendicular to the bones).

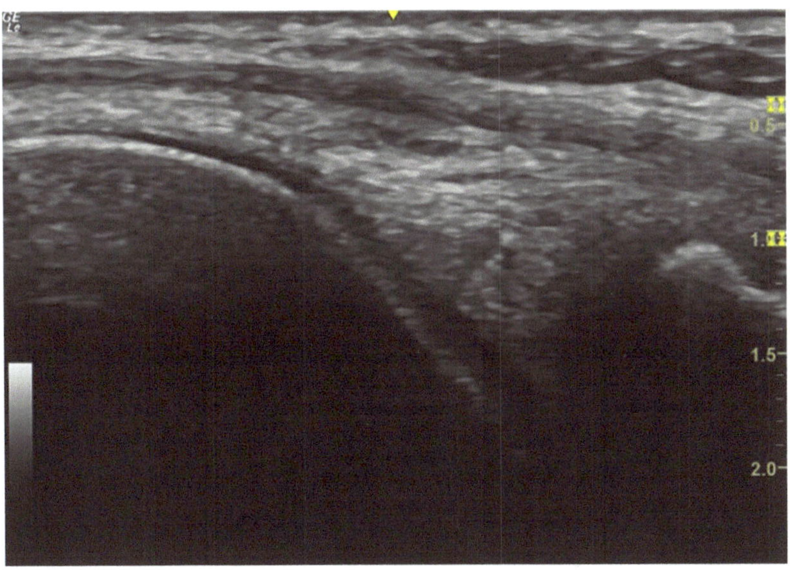

Figure 6-26c: In this view we can see the back of the medial femoral condyle, the medial meniscus and the tendon of semitendinosus (Figure 22: Line D but more posterior than in Figure 26a).

In extension, the semitendinosus tendon appears closer to the capsule than one would expect. But this subject is quite thin, and the top of the figure is the skin surface.

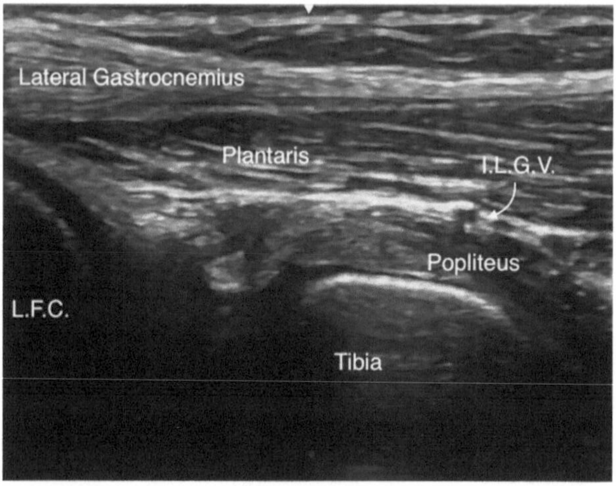

Figure 6-27a: On the lateral side posterior we can see the bones, the popliteus tendon, two muscles and the Inferior lateral genicular vessels (ILGV). When the vessels are anterior to the popliteus tendon they travel at the level of the lateral meniscus (Figure 22: Line E).

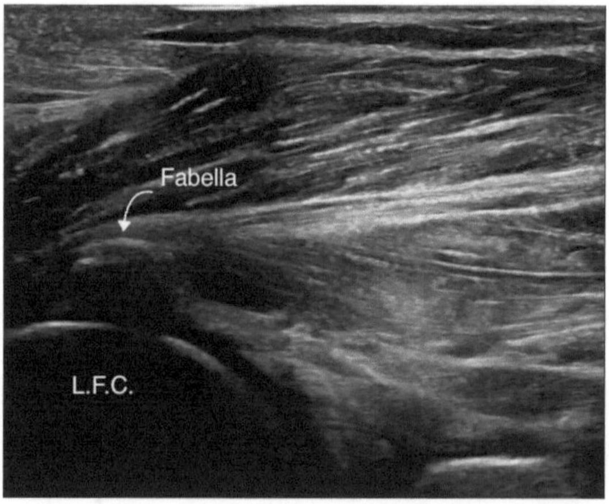

Figure 6-27B: A fabella can be seen articulating on the lateral femoral condyle and the back of the posterior tibia (Figure 22: Line E is more straight posterior than in Figure 27a).

Leg compartments

Ultrasound is especially easy in the lower leg. There is almost no obstruction of the view from air or bone. For larger legs you will have to use a lower frequency, especially with Doppler.

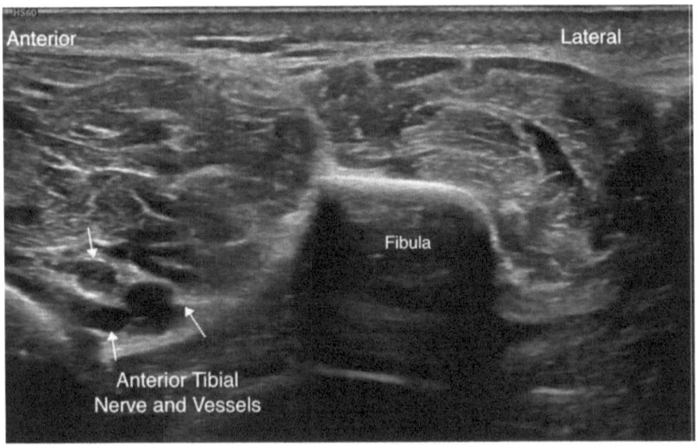

Figure 6-28a: A view of the anterior and lateral compartments of the leg. Almost nothing is obscured by bones. The interosseus membrane can be seen deep to the anterior tibial vessels and nerve.

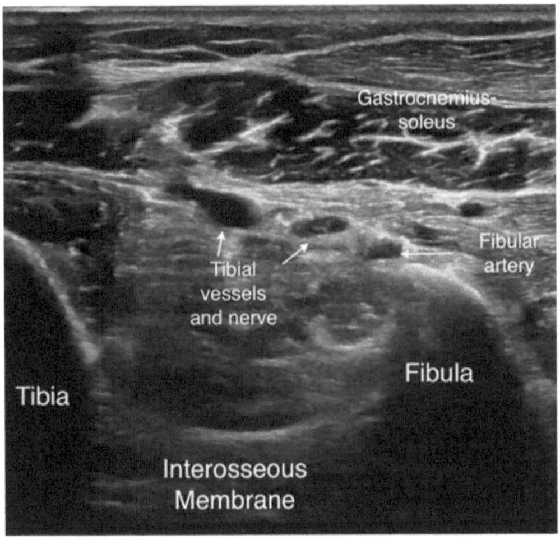

Figure 6-28b: A similarly clear view can be obtained in the posterior compartments. In individuals with more fat or muscle a curvilinear probe can be more useful especially when using the Doppler settings.

Office Work-Diagnostic

Many structures that are close to the skin and not obscured by bone are better observed in the office with ultrasound than by MRI. In addition, ultrasound allows some dynamic observations. This obviously excludes the cruciate ligaments and the menisci, in particular the interior or leading edges of the menisci.

MCL tear

A young adult male seen shortly after a valgus-stress injury to the knee. There is grade III laxity, and there is tenderness in the area of the origin of the MCL. Ultrasound was done to make sure there was no surgical lesion.

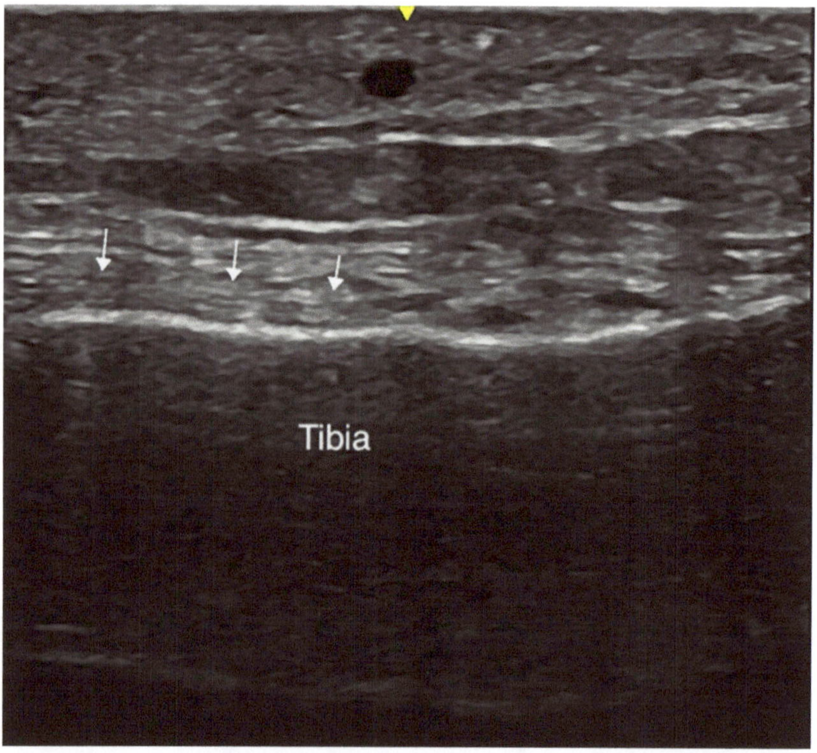

Figure 6-29a: Distally the MCL (arrows) is normal along the flair of the tibia.

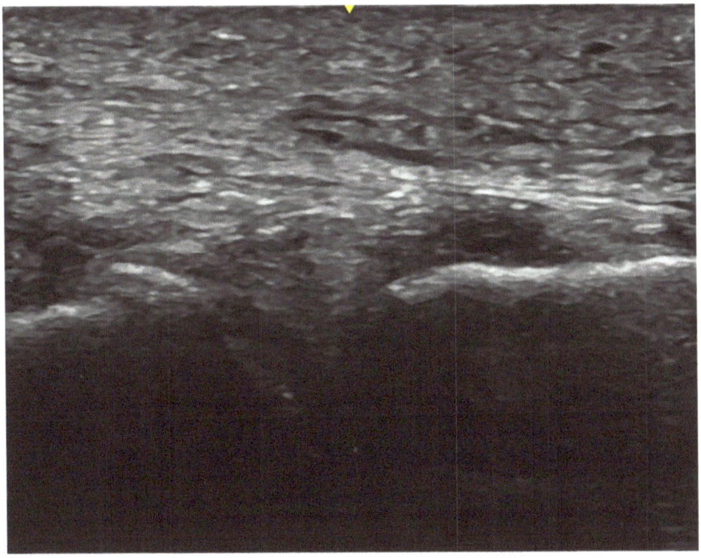

Fig. 6-29b: At the joint line the meniscus is normal for age. And there are no ligament parts stuck into the joint. An incipient osteophyte is seen on the femur on the left.

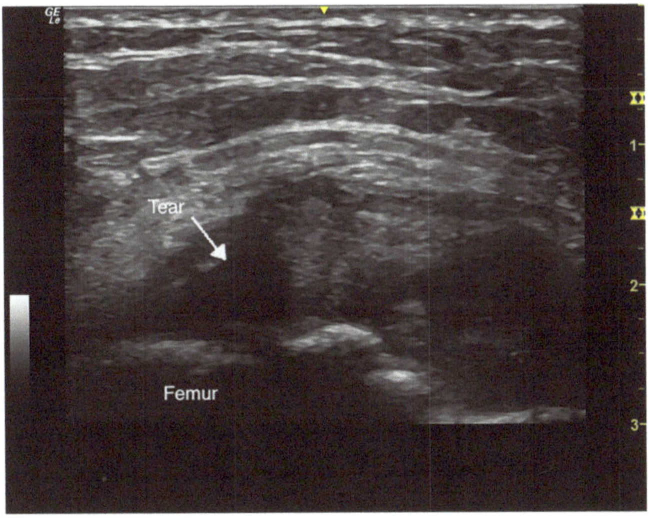

Figure 6-29c: The dark area is where we would normally see the femoral attachment of the MCL. It is hypoechoic, thickened and disorganized, but not so disrupted that surgery is necessary. Treatment was bracing with an excellent outcome.

Meniscus Lesion

Middle-aged male with pain and tenderness at the medial join line.

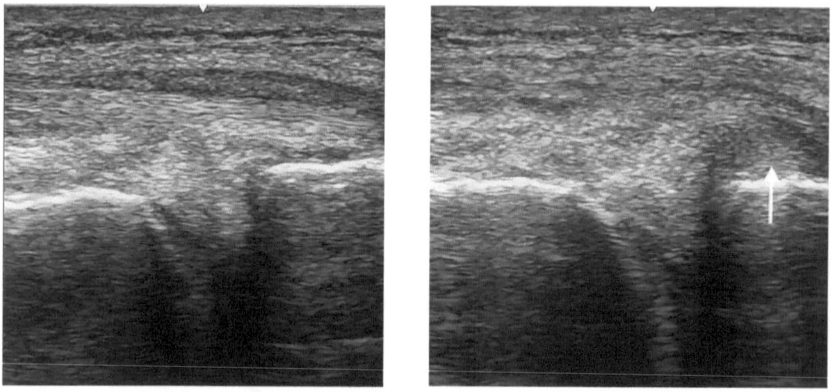

Figures 6-30 a & b: Meniscus fragment.

Figure 6-30a: An otherwise normal anteromedial meniscus with a little mucoid degeneration with a normal MCL over it.

Figure 6-30b: The same meniscus at the area of tenderness with a meniscus fragment between tibia and ligament.

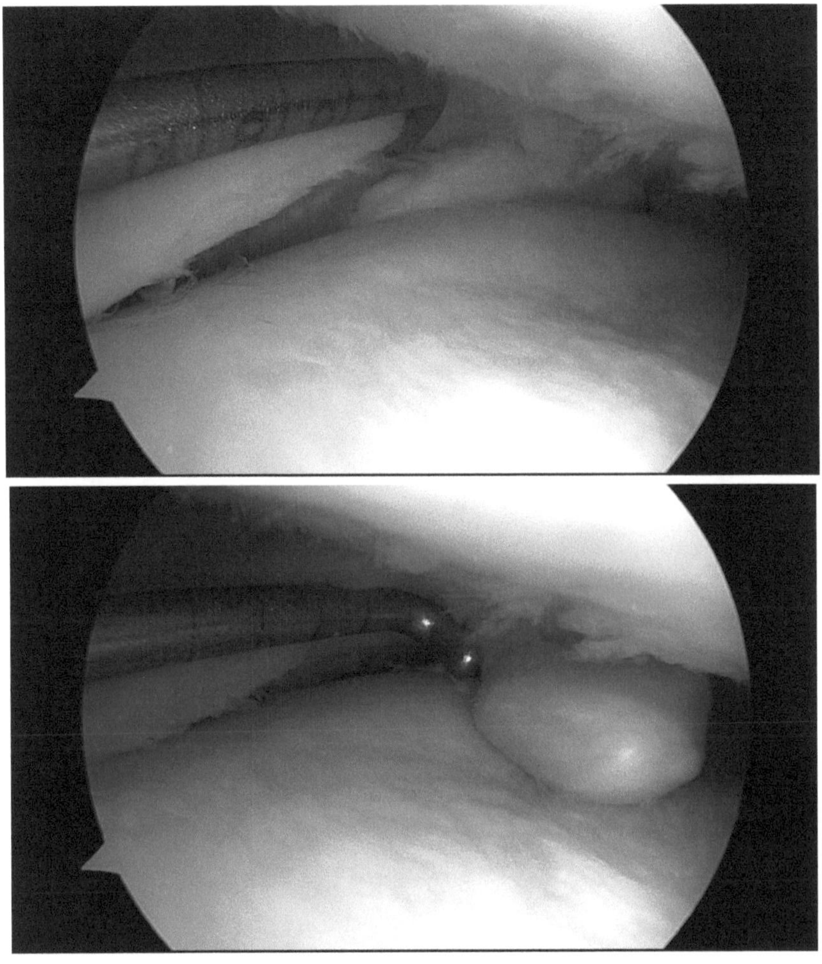

Figures 6-30c & d: Arthroscopic views.

Figure 6-30c: Initial view of the fragment under the medial meniscus.

Figure 6-30d: Fragment pulled into joint for excision and removal.

Snapping Lateral Plica

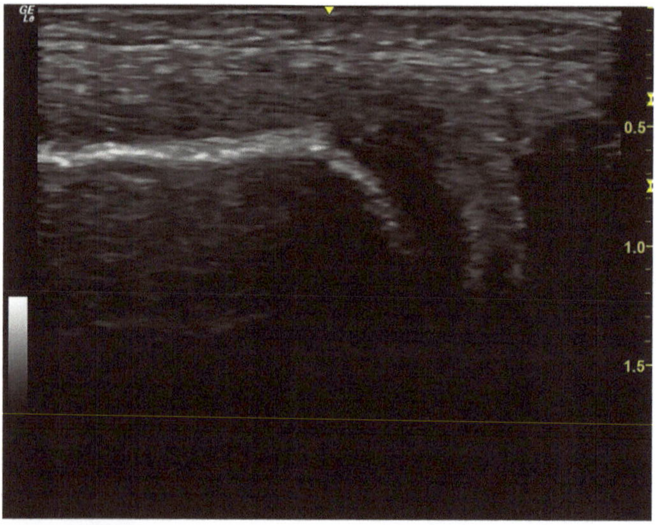

Figure 6-31a

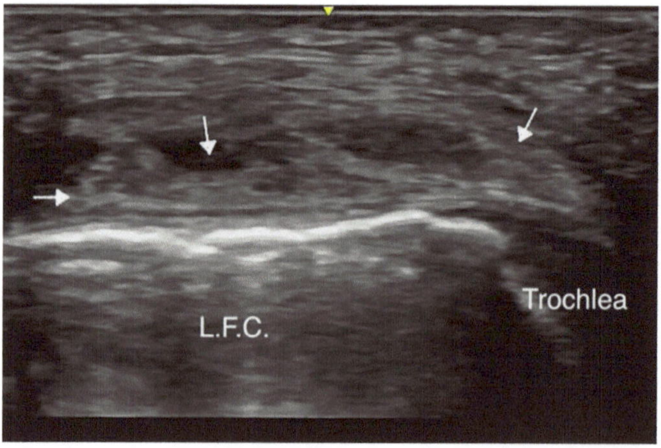

Figure 6-31b

Figures 6-31 a & b: Snapping lateral plica. Plica viewed from lateral. In Figure 31a the plica is resting on cartilage. In the second, Figure 31b, the plica is in the lateral gutter. The "snap" can be viewed dynamically with flexion-extension motion.

Effusions

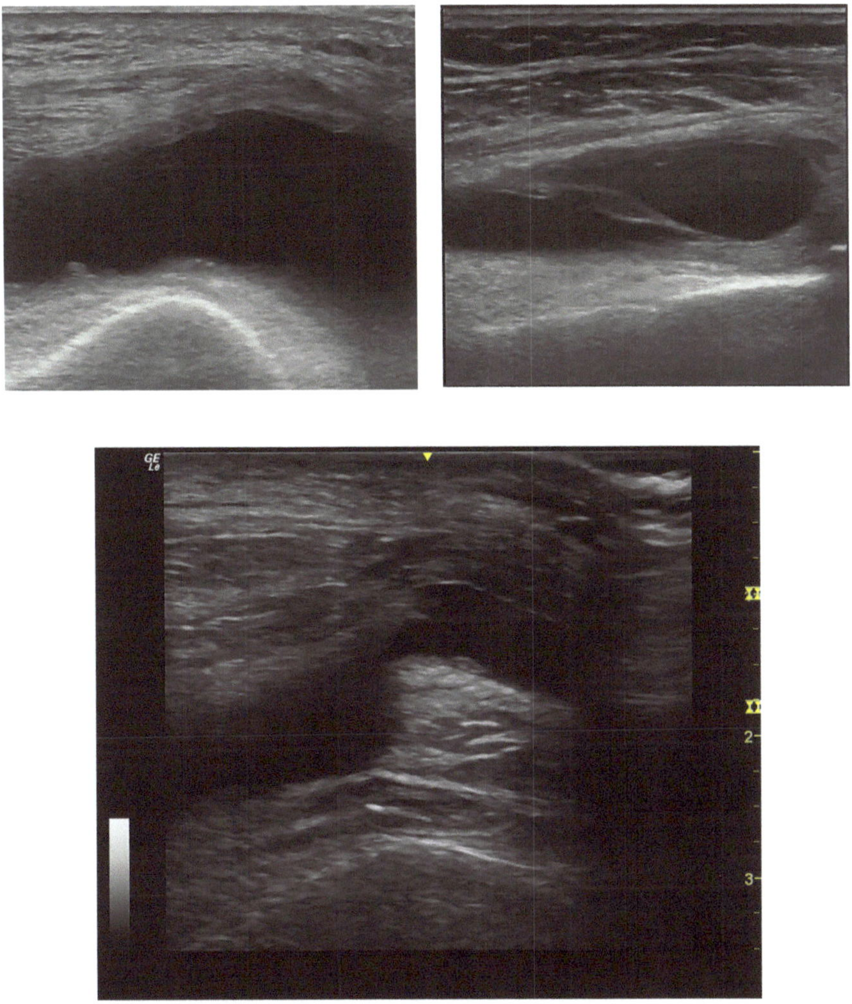

Figure 6-32: Effusions, serous, bloody and infectious. Knee effusions will offer some clues as to their content on ultrasound.

The first is completely anechoic and probably is a clear joint fluid.

The second is a little cloudy and has some fibrous bands and may be old blood. **The third shows how the fluid can act as a contrast medium. Back wall** enhancement shows the lateral fat pad which may obstruct the needle tip in injection or aspiration.

Post-traumatic Knee Effusion

This is a patient in her early 20s who was in an MVA. A knee effusion was noted on admission to the ER and a mild lateral tibial plateau fracture was found on X-ray. The CT shows a bilayer effusion of blood and fat, although we can see some early separation of the blood into two layers. The ultrasound was done two hours later, and shows the separation of the blood into the plasma and cellular layers. In addition, using the line of fluid separation as a level, comparing it to the cortex of the femur, we can see that the knee is more flexed.

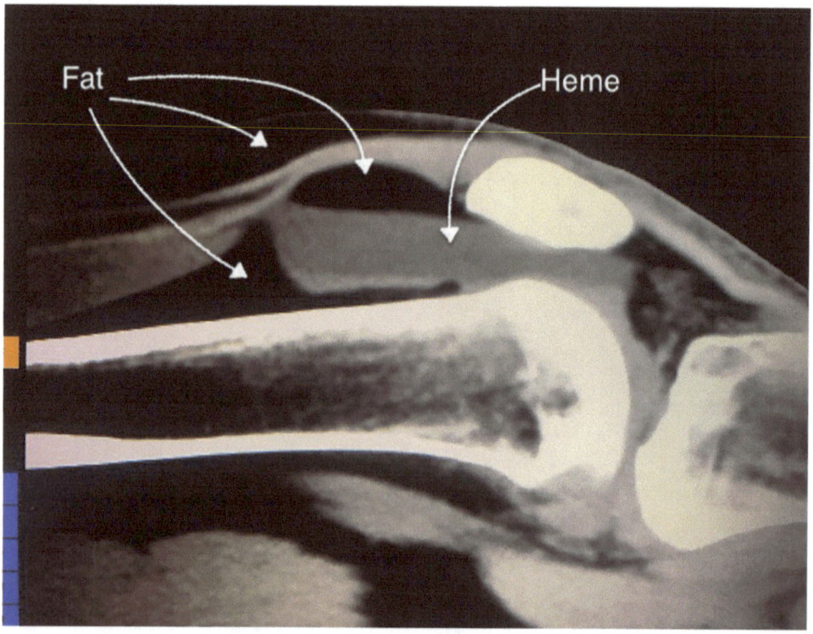

Figure 6-32.5 a: The intra-articular fat is on top of the blood layer. Even at this point the blood is starting to separate. As X-ray density is determined by the chemical make-up of a layer, it looks like the other fat collections. The tilt of the interface between blood and fat indicates that the knee is in slight flexion.

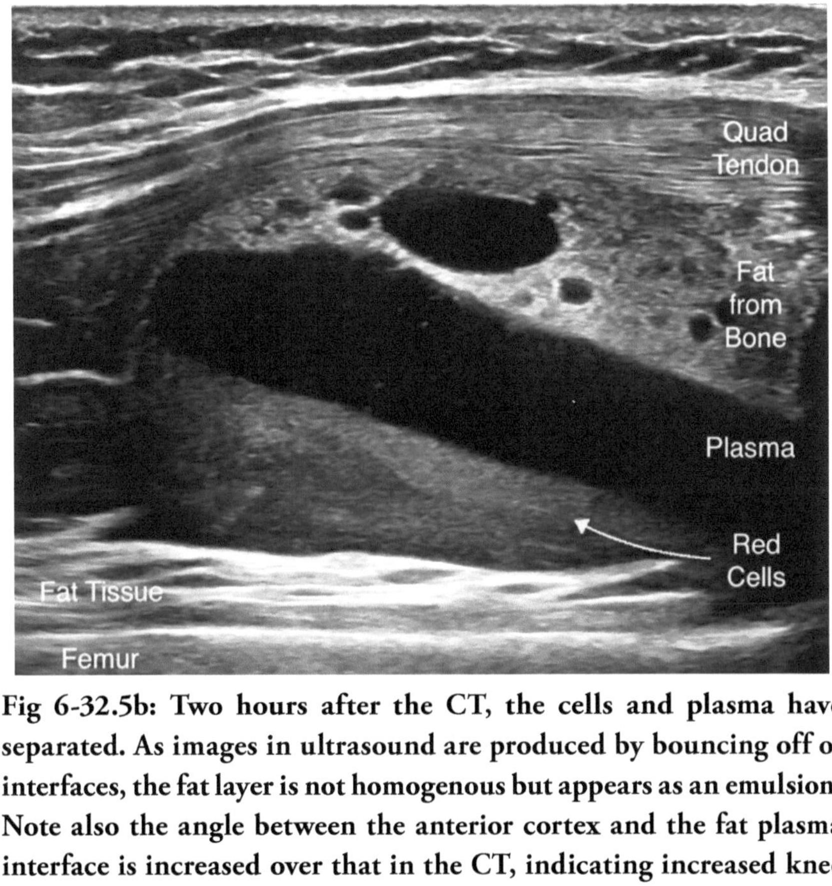

Fig 6-32.5b: Two hours after the CT, the cells and plasma have separated. As images in ultrasound are produced by bouncing off of interfaces, the fat layer is not homogenous but appears as an emulsion. Note also the angle between the anterior cortex and the fat plasma interface is increased over that in the CT, indicating increased knee flexion. In addition, at the top, as the fat coalesces it becomes a separate hypoechoic collection.

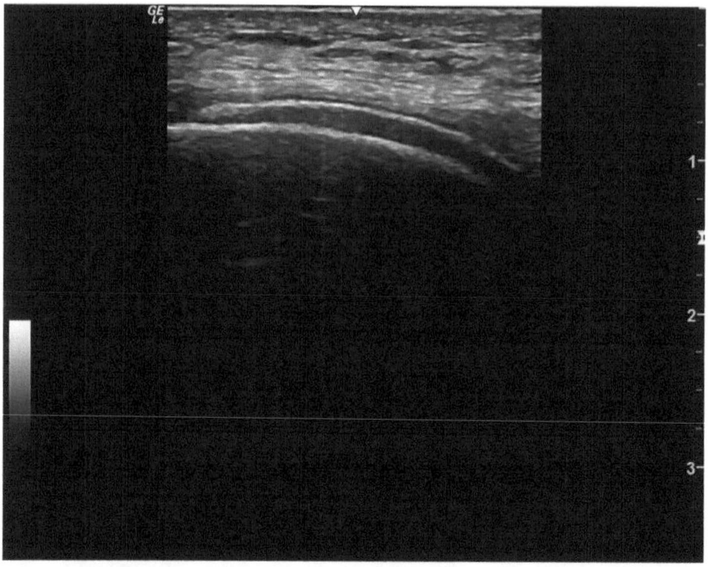

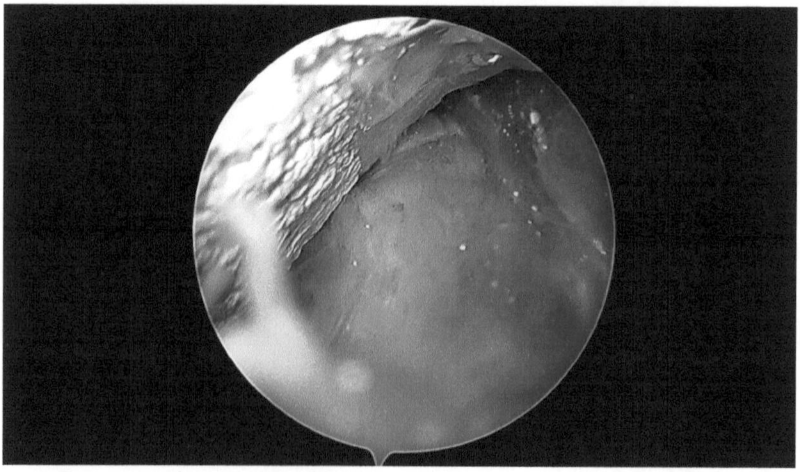

Figures 6-33 a & b: Crystalline arthropathy – gout. Ultrasound and arthroscopic views of "urate frosting". If there is crystal arthropathy and the crystals are on the surface of the cartilage that is gout as seen here. If the crystals are in the middle of the cartilage, that is calcium. There is a "double contour" to the femoral condyle. The outer layer is urate. The deeper layer is bone.

Cysts and cyst-like masses

On ultrasound, masses are assessed for echogenicity, back wall enhancement, and vascularity. A pure cyst, such as a ganglion, is very hypoechoic. In addition because the sound is so well transmitted the back wall appears brighter, 'back wall enhancement'. If there has been bleeding into the cyst there will be fibrin remnants in the cyst. If there is vascularity in the mass, this is not a cyst.

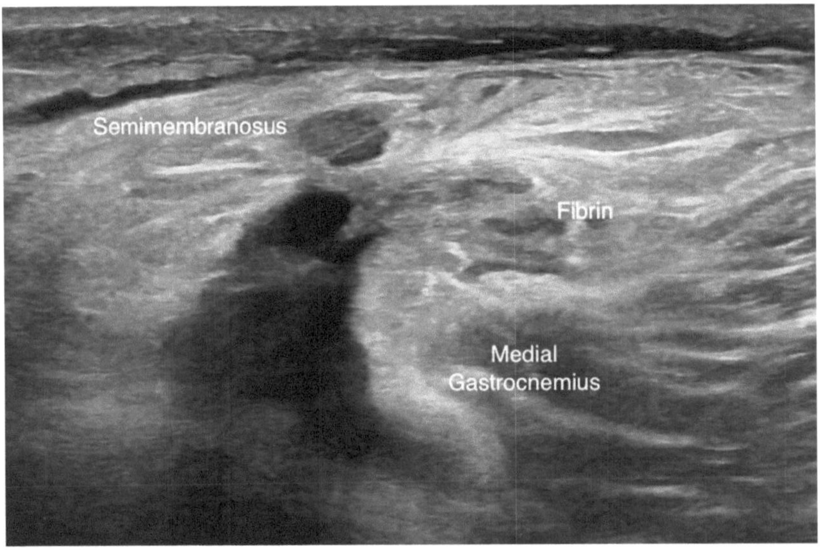

Figure 6-34a: The proximal end of a Baker's cyst that was causing a DVT-like clinical picture. On the medial side we see the anechoic fluid we normally see in cyst mixing with some weakly echogenic fluid, probably blood. The fibrin between the semimembranosus and medial gastrocnemius is an indication that this cyst has ruptured in the past. In addition, this does not appear to be large enough to mimic a DVT.

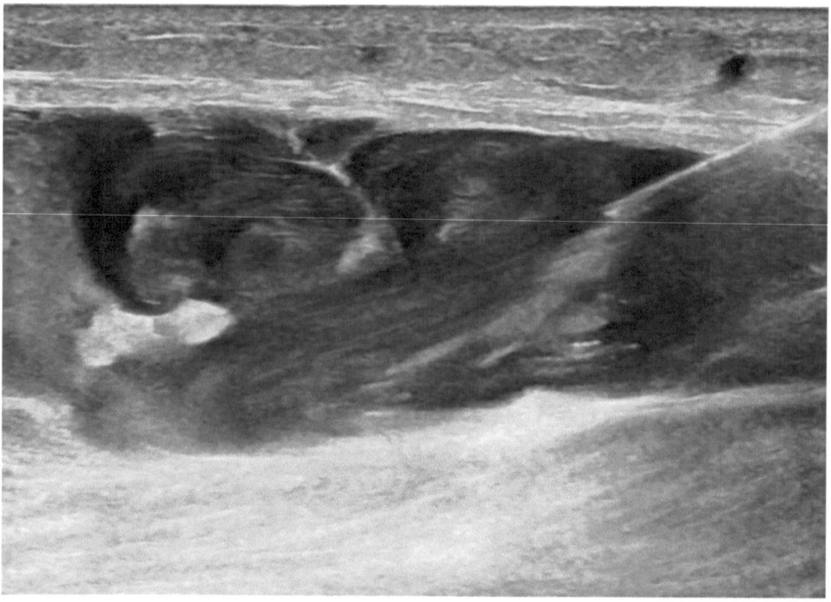

Figure 6-34c: The cyst shown above had dissected down the leg medial to gastrocnemius. The needle is aspirating 100mL. of an opaque, low viscosity, bloody fluid. The swirling debris causes a "Starry Night" appearance.

Cysts as a result of an implant

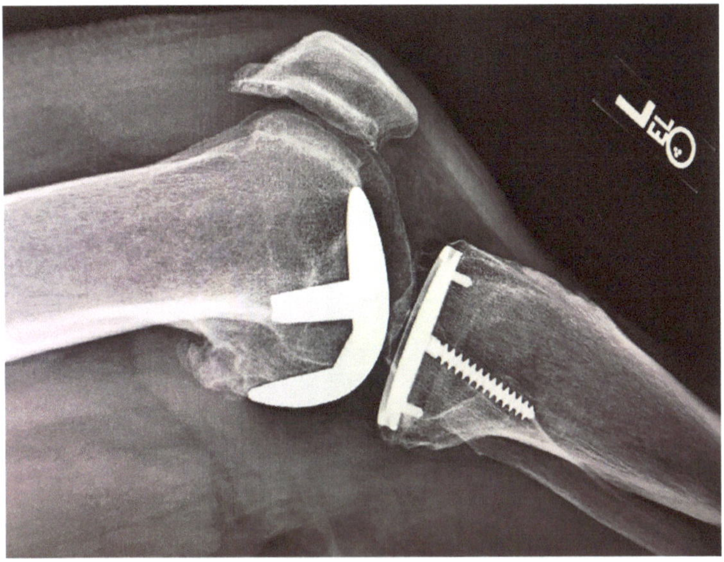

Figure 6-35a: A unicompartmental TKA placed 8 yrs ago. No radio opaque material is seen behind the knee. There is a one year history of a popliteal fullness. No radio-opaque material is seen in this view.

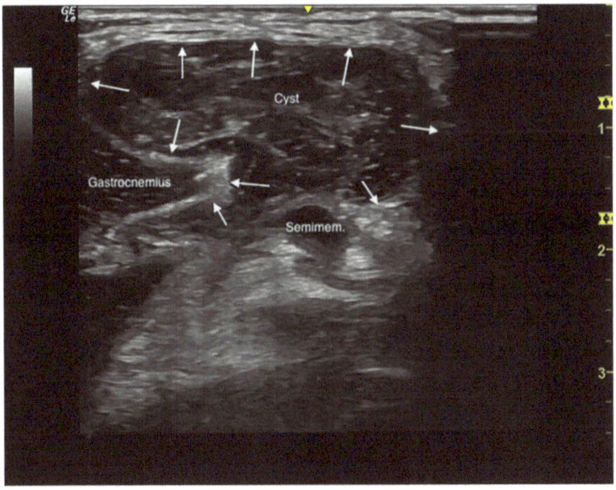

Figure 6-35b: This echogenicity suggests this cyst may be filled with wear debris.

Meniscus Cyst

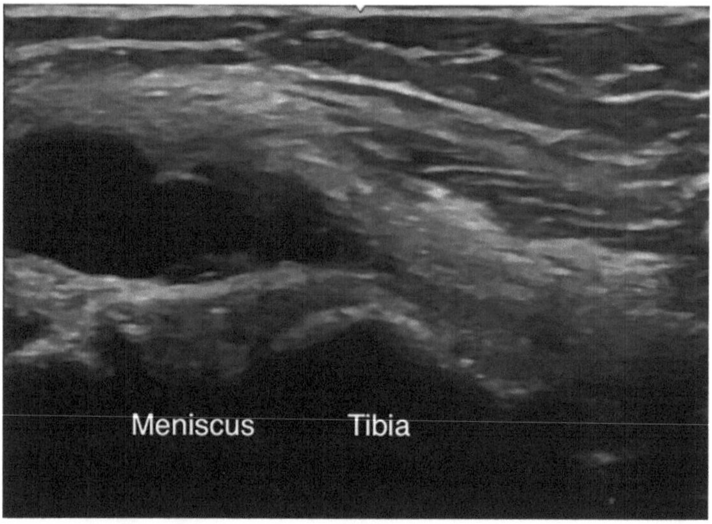

Figure 6-36a: A postero-medial cyst just to the outside of the meniscus and capsule. Note that this is in the region of the semimembranosus groove on the tibia.

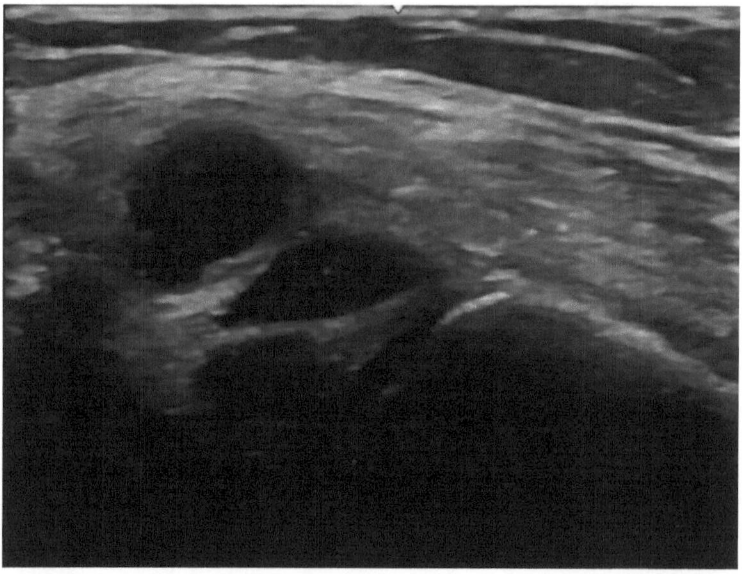

Figure 6-36b: The meniscal weakness and intrameniscal part of the cyst can sometimes be seen.

Cyst-like mass

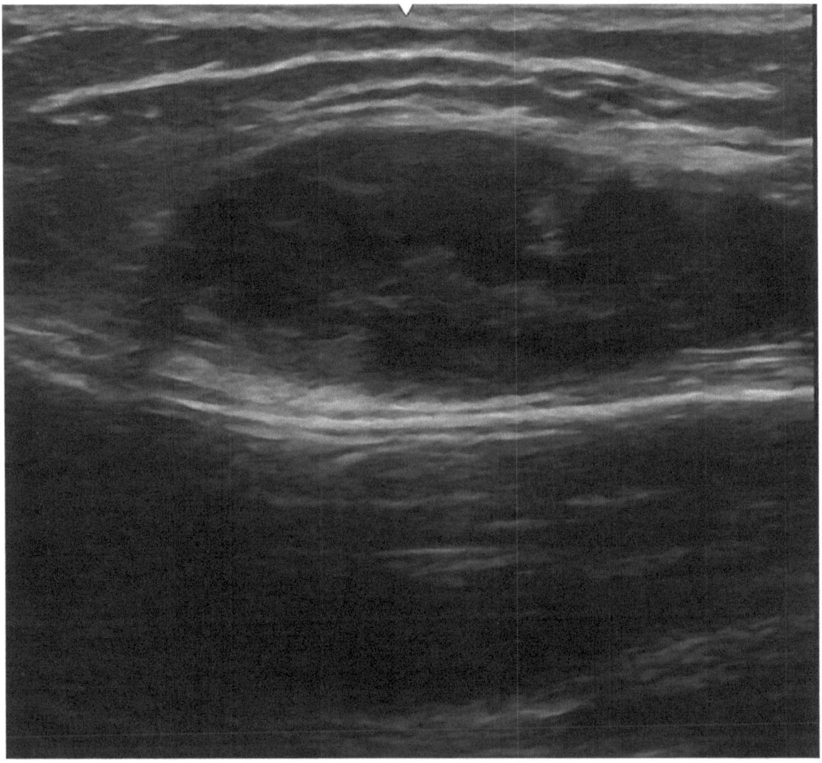

Figure 6-37a

Figures 6-37a & b: Assessment of masses.

Ultrasound is useful for assessing some superficial masses but for deeper masses, MRI with and without contrast will be required.

Figure 6-37a9a: This is mass over the medial tibia just at the flair. It is hypoechoic and not homogeneous. The patient is 16 and otherwise healthy.

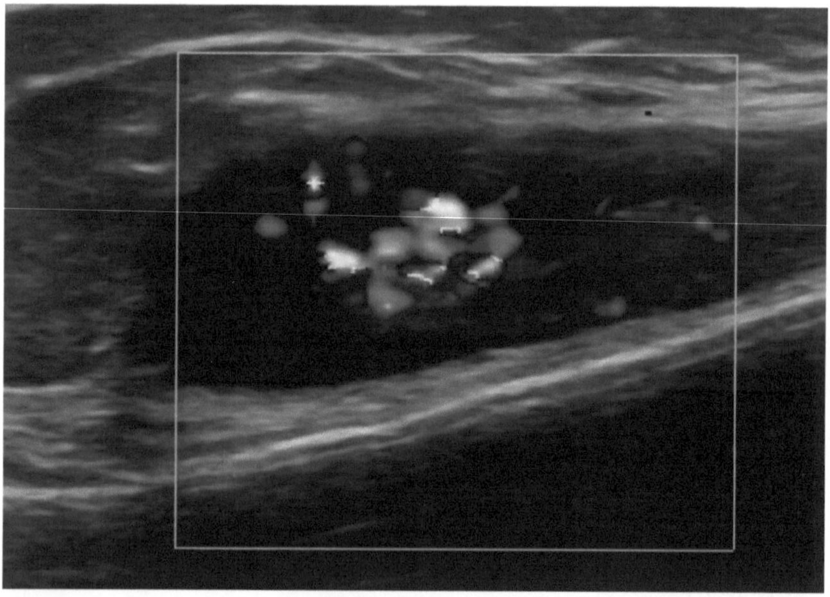

Figure 6-37b: Color Doppler shows vascularity within but no neovascularity at the periphery. MRI was done and at biopsy this turned out to be tenosynovial giant cell tumor (PVNS). Open resection was done rather than arthroscopy because of the proximity of the saphenous nerve.

Periarticular fungal growth

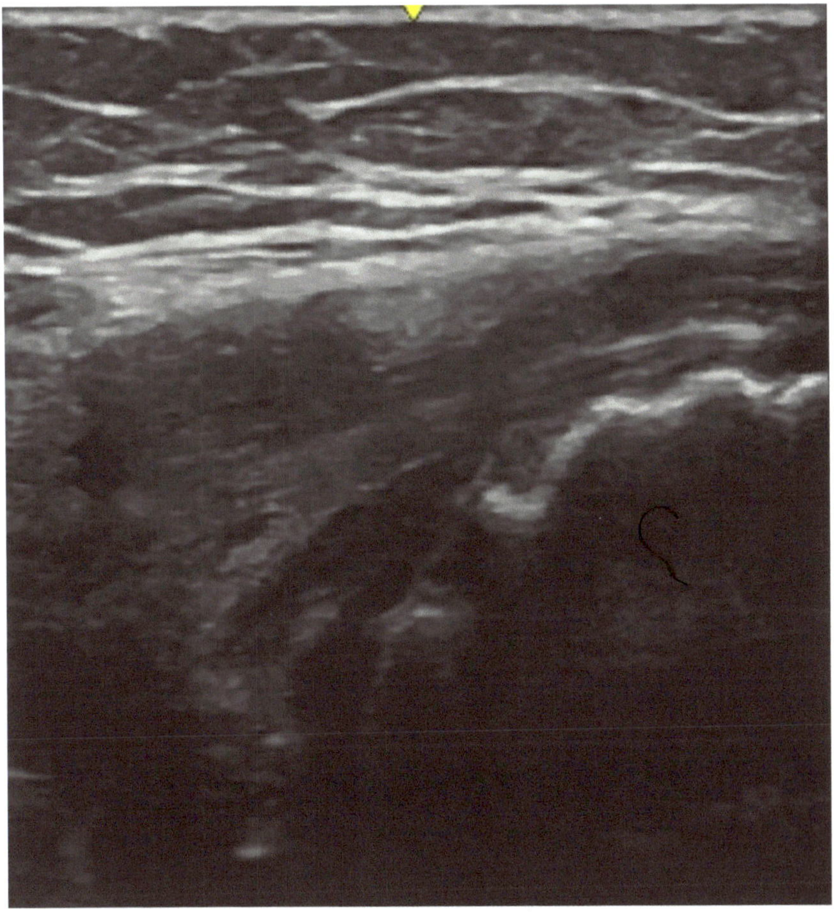

Figure 6-38a: Pre-op view of semimembranosus at the medial tibial insertion with synovitis on both sides of it. The pre-operative diagnosis was PVNS vs. Fungal synovitis on the basis of the MRI and previous fungal infection. This view taken in the OR prior to surgery showed the process was both inside and outside the joint.

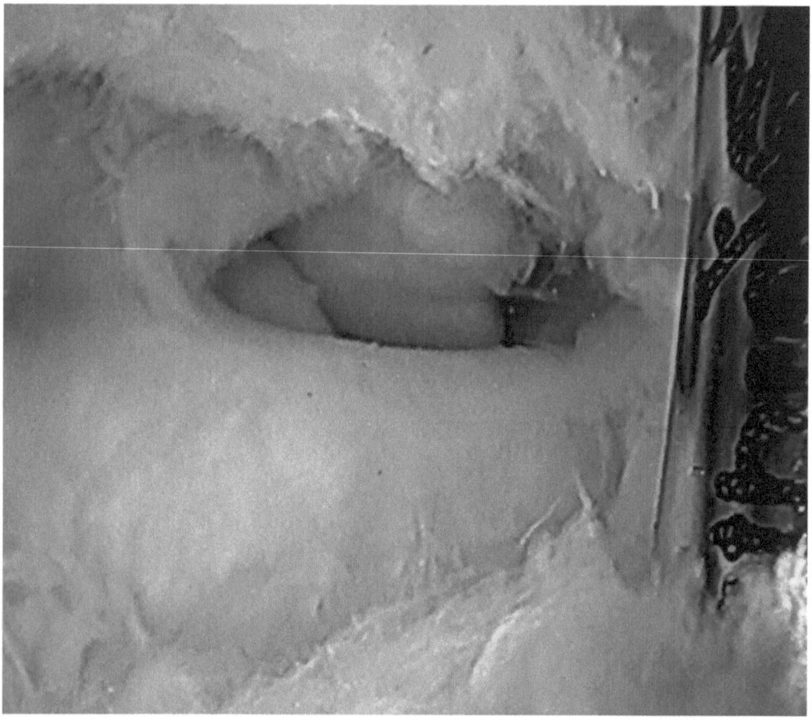

Figure 6-38b: View from inside the posterior medial knee over the semimembranosus to the fibrinous fungal material medial to the tendon. On biopsy and culture this turned out to be coccidiomycosis.

Quadriceps Rupture

Before the ready availability of MRI, quadriceps rupture was commonly missed in the acute period when repair would be so much easier and more successful. Patellar tendon injuries were never missed because that structure is right under the skin. Ultrasound allows the ER physician or orthopaedic surgeon to examine the quad mechanism in the early period.

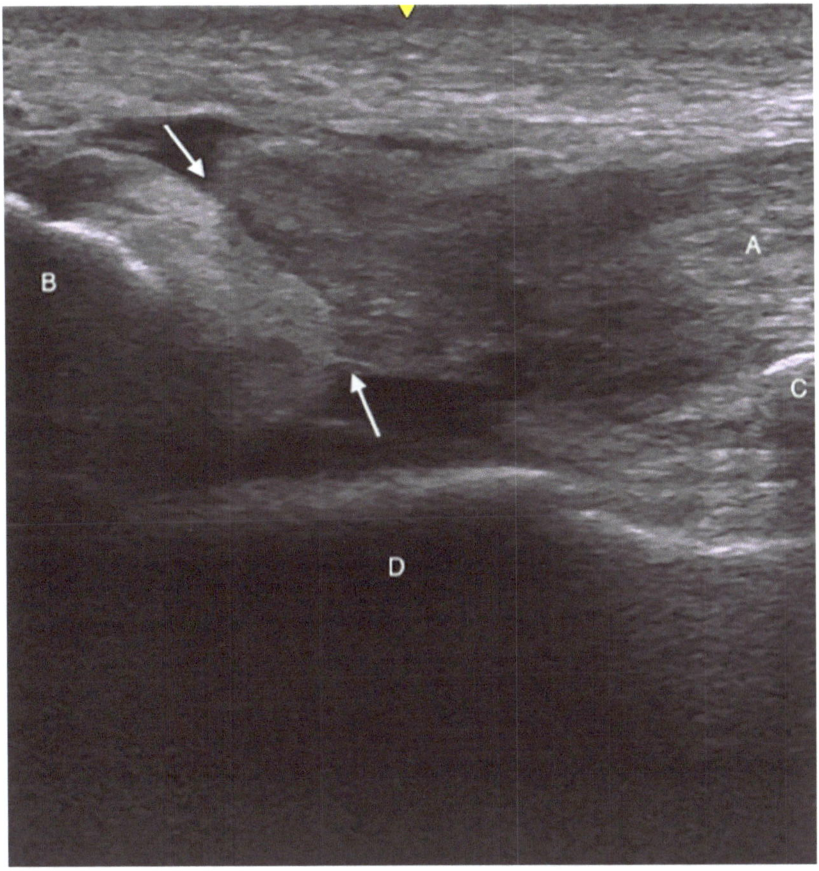

Figure 6-39a: Acute knee injury with moderate swelling. The arrows indicate the tear. The end of the quadriceps tendon and the tendon remnant on the patella are disorganized and hypoechoic showing what will be seen at surgery. In addition, there is a small patellar fragment on the right. A: Healthy region of quadriceps tendon. B: Patella. C: Retracted patella fragment. D: Femur.

Tendinosis

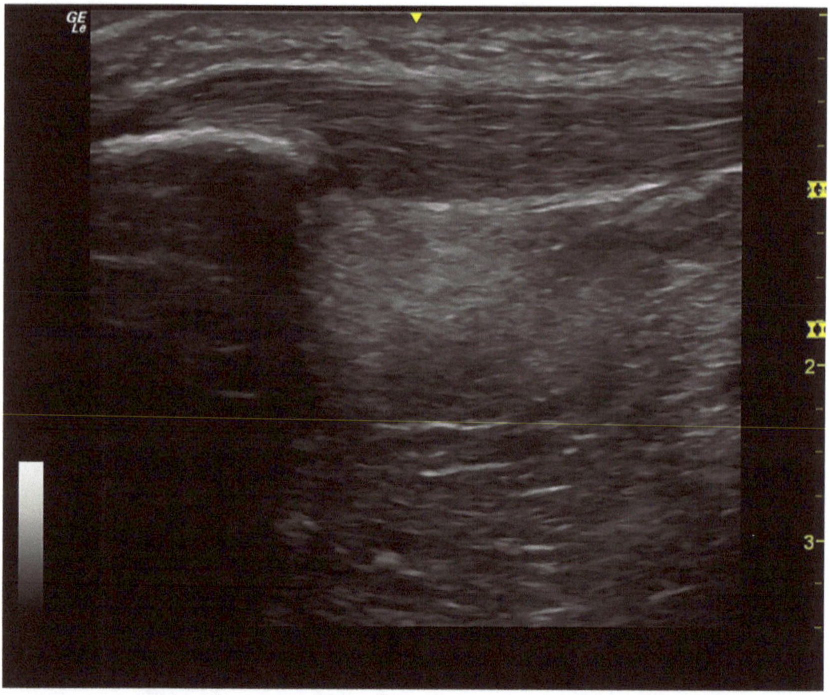

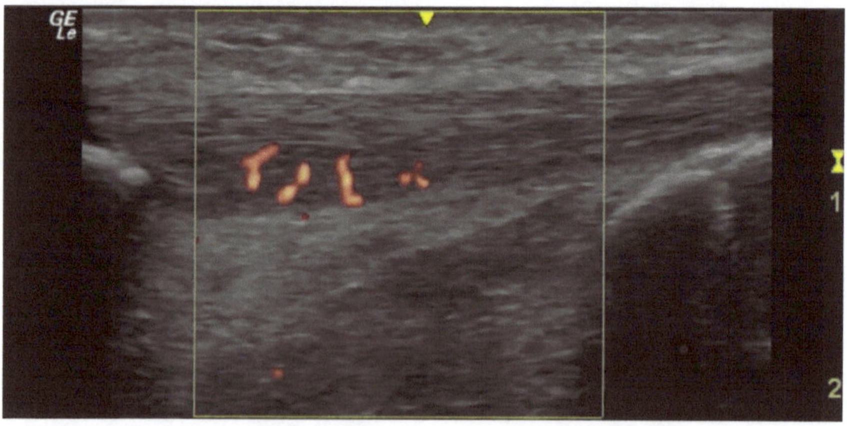

Figures 6-40a & b: Ultrasound views of tendinosis with and without Doppler. A relatively common picture in Patellar Tendinosis. The tendon is thicker just below the inferior pole of the patella. The loss of echogenicity is in the deeper layers, as is the increased blood flow.

Complete tendinosis

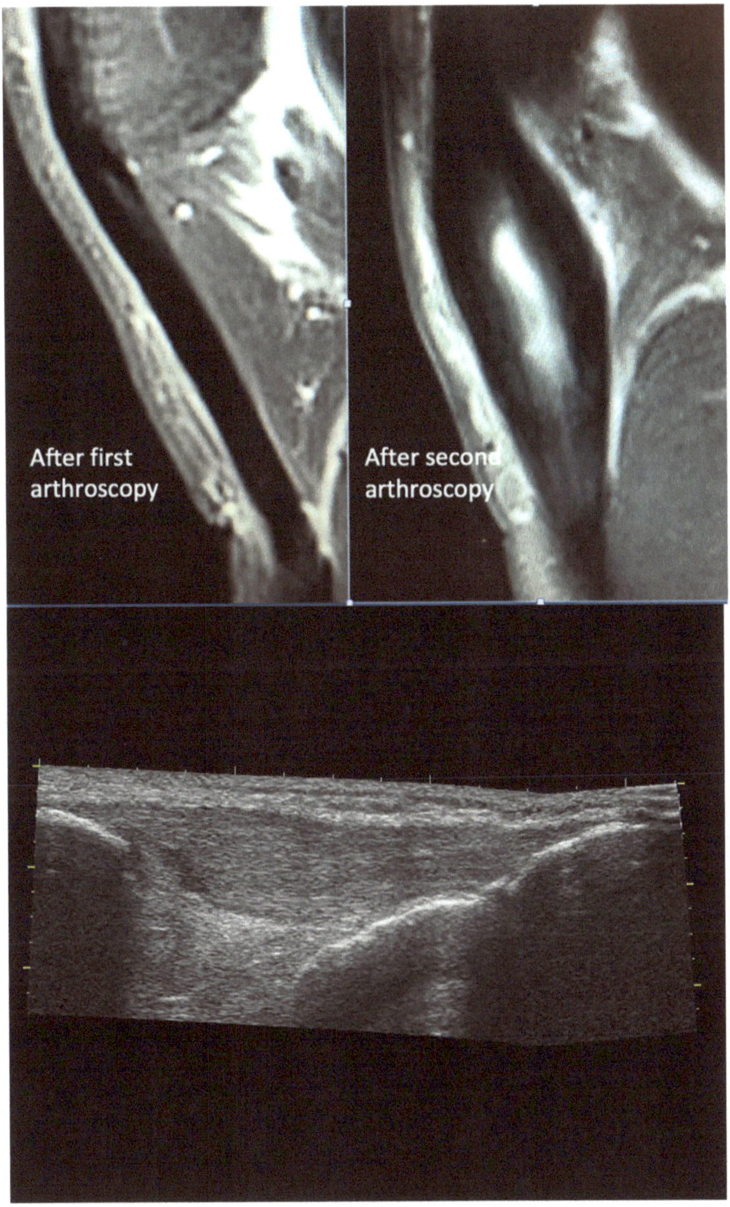

Figures 6-41a, b, b. This patient was seen for lateral compartment pain, not for pain in the patellar tendon region. The entire tendon was enlarged compared to the asymptomatic tendon seen below. There was also a decrease in echogenicity in the involved tendon.

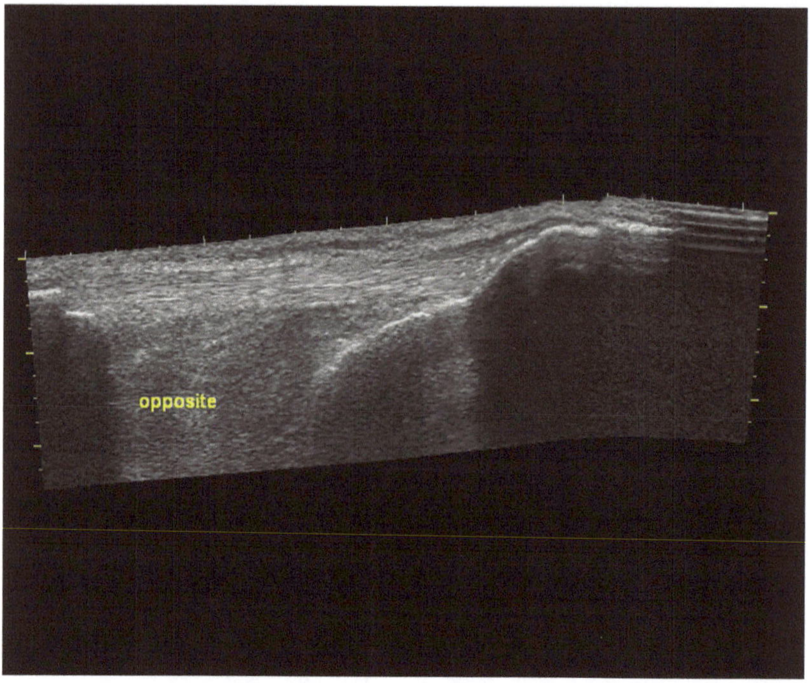

Figure 6-41d: An extreme example of complete involvement of the tendon with a comparison view of the opposite knee. What is ironic is that this was not the source of her pain but a concern in surgical planning for TKA. This is discussed below in the section on surgical planning. The patient had had two arthroscopies done by a fellowship trained surgeon that appeared to have been atraumatic. We thought that this tendinosis may have been a vascular event. It might be interesting to follow-up with ultrasound some of the rare large patella reconstructions done in TKAs.

This total involvement of the patellar tendon can sometimes be seen after TKA, and it may be painful.

Tendon pain after TKA (and normal thickening)

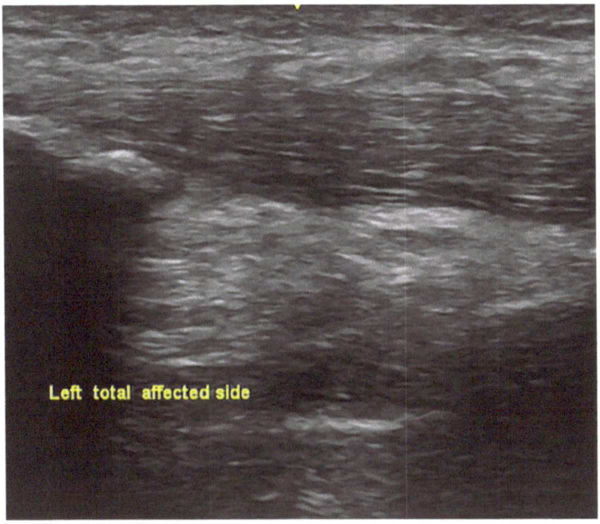

Figure 6-41e: Bilateral total knee. The left symptomatic patellar tendon is thicker than the opposite asymptomatic tendon, which is also thicker than normal.

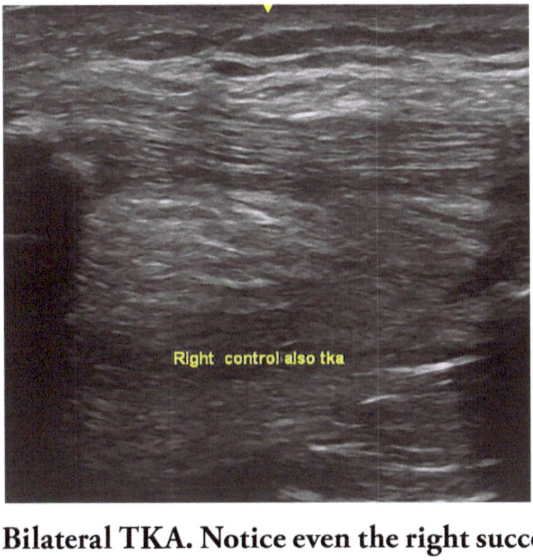

Figure 6-41f: Bilateral TKA. Notice even the right successful side has a thickened patellar tendon. This is normal in TKA. In the painful left side the affected tendon is even thicker and less echogenic.

Osgood-Schlatter's vs. enthesophyte

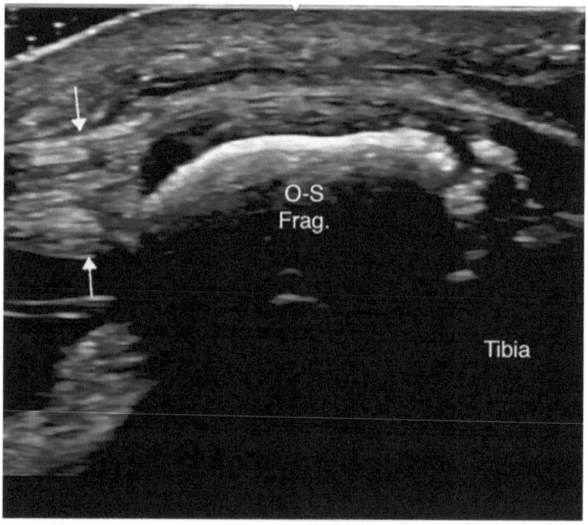

Figure 6-42a: A long axis view from left to right of the patellar tendon (arrows), insertion onto the tibial tubercle. Note that the extra bone is in the deep layer of the tendon.

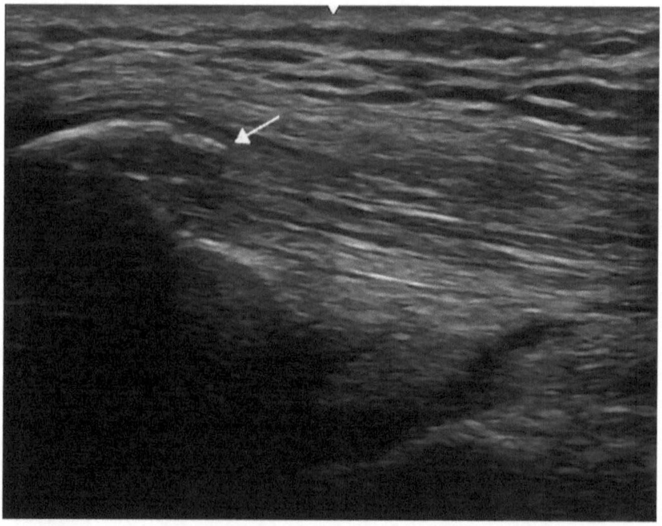

Figures 6-42b: An enthesophyte growing into the superficial layer of the patellar tendon.

Medial head of gastrocnemius tear

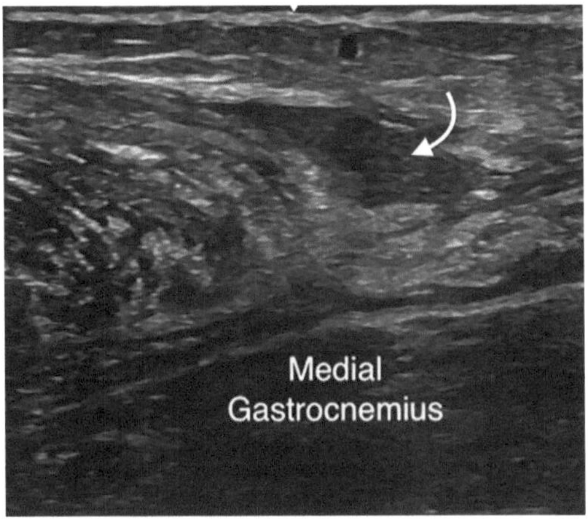

Figure 6-43a.

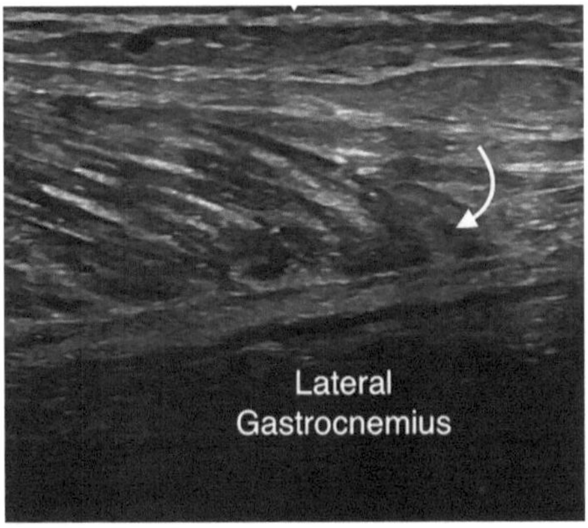

Figure 6-43b.

Figures 6-43a & b: Long axis views of partial tears of the gastrocnemius muscle, A, are almost always distal and on the medial head. B shows for comparison the normal lateral head. The arrows point out the distal insertions of the two heads onto what becomes the Achilles tendon. The curved retraction and fluid collection on the medial side can be compared with the nice "herring bone" pattern of the uninjured lateral head. This injury pattern is quite painful but resolves without surgery.

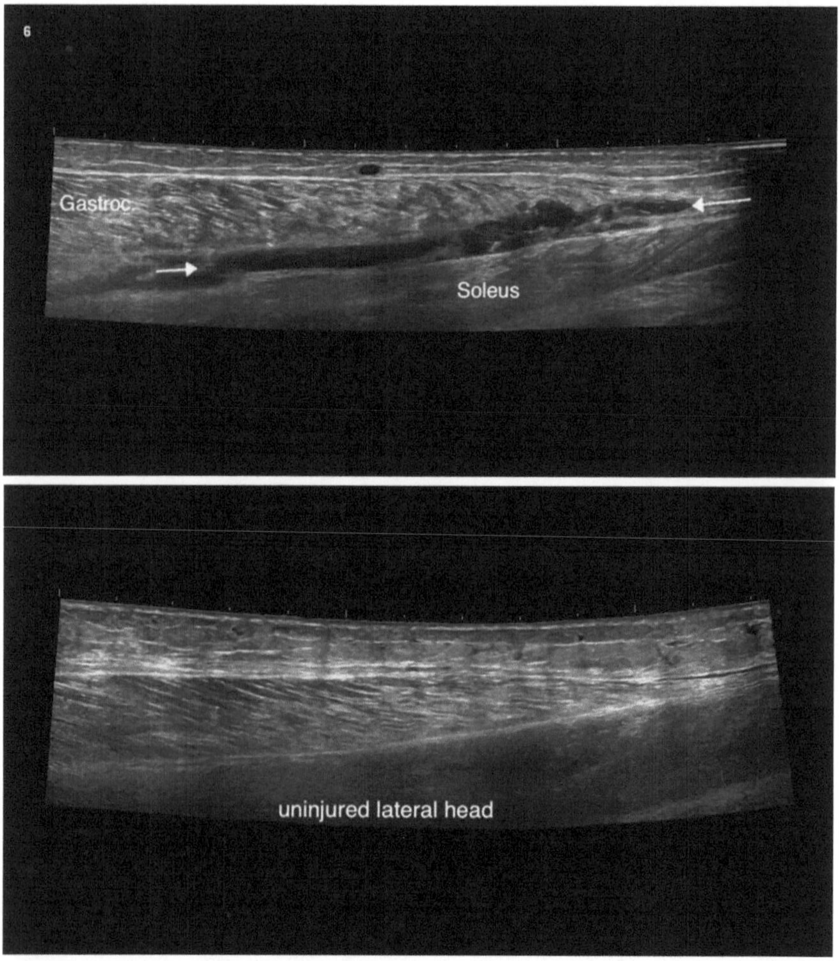

Figure 6-43c & d: This long medial gastrocnemius separation (arrows) from the soleus was paradoxically less painful than shorter partial tears. It would lead one to speculate that there is no point of increased stress, if the muscle is totally detached.

Office Work: Post-op Diagnosis

Postoperative Pain

Ultrasound can be used to investigate unusual sources of postoperative pain especially since these pains usually are in a tissue that is close to the skin and may be somewhat parallel to it.

Knee pain after IM nail of femur

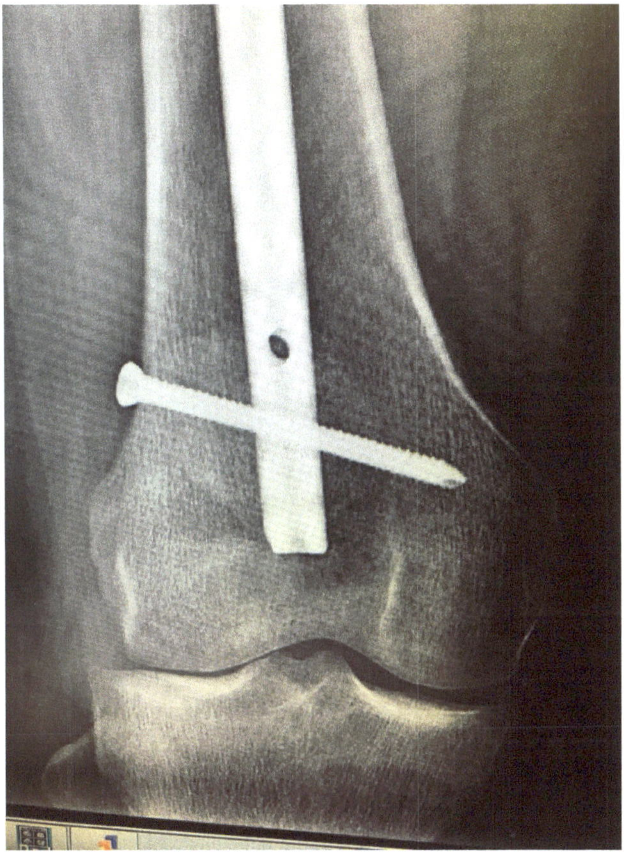

Figure 6-44a: The distal locking screw is no longer perpendicular to the rod. The tip may penetrate the anterior cortex of the medial condyle.

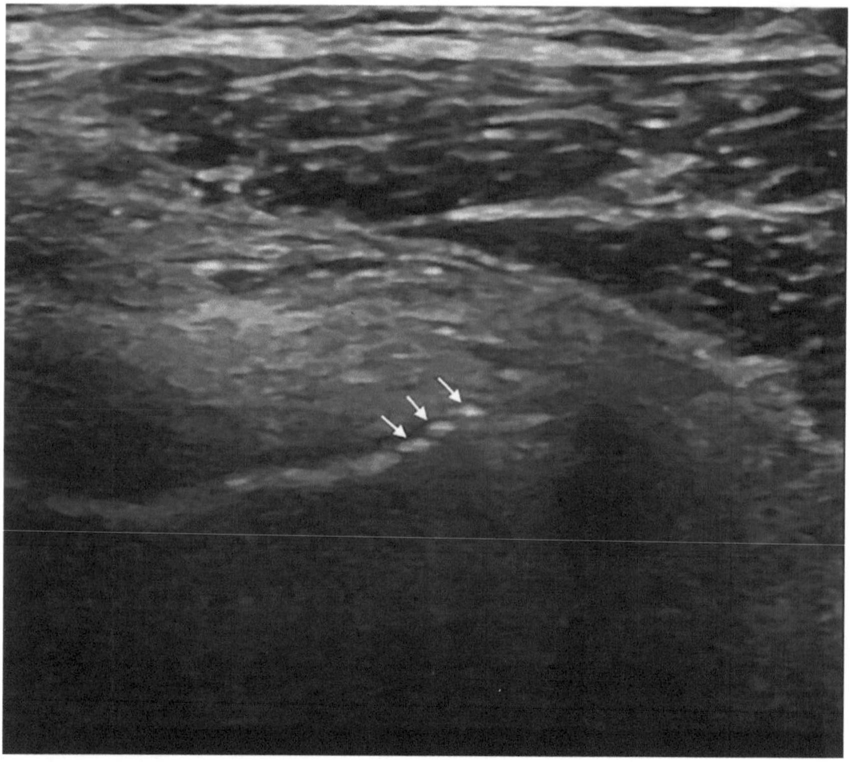

Figure 6-44b

Figures 6-44a & b: Six months after an IM nailing of a femur fracture there is pain and tenderness as well as some crepitus at the anterior superior knee.

Figures 6-47a and b show that the screw is no longer transverse but has angled inferiorly as the fracture healed.

Figure 6-47c: Three threads of the screw are now in the knee creating the painful reaction at the medial superior knee as the extensor mechanism rubs on the tip. Removal of the screw gave complete relief of pain.

Painful suture (meniscus repair)

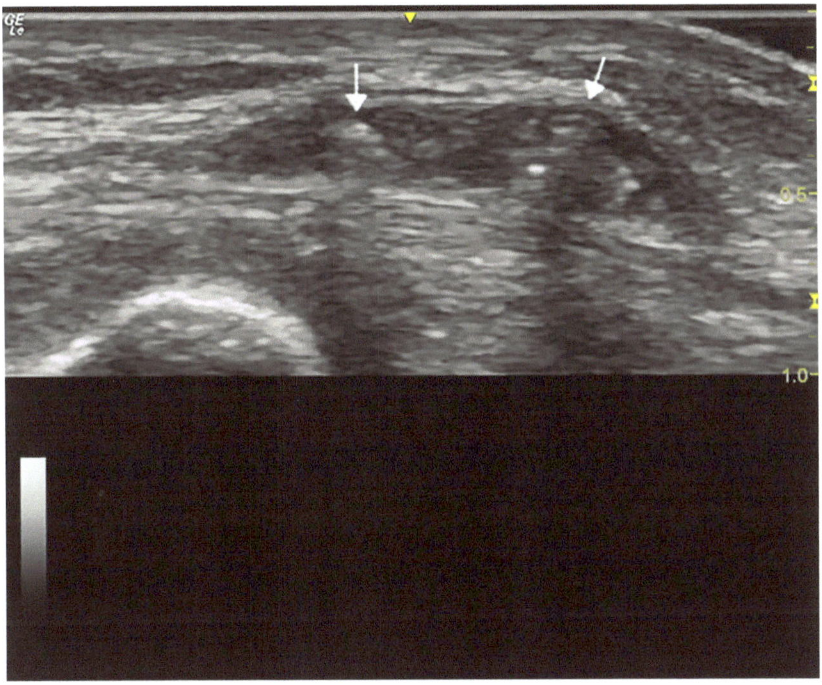

Figure 6-45: Ultrasound view of the suture in a meniscus repair in a preadolescent male.

Meniscus repair was done 6 months previously. Now he has pain and tenderness over the repair. The knots can be seen between the deeper tibial collateral ligament and the overlying retinaculum. This friction creates irritation. Removal of the suture gave complete pain relief.

Subluxing fabella after TKA

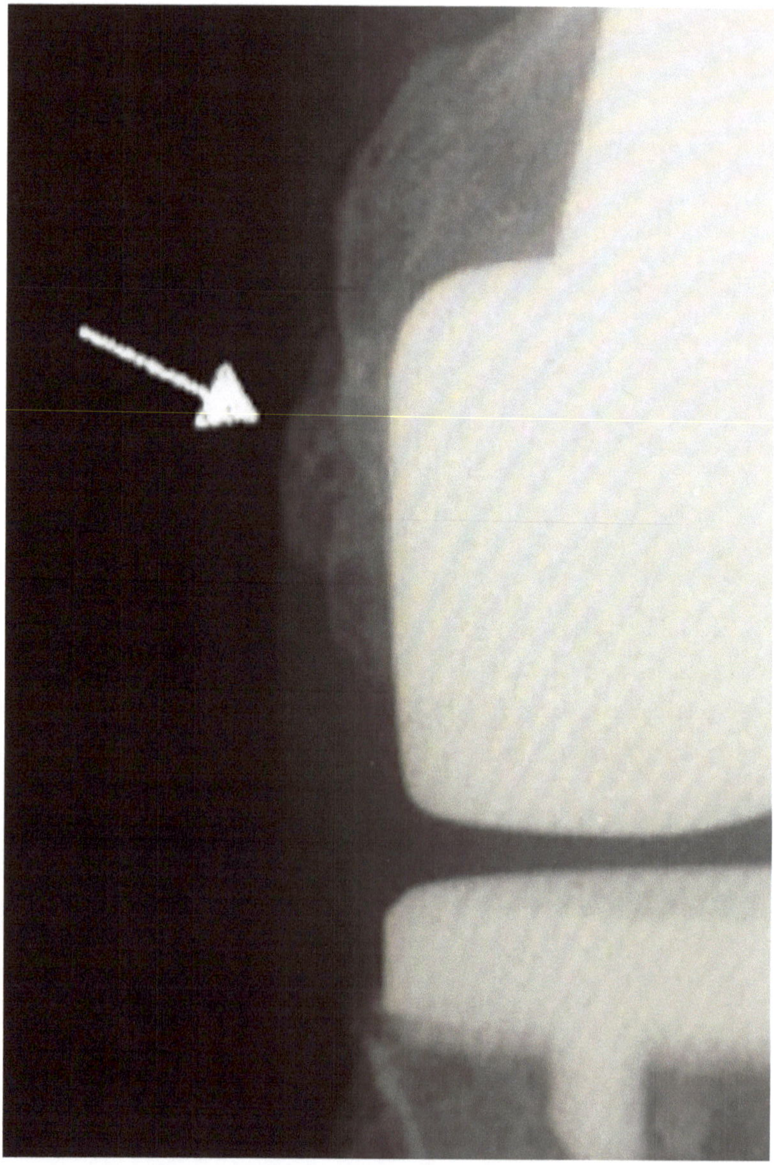

Figures 6-46 a & b: Views of a dislocating fabella.

Figure 6-46a: With the knee in extension the fabella can be seen just lateral to lateral condyles.

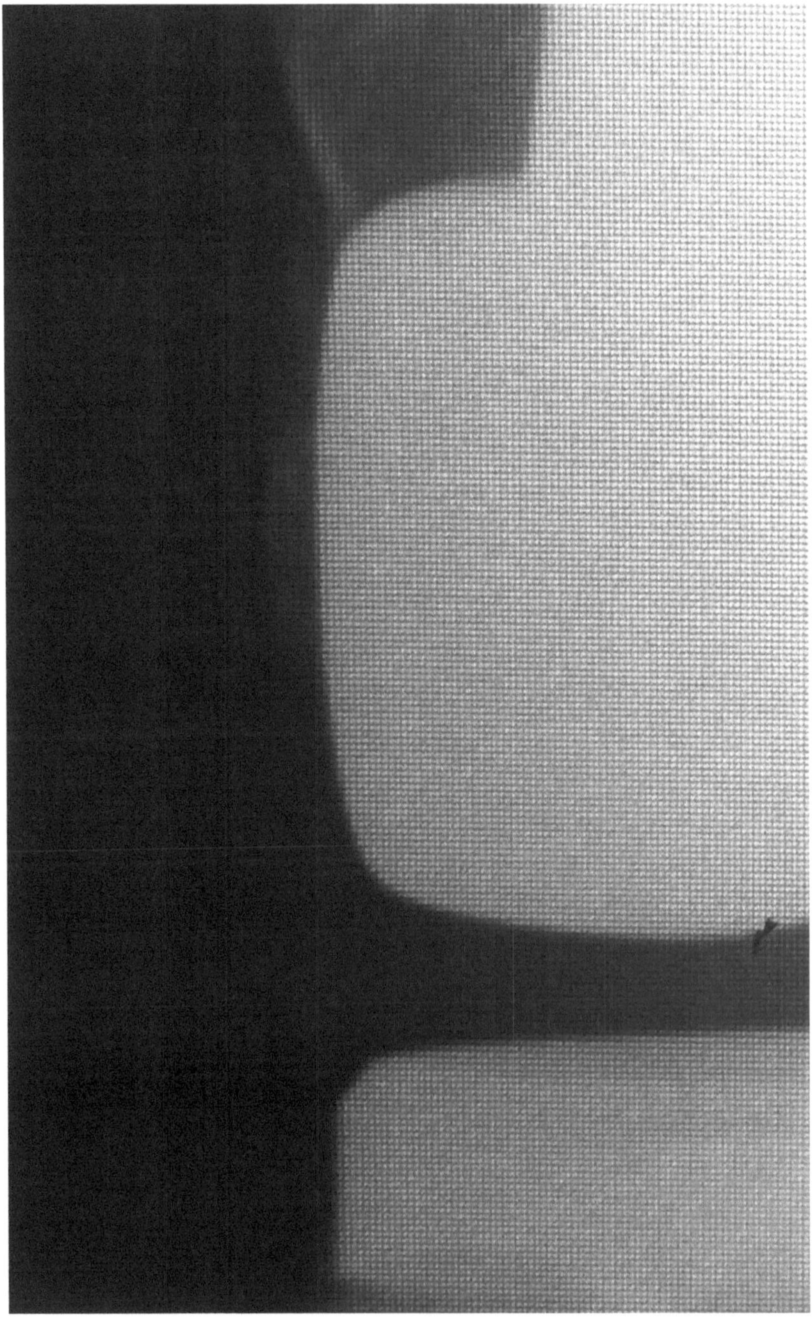

Figure 6-46b: In slight flexion the fabella is almost not seen. The patient walked in mild flexion and there was a palpable snap with he changed position from extension to flexion.

The patient is 2 years post TKA. He had a painful noise at the posterior lateral corner of the knee when he went between extension and flexion and as a result he walked with his knee in flexion. In the x-ray, in the extended position the fabella is more lateral than in the flexed position. It may be that in the extended position the condyle is more prominent and with the overlying biceps the pressure on the fabella-femoral joint is greater as is the pain. Fabellectomy yielded full pain relief and the patient was able to fully extend while walking.

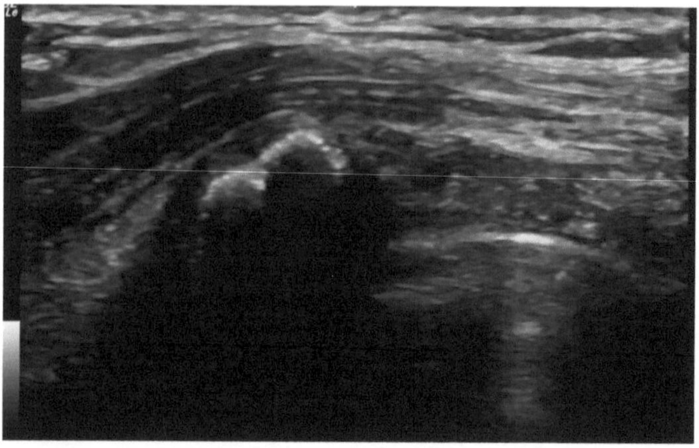

Figure 6-46c: In extension the fabella moves laterally and the biceps moves anterior-lateral to lie over the fabella.

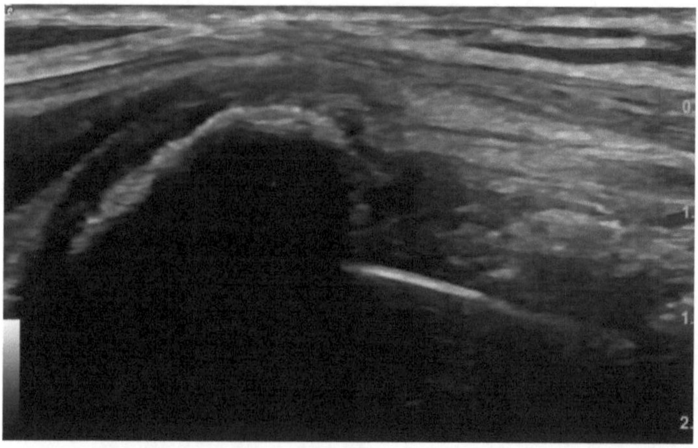

Figure 6-46d: In flexion in the ITB drops back to cover the area.

Loose PMMA after TKA

PMMA can, like bone, be a source of pain either by friction or as a loose body.

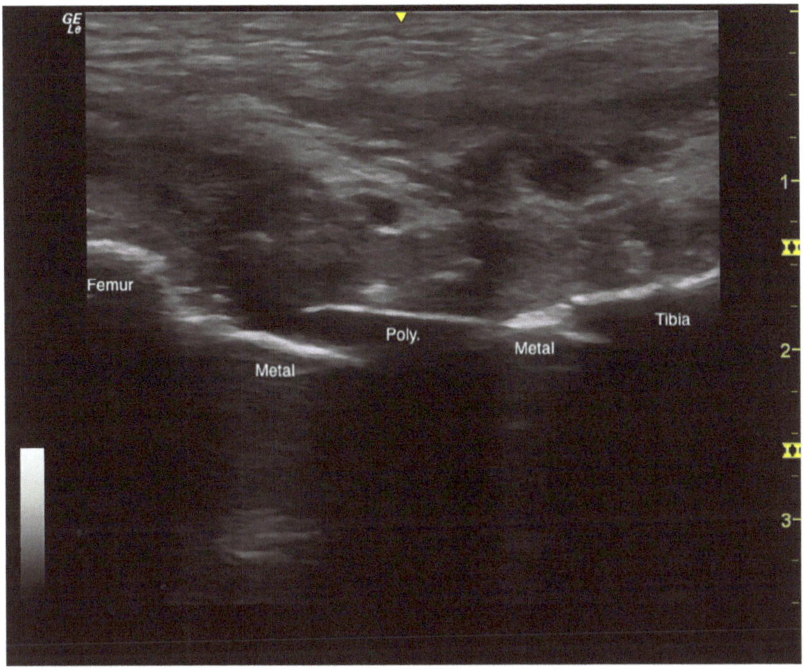

Figures 6-47: Ultrasound view of PMMA in the lateral gutter of a total knee arthroplasty.

Figure 6-47a: This is a normal lateral view of a TKA with the lateral inferior genicular artery seen as the dark circle in the center.

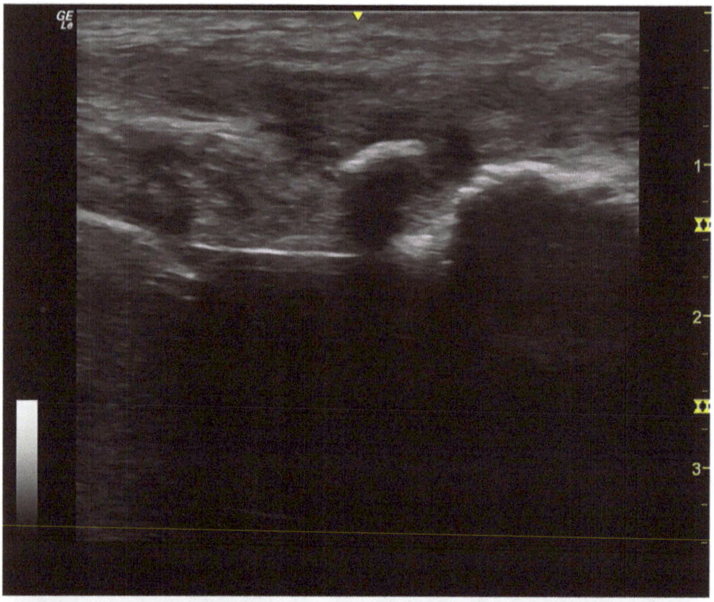

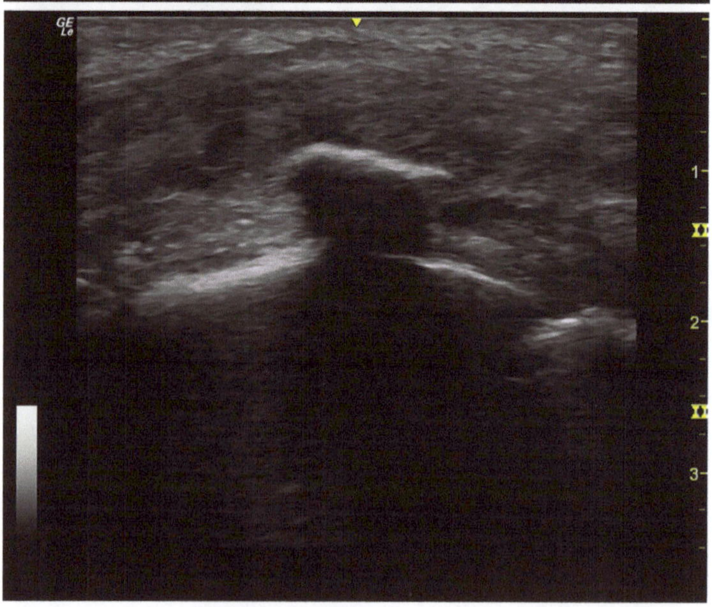

Figure 6-47b: The second is a slightly different probe position. A bit of PMMA creates a shadow over the metal of the tibial module.

Figure 6-47c: The third shows PMMA proud over the femur and its prosthesis.

Office procedures – aspirations and injections

Many injections are done without ultrasound, particularly in thin people. Ultrasound uses the same anatomic landmarks but is useful in deeper areas and in patients in whom bony structures have been obscured by swelling or fat. The operator selects an approach that will allow the needle to be perpendicular to the beam of the probe for greater visualization. The needle enhancement setting on the ultrasound machine is also useful. For especially deep structures, special needles that are designed for ultrasound use can be used. These are also useful if one is going to inject close to a nerve as the tip of the nerve block needle has a 45° bevel, as opposed to the 18° bevel of the needles we usually use in the clinic.

An interesting effect that we see in the knee in the overweight patient is the result of the differing indices of sound refraction. Sound travels through fat slower than it does through muscle and in the approach to the knee the needle appears to bend on the screen. I call this the "Uri Gellar" affect after the famous mentalist who would bend spoons with his mind.

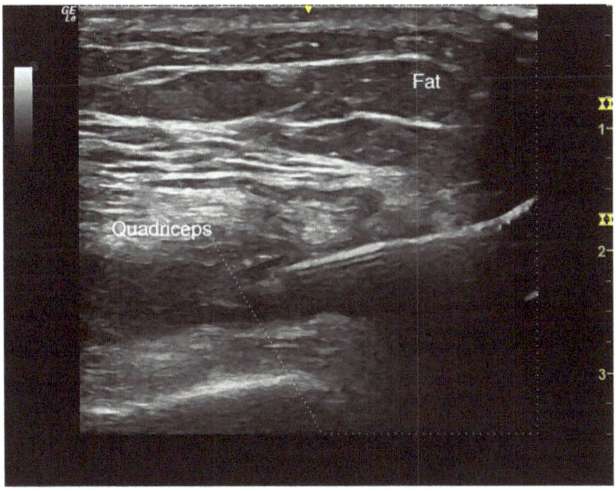

Figure 6-48: "Uri Geller Effect." A difference in speed of sound between fat and tendon creates an apparent bend in the needle, which 'magically' straightens as the needle is withdrawn. The effect in this patient is accentuated by the combination of a thickening water density and a diminishing fat layer.

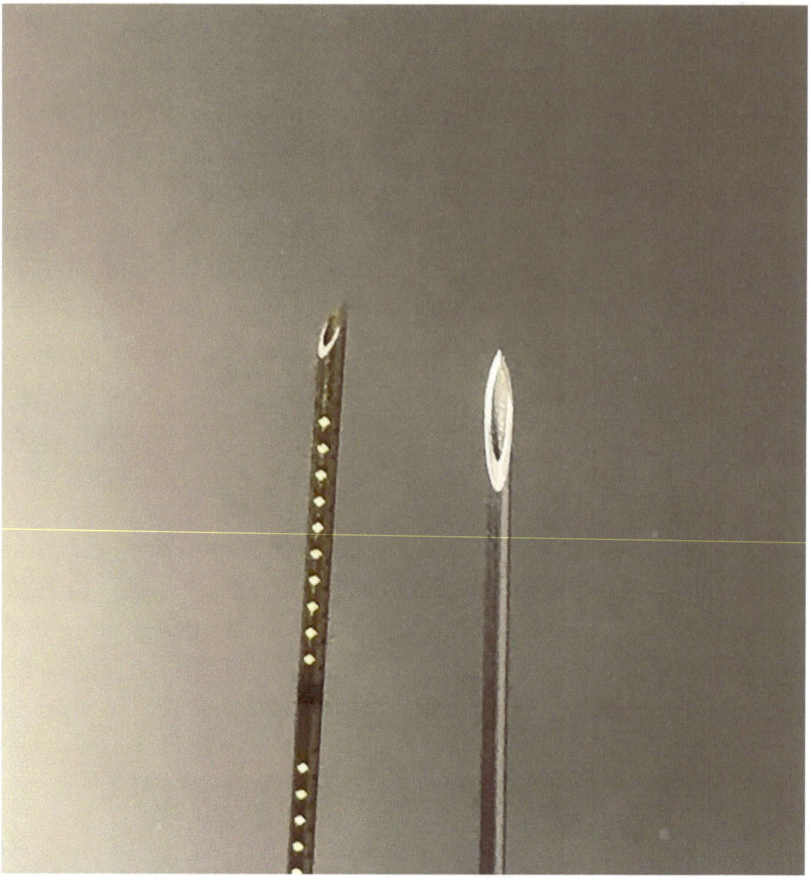

Figure 6-48: Photo of needle tips. On the left is a nerve block needle and on the right is one of the usual needles we have in clinic. The bevel of the nerve block needle is 45º while the normal needle is a much sharper 18º. In addition, the shaft of the nerve block needle has been modified to make it echogenic even at steeper angles.

Appearance of injections on ultrasound

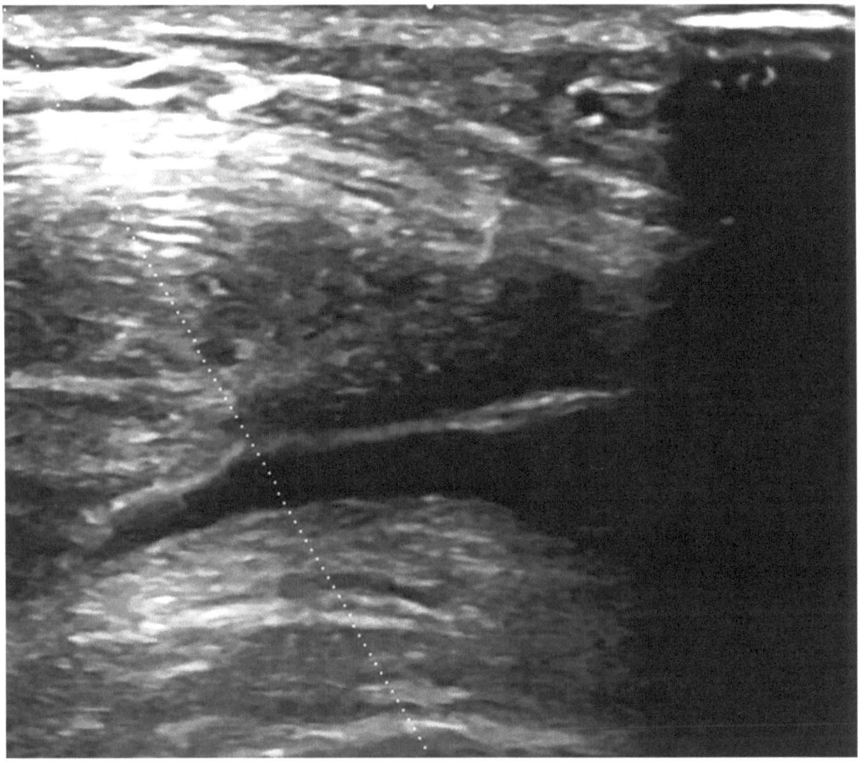

Figures 6-49a & b: Ultrasound view of injection of the knee – steroid and visco-supplementation.

Figure 49a: Steroid injection the starch granules create a trail across the knee. The knee is in extension.

The approach is from the lateral side in the short axis. If there is an effusion, the injection is best done with the knee in extension over the femoral fat. If there is no effusion, knee flexion allows the use of trochlear cartilage to make joint space more visible.

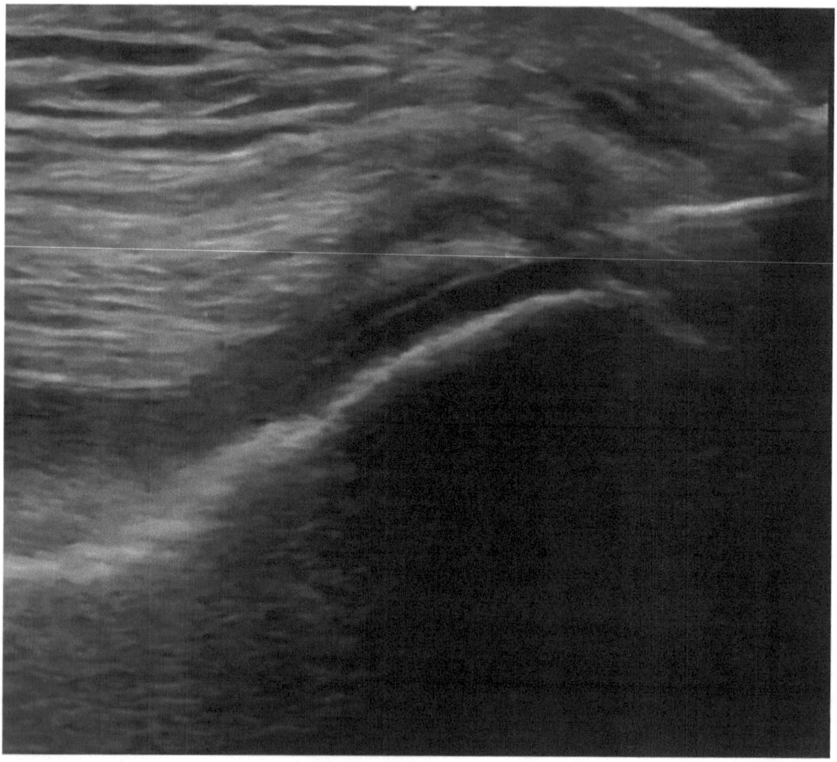

Figure 6-49b: Visco-supplementation is, of course, more viscous. There is no turbulence on Doppler and no starch granules. The knee is in flexion. The fluid emphasizes the surface of the trochlear cartilage.

Knee injection in morbid obesity and fat refraction

In obesity we need, a longer needle, lower frequency and a steeper approach. Together this indicates the use of the modified ultrasound needles mentioned above. The patient is seated with the knee flexed, so that we can use the trochlea as our target.

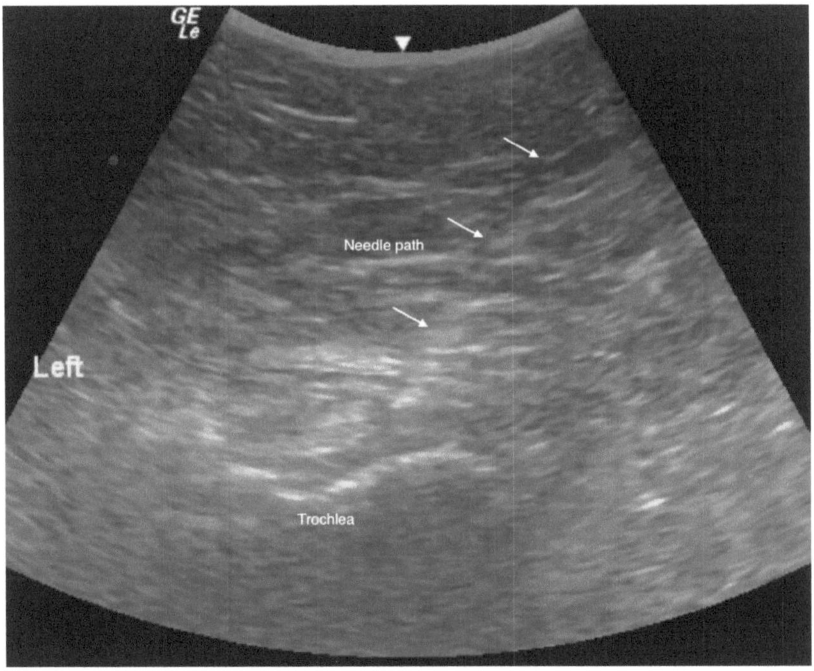

Figure 6-50: Morbidly obese patient with osteoarthritis. The patient is seated with the knee flexed about 90°. The needle is a 100mm nerve block that is used by the anesthesia service.

Needle approach to tendinosis

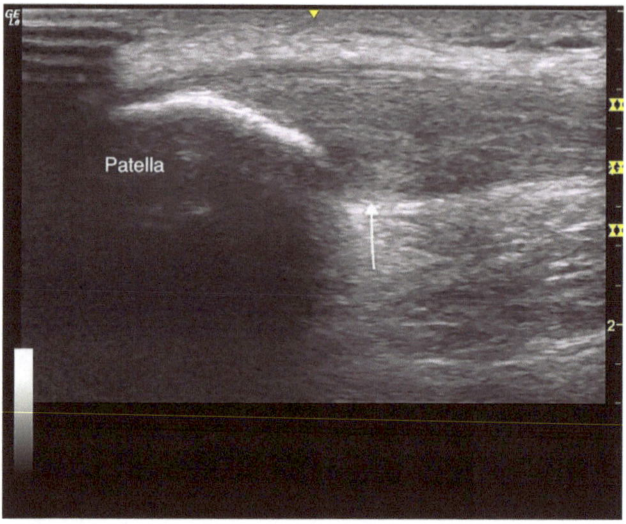

Figure 6-51a & b: Ultrasound view of the needle approach to tendinosis: appropriate for dry needling or PRP.

Figure 6-51a: Tendinosis as described in the diagnostic section. The tendon is thicker here at the patellar end and the deeper portion is less echogenic. Therefore our target is the deeper area of the patellar origin.

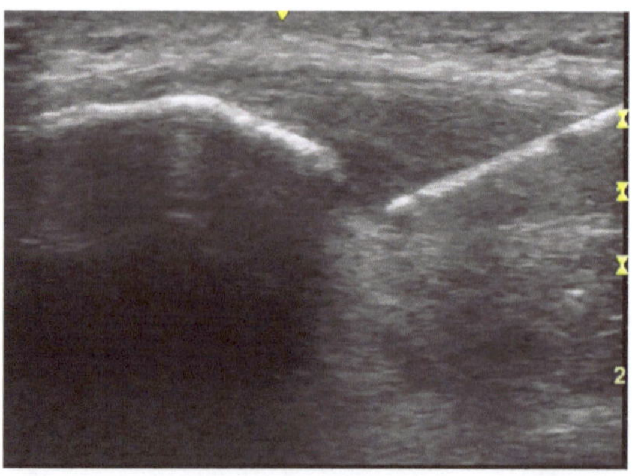

Figure 6-51b: The needle goes to the deep layer of the origin. In this low angle approach a modified needle is not required.

Bursa aspiration

Prepatellar aspiration is usually for a clear serous or serosanguinous fluid. Use of the ultrasound can allow viewing the needle tip to avoid sucking up synovial lining and plugging the needle.

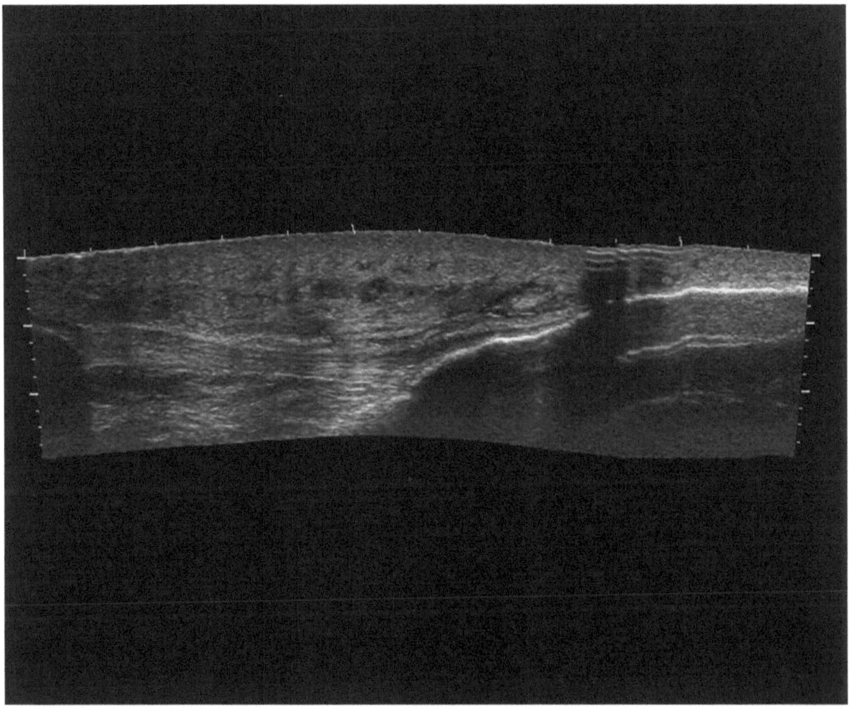

Figure 6-52a-d: Ultrasound view of the aspiration of a prepatellar bursa: old and new.

Figure 6-52a: A chronically thickened bursa without any fluid to drain. No aspiration was attempted

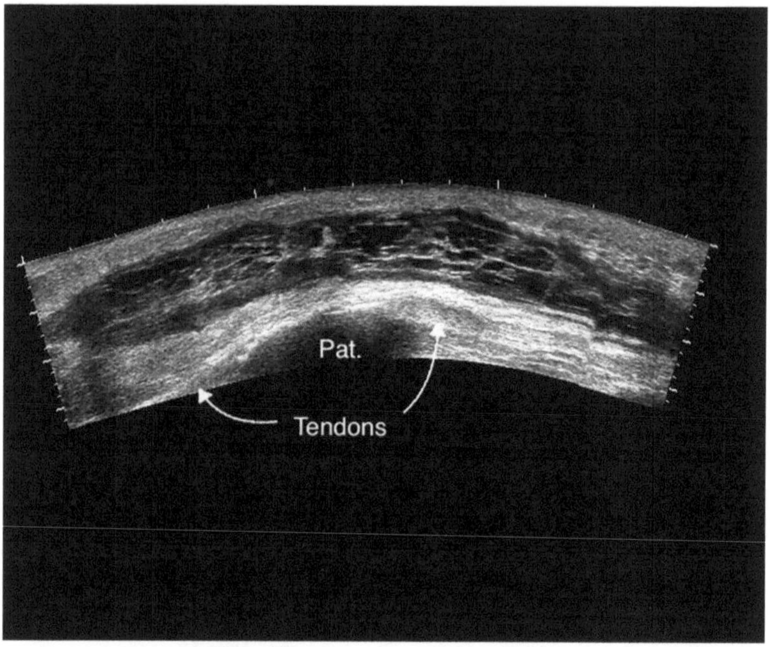

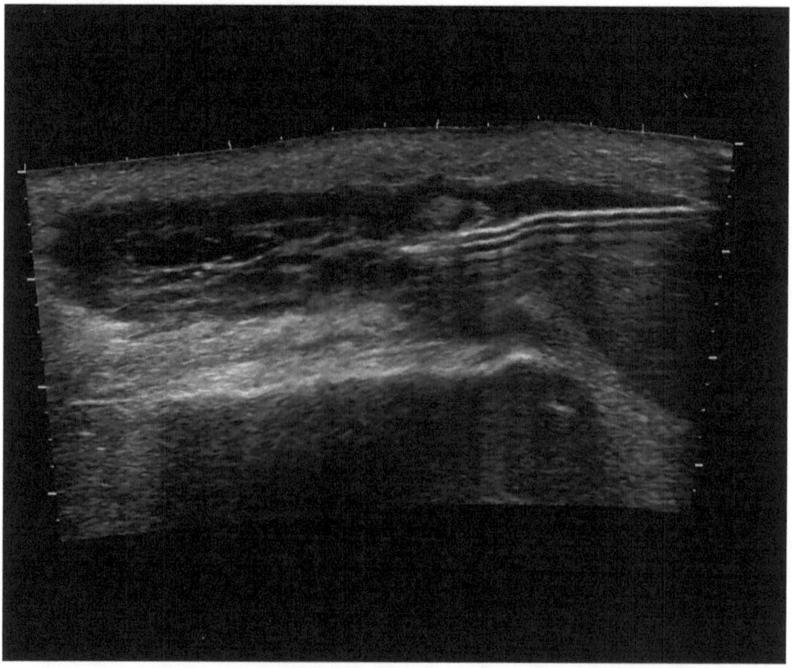

Figure 6-52b: An infected bursa with loculations, which can be broken up with the needle.

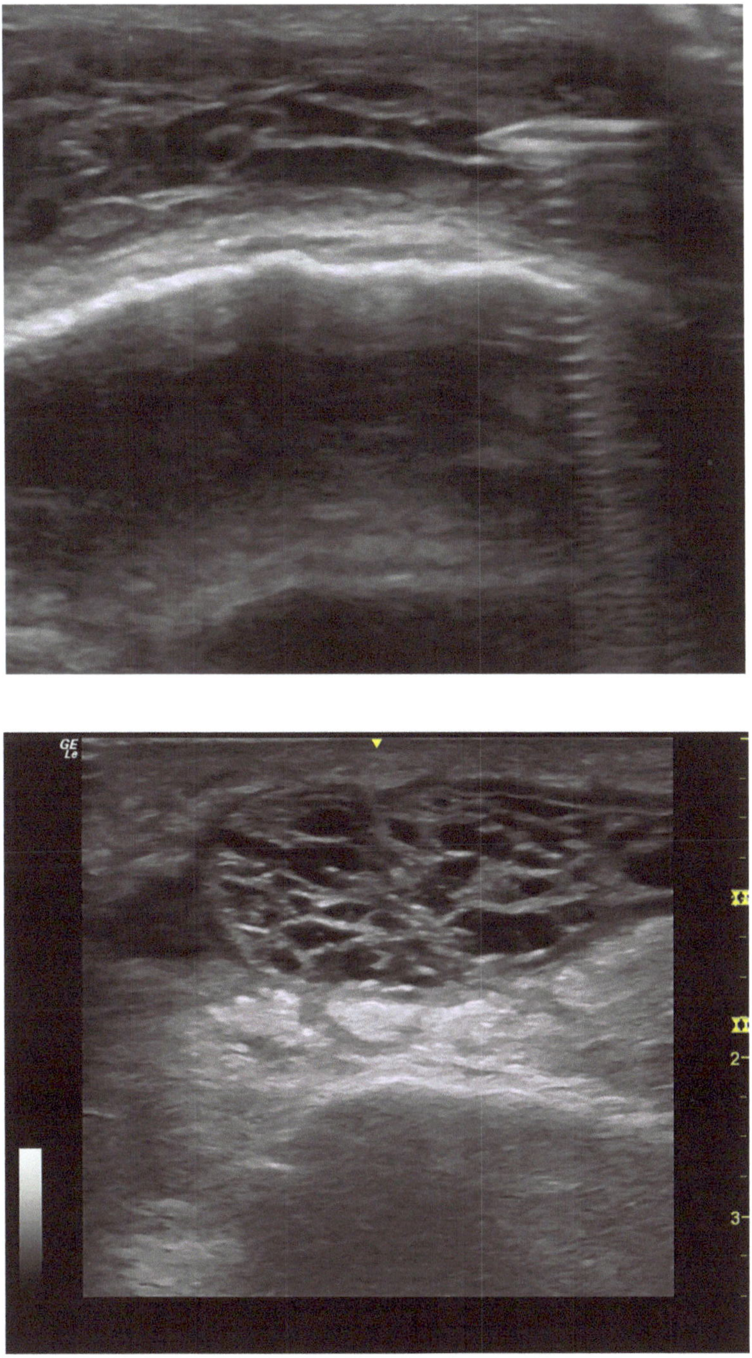

Figures 6-52c & d : Some hemorrhagic bursae require breaking up with a needle as well. A chronic hemorrhagic bursa at two months.

Differentiating cellulitis from bursitis.

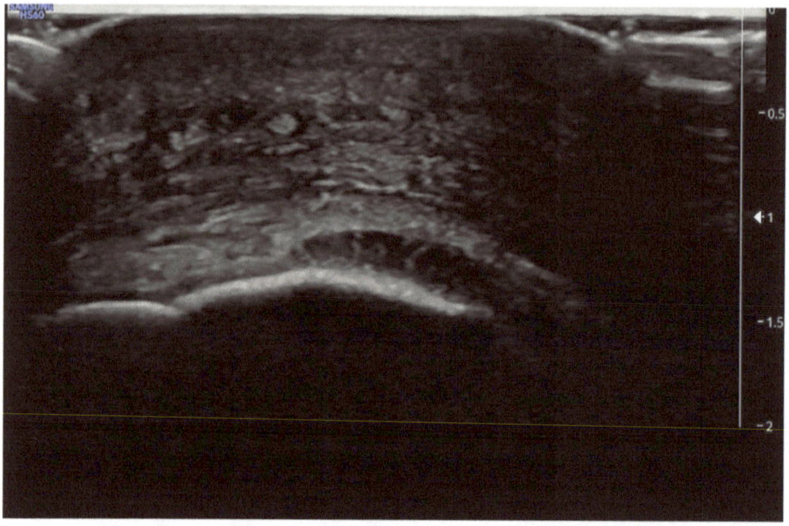

Figure 6-53: Prepatellar cellulitis. Ultrasound was done on this ICU patient to rule out an abscess or any other fluid. Subcutaneous tissue edema was seen without fluid abscess. As a result of this ultrasound the patient was not taken to surgery. He recovered with antibiotics alone.

Ultrasound use in operative procedures

The placement of the arthroscope without the ultrasound is done on the basis of bony landmarks. These landmarks can be obscured in cases of obesity. In addition, when the surgeon is accustomed to using the ultrasound probe additional or rarely use portals can be developed, portals which are routinely overlaid with soft tissue, in particular the posterior knee.

Portal placement in obesity

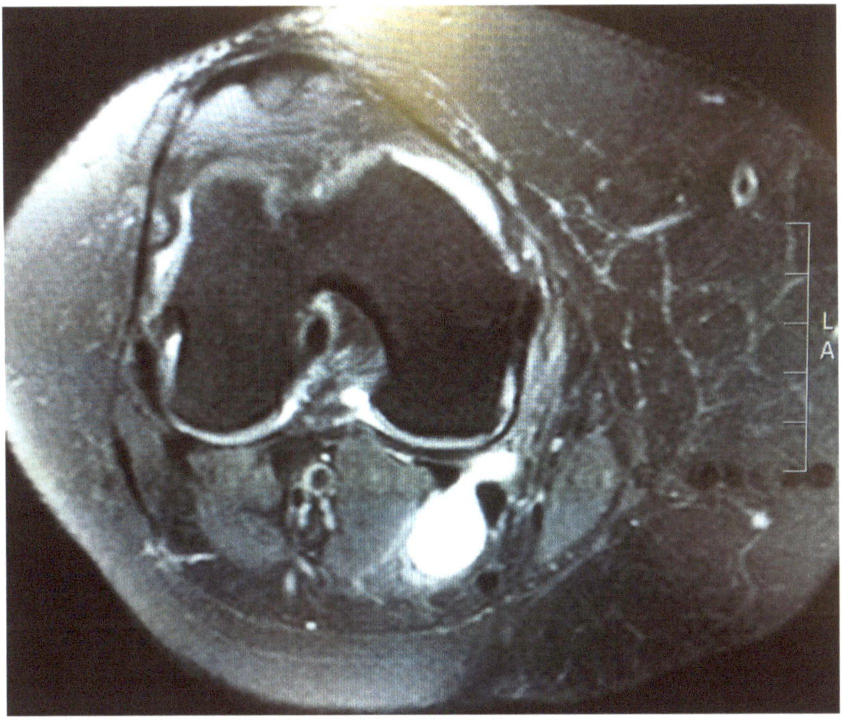

Figure 6-54: Ultrasound posterior medial portal placement in an obese patient.

Figure 6-54a: In the obese patient there is often only a small increase in subcutaneous fat on the anterior knee, but in the posterior and medial knee where the surgeon may want to make a posterior medial portal it can be inches thick and obscure the bony landmarks. The anterior portals were developed in the usual fashion.

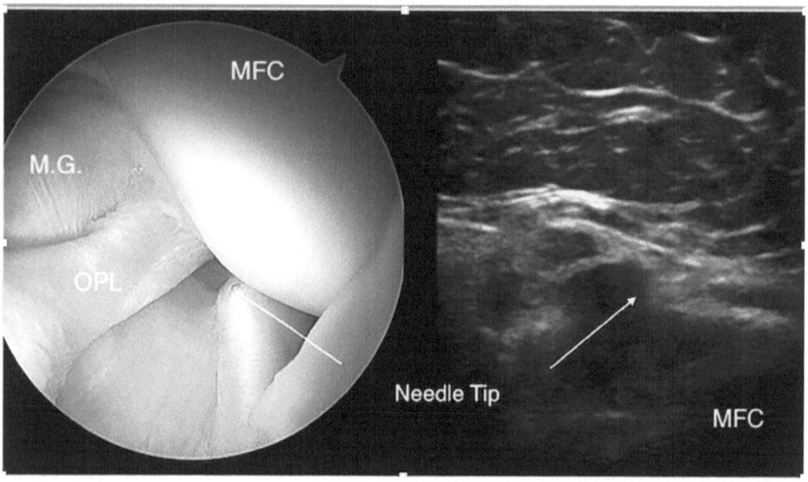

Figure 6-54b: In this dual projection ultrasound restores some of the landmarks. In the arthroscopic view a 70° scope has been inserted through the anterior lateral portal, then between PCL and the MFC, into the posterior knee, while the knee is held in 90° of flexion. The ultrasound probe on the other hand is on the medial surface of the knee. We see the needle tip entering between a band of the oblique popliteal ligament, OPL, and the medial femoral condyle. The ultrasound probe on the other hand is on the medial surface of the flexed knee. The needle is better visualized in a dynamic ultrasound view than in this static view. The condyle is to the right of the needle and the two small dark circles to the left are portions of the cyst.

Ultrasound guided posterior portal placement (PVNS) (especially posterolateral)

Posterior portals are not commonly used in arthroscopy of the knee. One of the major factors in this is that the major nerves and vessels are close to the posterior capsule. The most at-risk structure is the peroneal nerve, so we will use it to demonstrate how ultrasound guidance can eliminate some of the risk. The portals are developed by passing a needle under ultrasound guidance through the posterior compartments from lateral to medial. A wire is passed and then the cannulae are passed over the wire using a modified trochar. The needle is passed with the knee in medium flexion, a compromise, so that condyles can be seen (best in extension) and the peroneal nerve has dropped back (best in full flexion).

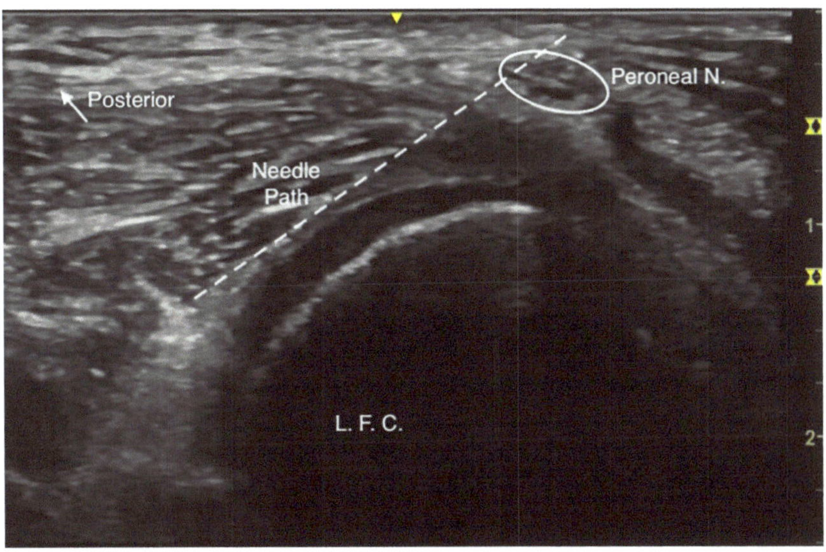

Figures 6-55a.

In full extension one can see both the peroneal nerve and the back of the lateral femoral condyle. In this particular patient a posterolateral portal, dotted line, would go right through the nerve.

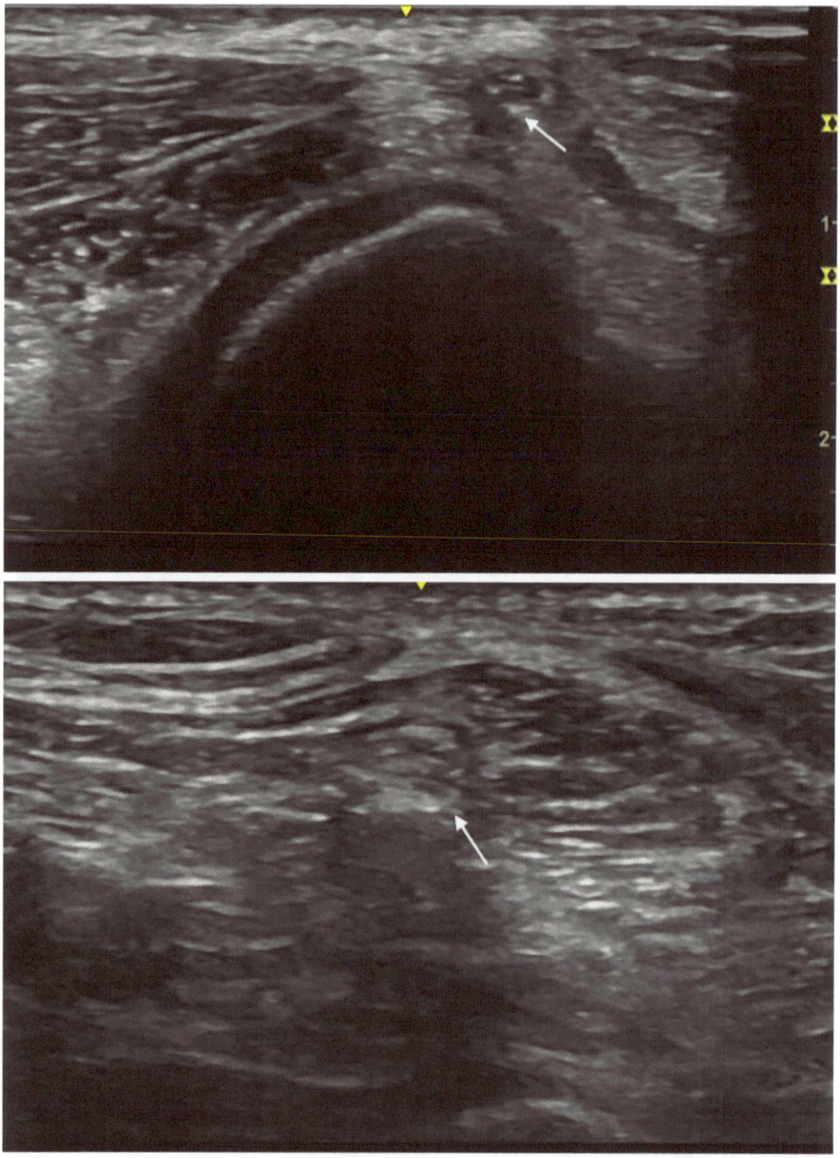

Figures 6-55b & c : As flexion begins, B, the nerve moves a little posterior to the condyle. In deeper flexion, C, the nerve and the adjacent biceps move to a safe distance, but the condyle is less well seen. So, the optimum flexion is the position in which the surgeon can see the back of the condyle and that the nerve is at a safe distance. Having the knee filled with arthroscopy fluid helps with visualization and with moving nerves and vessels away from the condyles.

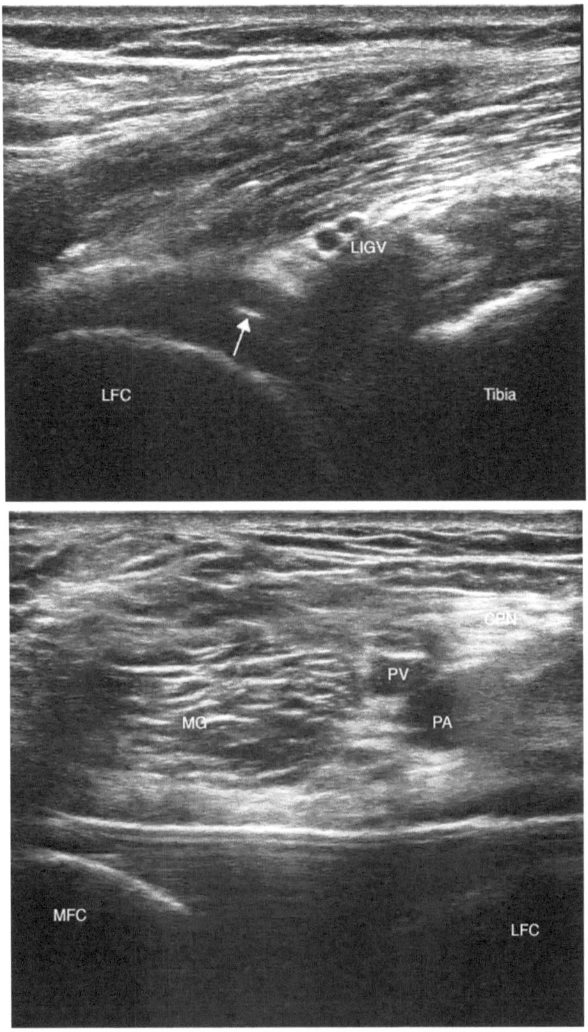

Figures 6-55d and e. Figure 55d: Long axis of limb and Figure 55e: Short axis of limb. In mid-flexion, about 70°, there is room behind the knee for the ultrasound probe. While at the same time both the condyles and the nerves can be seen. The needle (arrow) is placed below the condyle and above the meniscus. The needle is continued across the knee to a similar position with respect to the medial structures and then out the medial skin. A wire placed through the needle allows the placement of cannulae over cannulated trocars. LFC, lateral femoral condyle; LIGV, lateral inferior genicular vessels; MFC, medial femoral condyle; MG , medial gastrocnemius; PA popliteal artery.

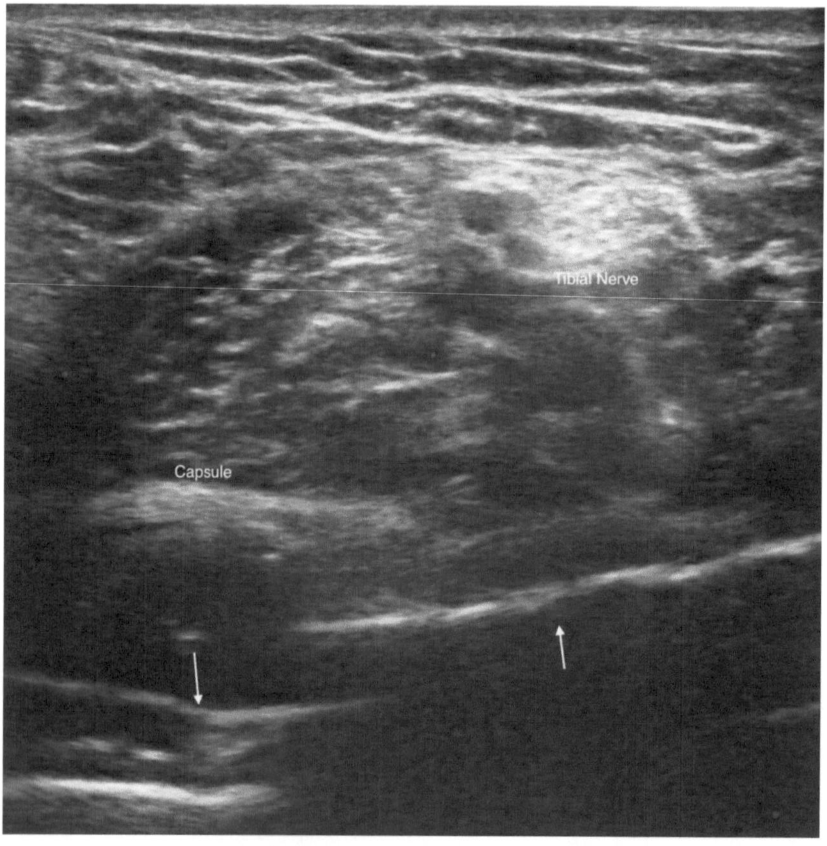

Figure 6-55f: In full 90º flexion and with arthroscopic fluid there is ample room for the instruments (arrows). But the distance from capsule to nerve stays the same.

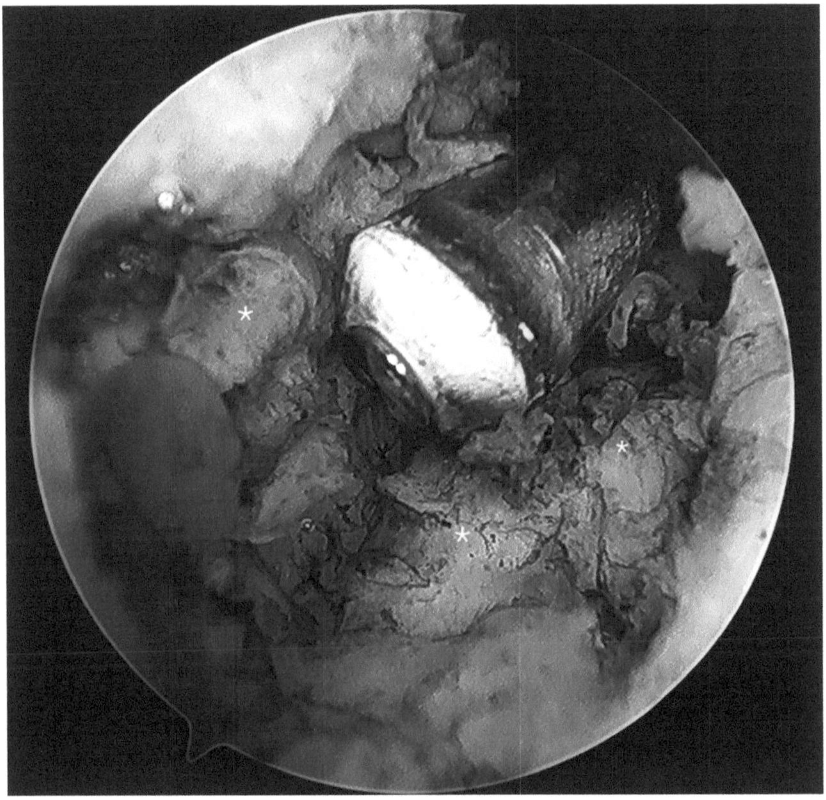

Figure 6-55g: There is adequate room to work on the PVNS. In this picture the electrocautery is opening a little of the popliteus fascia to expose some nodules which grew down the sheath. The scope is in the posteromedial portal. Note how in flexion the portals move posteriorly so we get a better view and more instrument mobility.

Posterior lateral portal in loose body retrieval

Ultrasound can be used to locate a truly loose body. This 32 y.o. woman had a history of internal derangement of the left knee and imaging that was negative for everything but a sessile body seen at the base of the ACL. At surgery her knee was in excellent condition, but the loose body could not be found. Ultrasound was used to see if she had a Bakers cyst which the body might be hiding. The loose body was spotted in the posterior lateral compartment above the lateral condyle. Ultrasound was used to make a posterior lateral portal through which the loose body was retrieved.

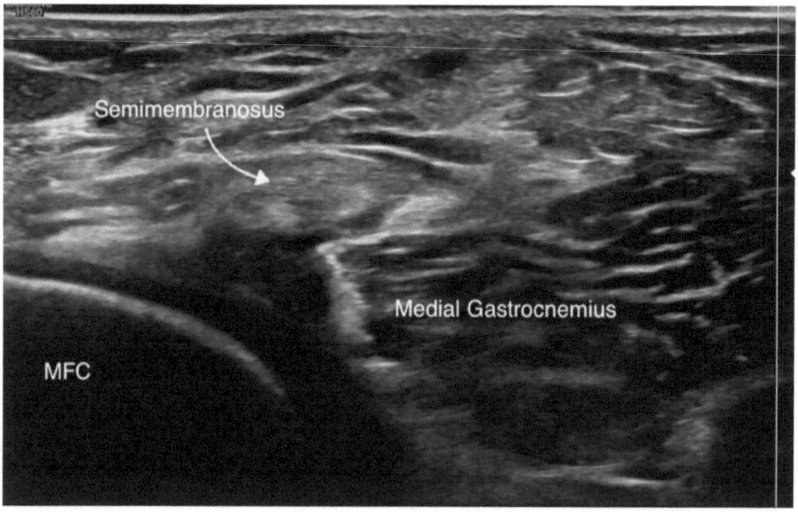

Fig. 6-56a: No cyst was found in this posterior medial corner view. A Baker's cyst would be found between semimembranosus and medial gastrocnemius.

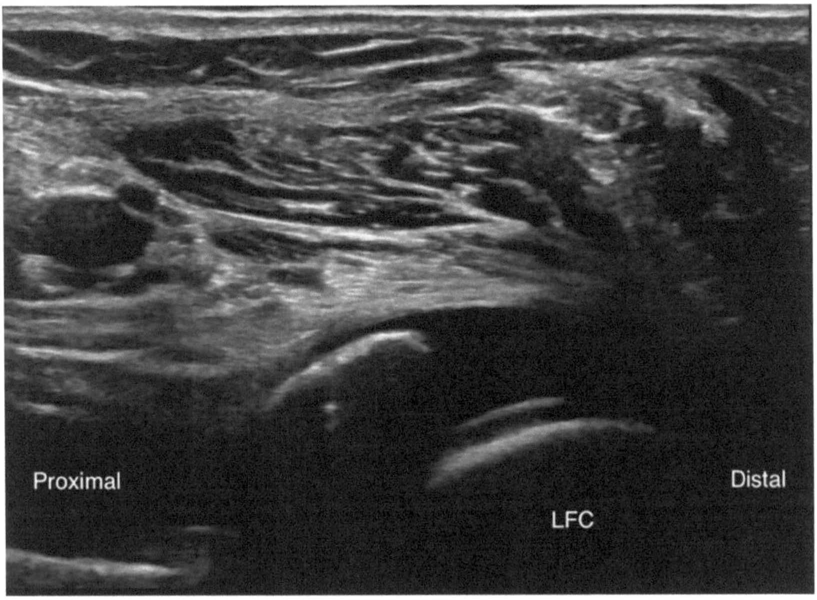

Fig 6-56b: A long axis view of the posterior lateral compartment. In sweeping the back of the knee, in short axis, we spotted the loose body. This long axis view shows the body hidden above the lateral condyle.

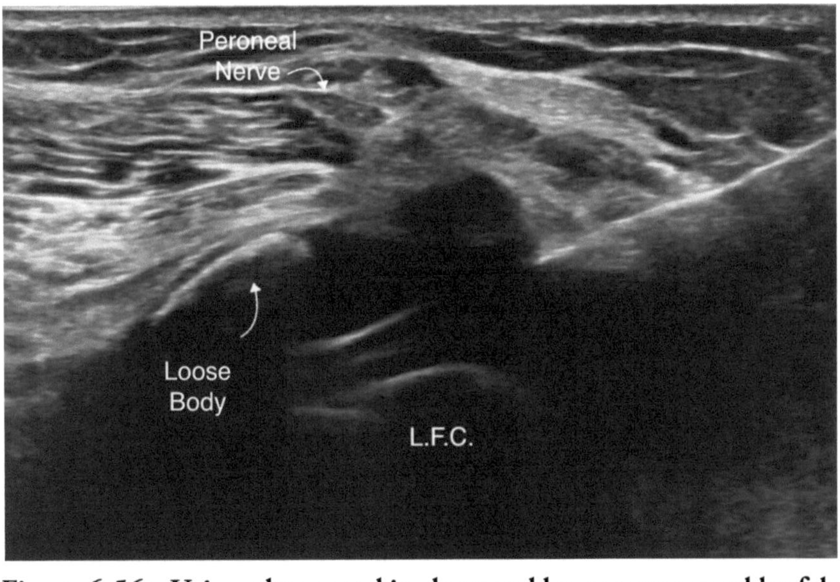

Figure 6-56c: Using ultrasound in short and long axes we could safely select our portal with a needle. This is a short axis view.

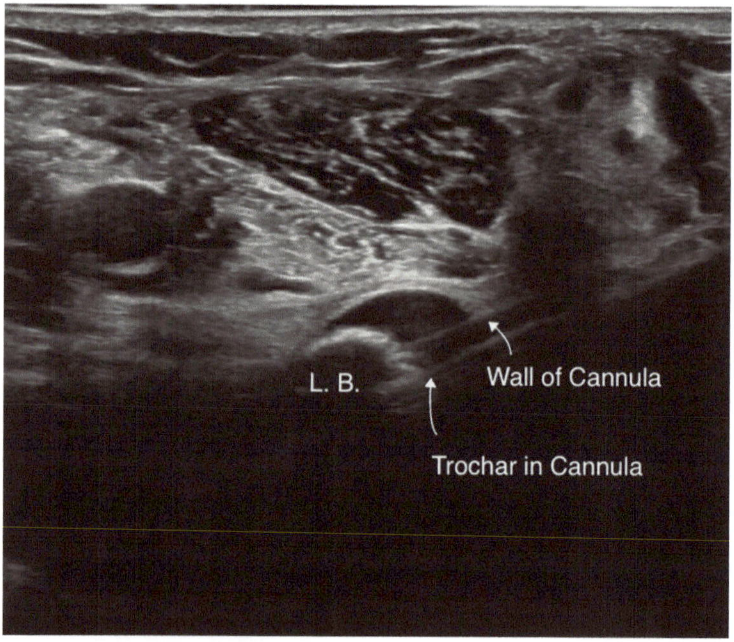

Figure 6-56d: Cannula placement.

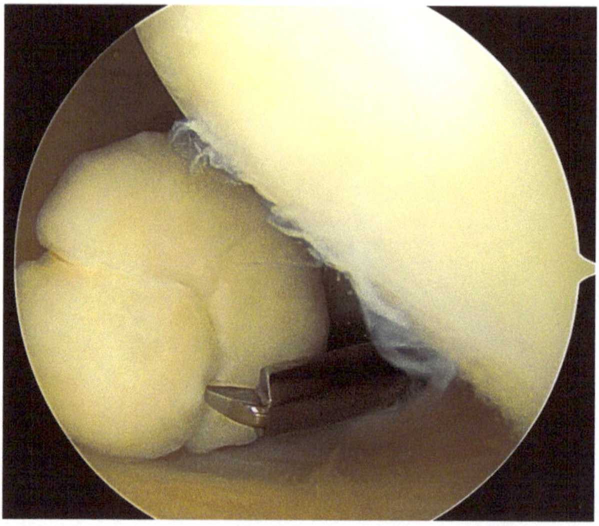

Figure 6-56e: We viewed through the anteromedial portal, so we did not make a posteromedial portal. We could place the grasping instrument but could not retrieve through the cannula, so loose body, instrument and cannula were removed together.

Sciatic nerve block at the knee

The sciatic nerve and its two main branches are readily visible by ultrasound in the popliteal fossa. Perinervous hydro-dissection can produce a profound anesthesia in the lower leg, ankle and foot. This is useful for foot and ankle fractures and other emergency treatment especially if the patient's condition makes deeper anesthesia undesirable. The approach is from the lateral side, with a needle that has a 45° bevel (as opposed to the 18° bevel standard needles have). This makes the needle less likely to puncture nerves, but it does make skin penetration a little more difficult. As the needle approaches the nerve the local anesthetic is injected to dissect the soft tissue off of the nerve and create a 'donut' of anesthetic around the nerve. Injecting around the tibial and peroneal branches offers a little more surface to the anesthetic for absorption as opposed to the main nerve, but the choice is most often made on the basis of visualization. Because of the thickness of these nerves, allow some time to pass for the anesthesia to take effect.

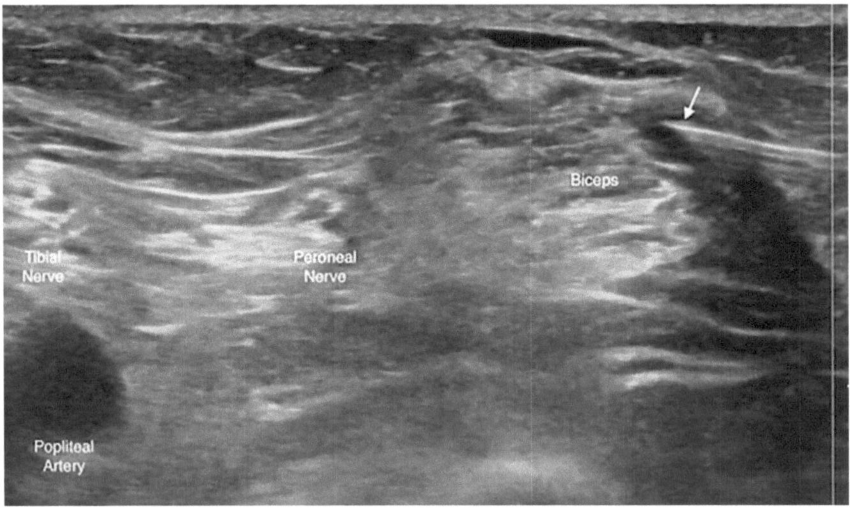

Figure 6-57a: The needle (arrow) is brought in from the lateral side. In this example the initial direction is a little too dorsal or superficial. The needle is redirected toward one and then the other branch. Further down the limb the peroneal nerve is much closer to the biceps.

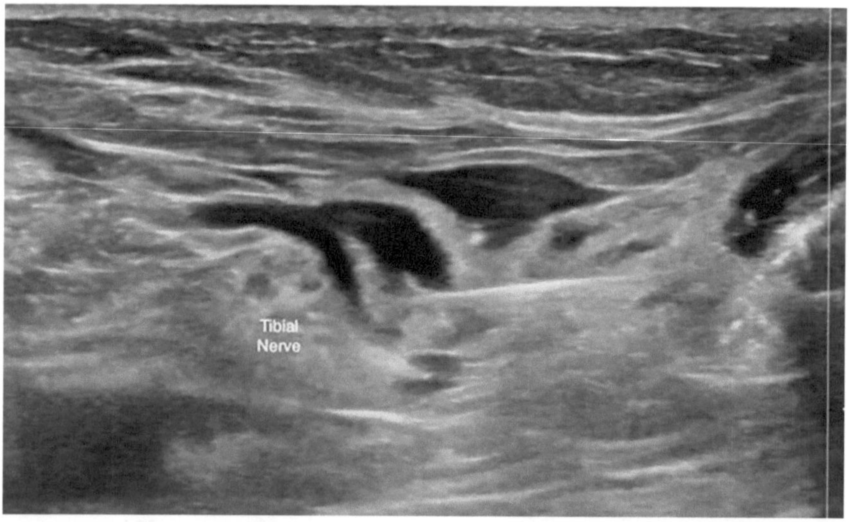

Figure 6-57b: Initial hydro-dissection at tibial nerve. The anesthetic is the dark area on the upper and right sides of the nerve. The needle is then moved to a deeper surface and more anesthetic injected.

Abscess drainage in the O.R.

Ultrasound allows the surgeon to observe an abscess in real time. The result is that one can exam all of the recesses of the fluid collection and ensure complete drainage without making an even larger incision. We still need to have adequate drainage.

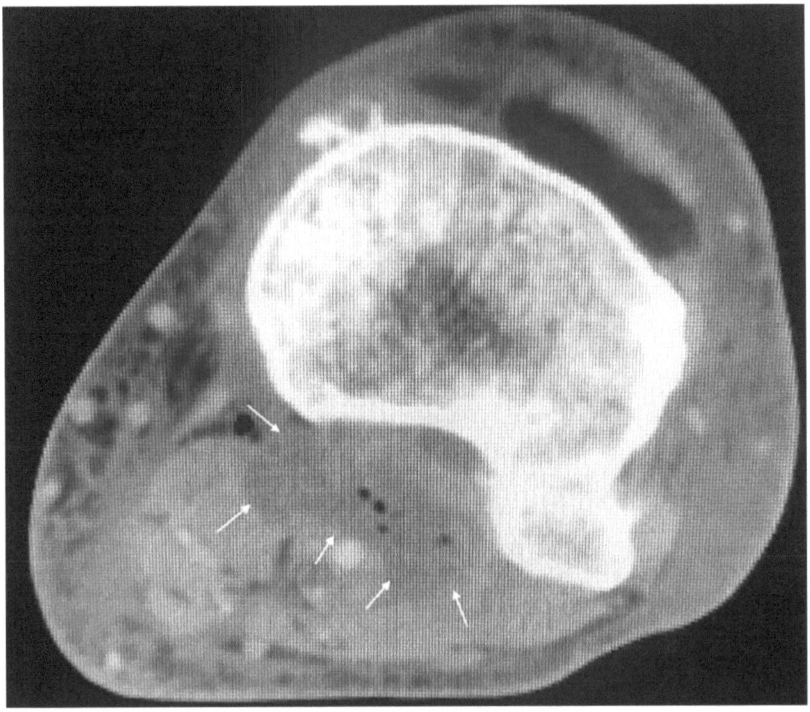

Figure 6-58a-e: CT and ultrasound views of an abscess behind the knee and exploration thereof. The patient was a chronically ill man with arthritis of the knee who appeared in the ER with infection behind rather than within the knee.

Figure 6-70a: A contrast CT scan just below the knee shows the abscess with small air bubbles between the tibia and the contrast in the popliteal artery.

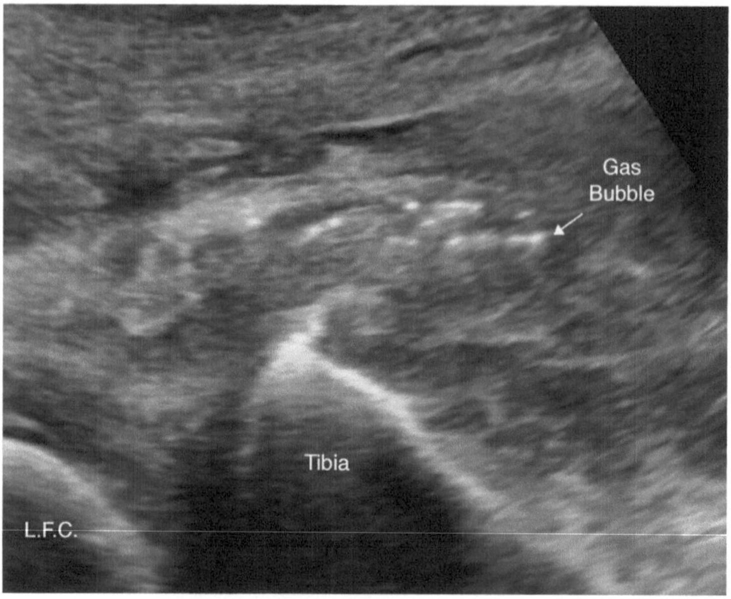

Figure 6-58b: Long axis ultrasound view behind the knee shows the disturbed area with small hyperechoic gas bubbles.

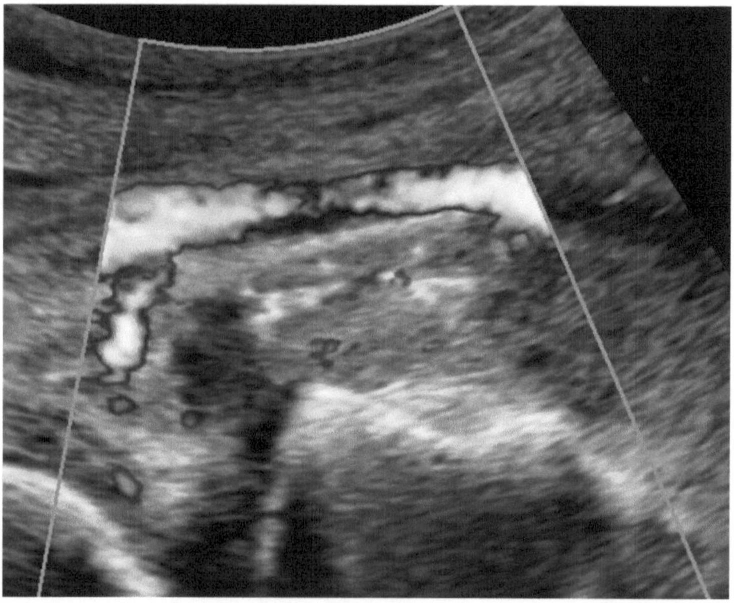

Figure 6-58c: Ultrasound Doppler will show the popliteal artery and the abscess perhaps even more clearly.

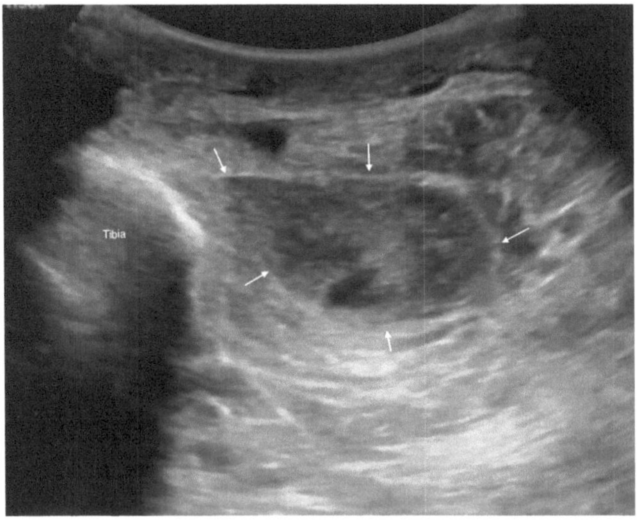

Figure 6-58d: The abscess can be traced distally down the back of the tibia.

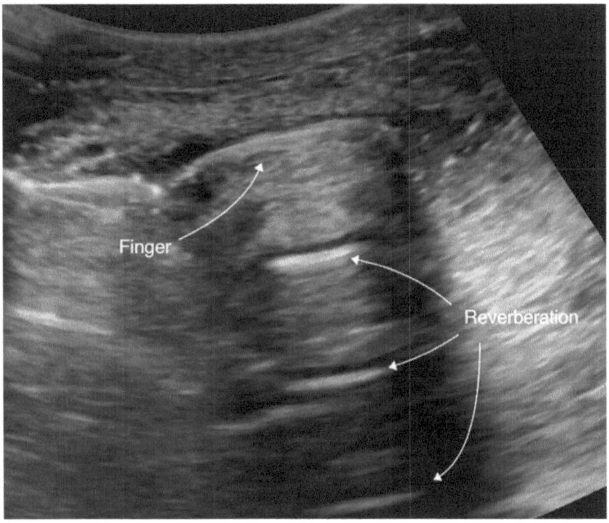

Figure 6-58e: During the surgery the surgeon's finger can be followed, here seen near the skin in the lower abscess. Drain or packing placement can also be followed. In this last figure one can see the surgeon's gloved index finger with three reverberation or artifact lines deep to it. Adequate drainage is obtained without having to do even more dissection to ensure the safety of nerves and vessels

Abscess in BKA stump (late)

In the event of an actual infection, ultrasound can determine the likelihood of infection and help with surgical planning. This patient was 5-years from his amputation. He thought he was doing well with his prosthesis until he developed pain, swelling and fever. The skin at the distal stump was lichenified indicating that his weight was not evenly distributed.

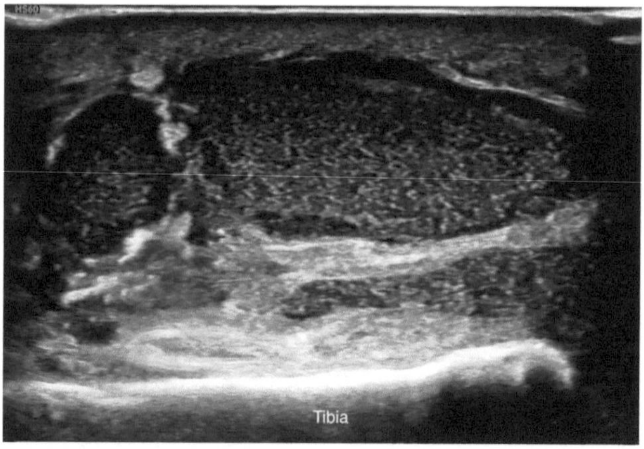

Figure 6-59a: Three portions of the abscess are seen over the distal anterior tibia. It is a complex yet uniform fluid. The three sections proved to be all one collection on ultrasound.

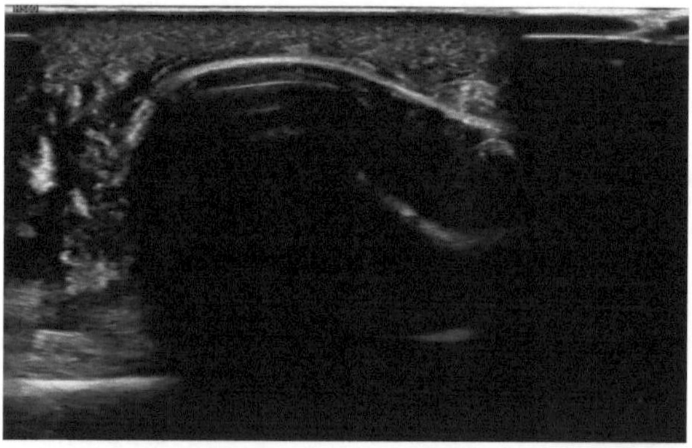

Fig 6-59b: During the surgery, the position of the surgeon's finger can be followed to ensure that the entire abscess is explored.

Multiple puncture wounds

In these cases we need to make sure that none of these wounds injure a nerve or vessel. When the patient is undergoing wound irrigation, each wound can be explored with a finger and the proximity of the finger to the vessels observed on Doppler. Since nerves tend to travel with vessels this allows us to assess deeper nerves which may not be visible on ultrasound in the trauma setting. In a heavier or more muscular individual this will involve use of the curvilineal, lower frequency probe. More superficial nerves such as the common peroneal can be observed directly with a linear probe.

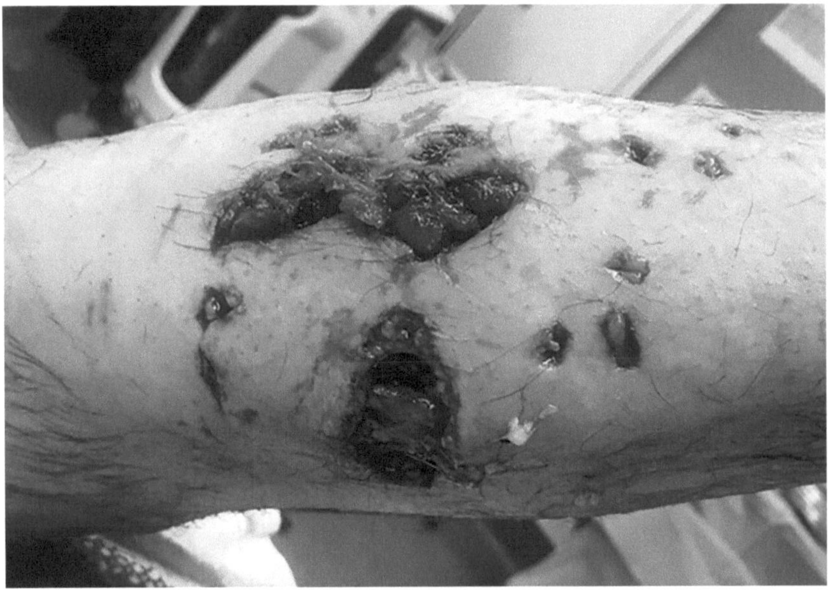

Figure 6-60a: Police dog bite of the calf. Nerves and vessels are intact on physical exam.

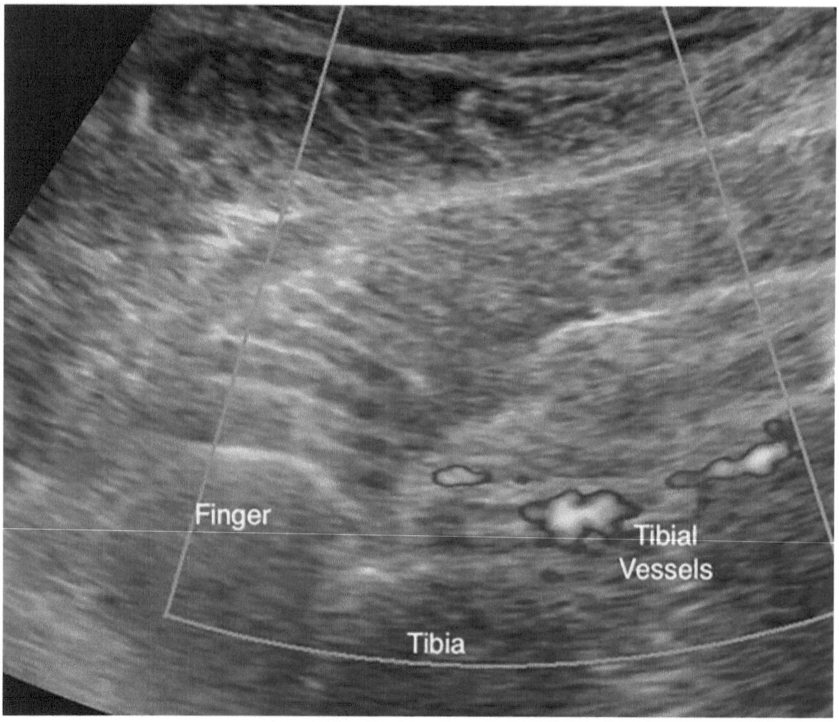

Figure 6-60b: After irrigation and debridement, each puncture can be digitally explored to ascertain if the depth of the wound comes close to the vessels and their associated nerves. In the more muscular or heavier patients the lower frequency curvilinear probe gives a better Doppler picture at depth.

Ultrasound use in preoperative planning

Ultrasound can also be used in assessing the anatomy of the knee that is affected by a previous surgery. In the case below the patient had two previous arthroscopies on the lateral joint space but continued to experience sufficient pain in the lateral joint that she required a total knee arthroplasty. Ordinarily one would not do an ultrasound in preparation for a total knee replacement, especially in someone who had had so little manipulation of the tissues in her previous surgeries. But on the most recent MRI, she was noted to have considerable swelling of the entire patellar tendon. As her previous surgery had not traumatized the tendon, we decided that this must have been a circulatory problem of the tendon.

We did a Doppler assessment to see what the current vascular situation was and found that the tendon was largely dependent on the recurrent anterior tibial artery and the lateral inferior genicular artery. We used the usual medial approach, but we were very protective of those two arteries.

At two years the arthroplasty was doing well, and the tendon was closer to normal in thickness and echogenicity as well as vascularity.

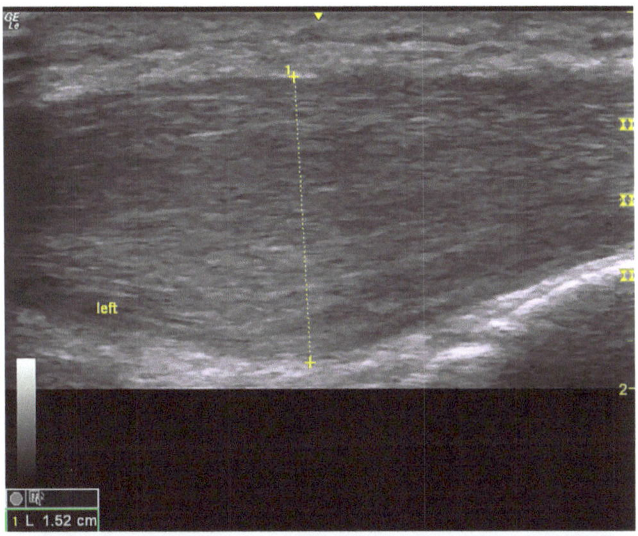

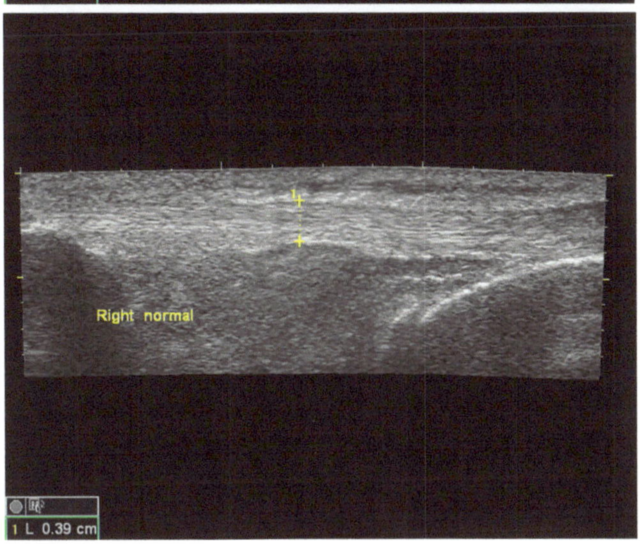

Figures 6-61a-i: MRI and ultrasound pre-and postoperative left total knee arthroplasty.

Figures 6-61a & b: Ultrasound imaging demonstrates complete involvement of the patellar tendon on the left compared to the normal right. The left patellar tendon is thicker and hypoechotic.

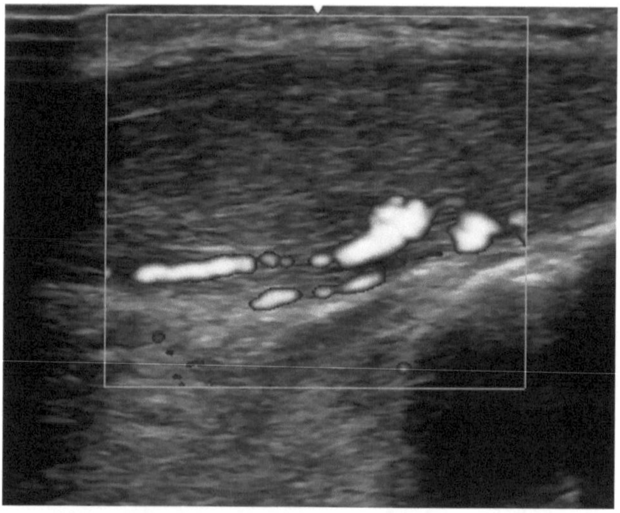

Figure 6-61c: Doppler of swollen tendon and vessels on the deep surface.

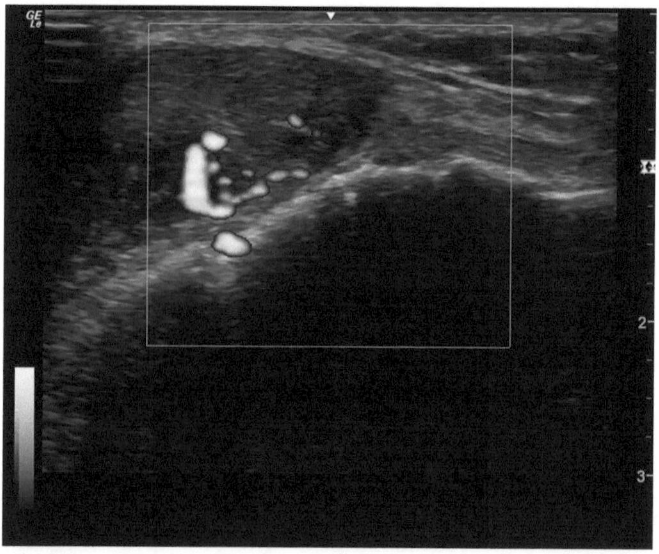

Figure 6-61d: Dilated vessels come from the deep and from the lateral side.

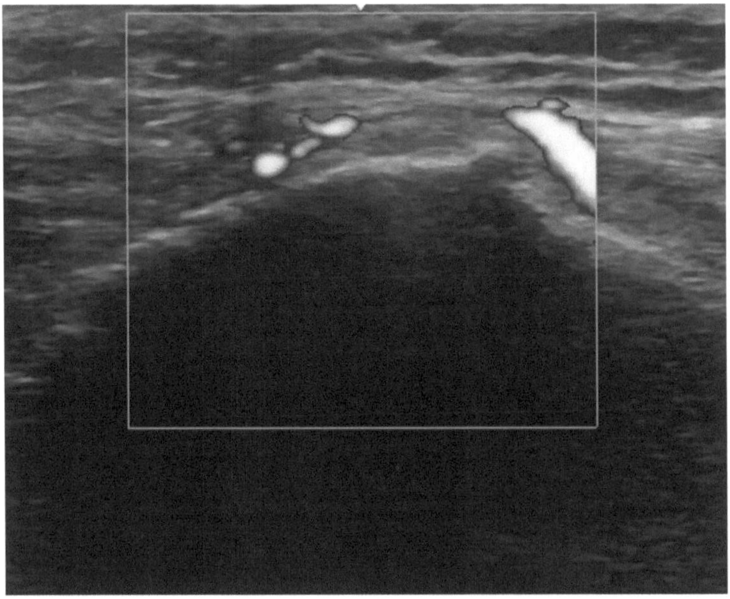

Figure 6-61e: Doppler of dilated recurrent anterior tibial artery.

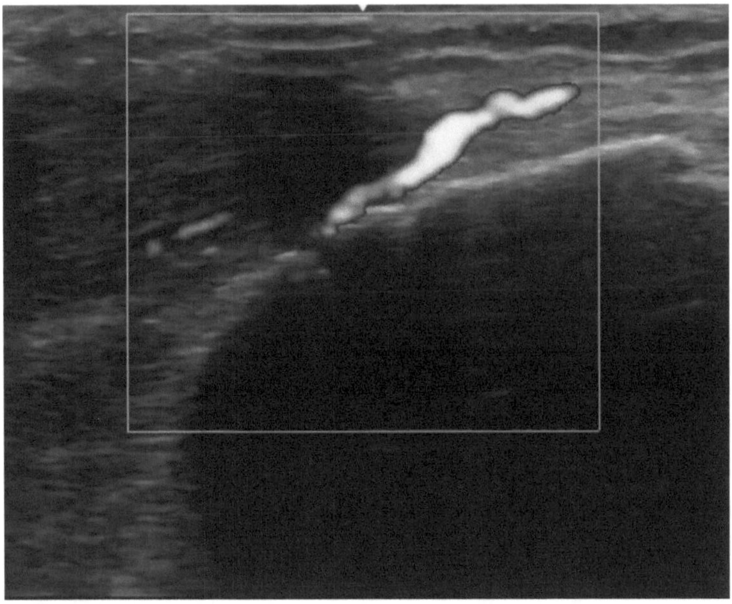

Figure 6-61f: The recurrent anterior tibial artery coming anterior to Gerdy's tubercle was dilated more than normal as was the lateral inferior geniculate artery.

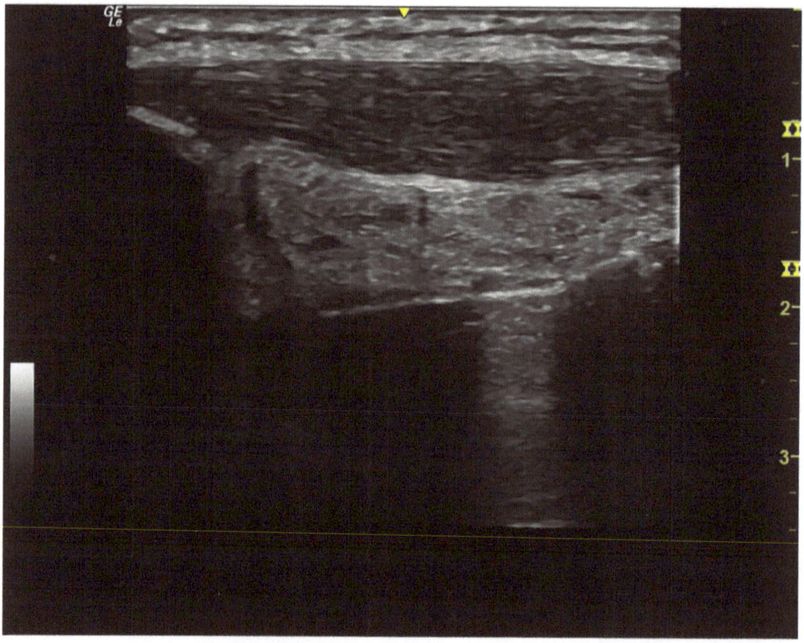

Figure 6-61g: Two year follow-up ultrasound shows improvement.

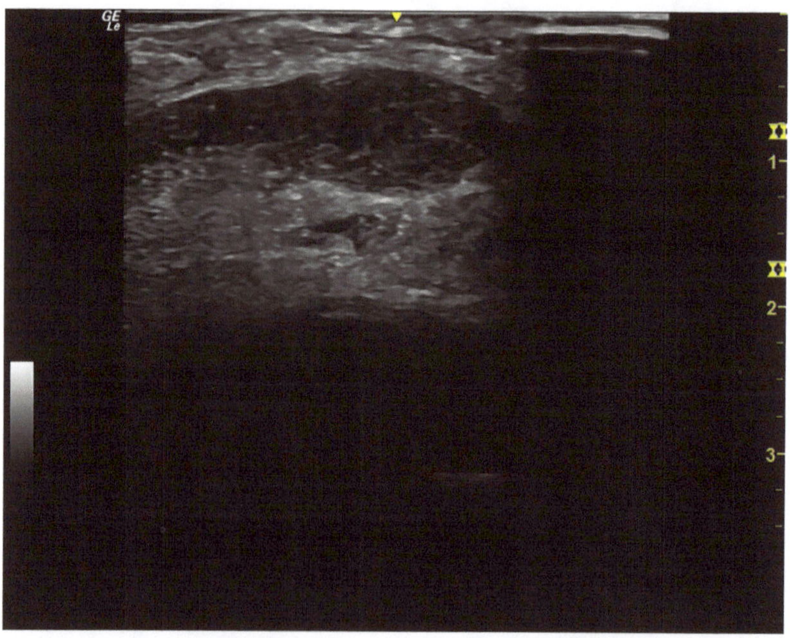

Figure 6-61h: Short axis at 2 years. The tendon is thinner and more echogenic.

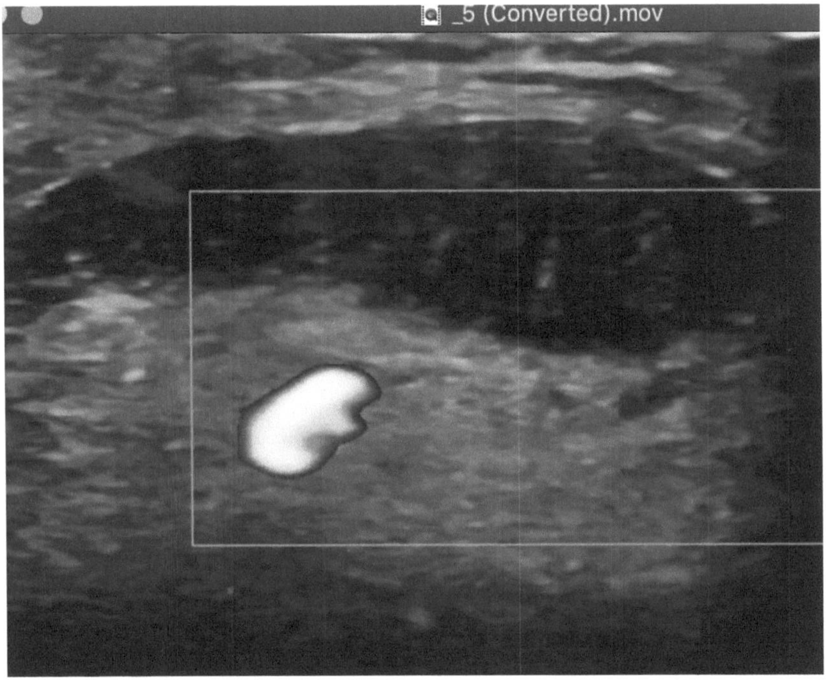

Figure 6-61i: Doppler Two years after surgery also shows less vascularity.

Summary and predictions

If we omit cruciate ligament injuries and meniscal tears, ultrasound can contribute tremendously to knee evaluation and management, because so many important structure are close and parallel to the skin.

In the future surgeons with ultrasound skills will use ultrasound to make advances in diagnosis and in procedures. We will develop more diagnostic capability especially with dynamic examination. In the OR we will add instrument placement skills and even new instruments.

Further Reading

Jacobson JA: Fundamentals of musculoskeletal ultrasound, Third Edition, Elsevier, Philadelphia, 2018

A classic introductory text. I used the second edition to prepare for the RMSK certification.

Van Holbeeck M., Introcaso J: Musculoskeletal ultrasound. https://books.apple.com/us/book/musculoskeletal-ultrasound/id991915241

An encyclopedic text, which I keep on my iPad.

Chapter 7 Foot and Ankle

- Alyssa Speciale, MD;
- Tyler Fraser, MD;
- Christopher Kreulen, MD
- Rosa Magana;
- Eric Giza, MD

Introduction

Ultrasound is an invaluable modality, both diagnostic and therapeutic for a foot and ankle surgeon. Ultrasound of the foot and ankle offers low cost, in-office real-time dynamic imaging without radiation. Given the complex and relatively smaller size of the many joints of the foot, ultrasound guidance can increase the accuracy of intra-articular aspirations and injections. Ultrasound detects pathology in the posterior tibial tendon, peroneal tendons and lateral ankle ligaments with similar sensitivities and specificities as MRI[1]. Another benefit of ultrasound includes the ability to see tendinous structures near previously placed surgical hardware without the artifact seen on CT or MRI. Limitations include operator dependence and variability with foot and ankle ultrasound, limited penetrance in a wider soft tissue envelope, as well as anisotropy giving a false sense of tissue pathology. Other small but relevant limitations to ultrasound in the foot and ankle include the need for the probe to be physically touching an area that may be tender, or be precluded by overlying casts or splints. Besides its use for clinical diagnostic and therapeutic purposes, ultrasound guidance is the gold standard for peripheral nerve blocks for a significant number of foot and ankle surgeries. Whether helping to establish a diagnosis, aid in non-operative treatment or localize anatomy for postoperative pain control, ultrasound is an invaluable imaging technique for a foot and ankle surgeon.

Diagnostic exam

a. Anterior Ankle:

For sonographic evaluation of the anterior ankle, the patient should be lying supine on the exam table with the foot slightly plantar flexed or with the knee bent and foot flat on the table. The examiner should be seated to the side of the foot with the ultrasound (US) machine in direct line of vision. A linear high frequency transducer is recommended, as most of the structures of the foot and ankle are superficial. The primary structures for evaluation include the anterior joint recess of the tibiotalar joint, tibialis anterior tendon (TA), extensor hallucis longus tendon (EHL), dorsalis pedis artery, deep peroneal nerve, and extensor digitorum longus tendon (EDL).

Start with the probe in the sagittal plane over the tibiotalar joint (Figure 7-1), just medial to the TA tendon. The tibia and talus bones will be hyperechoic with hypoechoic hyaline cartilage lining the surface of the talus. The fat pad of the anterior recess will also be hyperechoic (Figure 7-2). Evaluate for joint effusion and abnormal bony contour consistent with osteoarthritis. The probe should then be rotated 90 degrees to the transverse plane at the level of the talus to evaluate the tendons which will demonstrate uniform hyperechoic fibrillar echotexture[2] (Figure 7-3). Tendons are subject to high anisotropy if the ultrasound beam is not directly perpendicular to the tendon collagen fibers. To eliminate anisotropy, toggle the transducer to bring the hyperechoic tendon into view when in transverse axis[3]. The TA tendon will be the largest and most medial tendon followed by the EHL laterally. The EHL muscle extends more inferiorly than the TA and appears more hypoechoic compared to the tendon. The dorsalis pedis artery which is a continuation of the anterior tibial artery will be seen running with the deep peroneal nerve, lateral to the EHL tendon. The artery will appear as a hypoechoic pulsatile round structure while the nerve demonstrates a honeycomb appearance and crosses from medial to lateral over the artery as the probe is translated distally. The next structure laterally will be EDL tendon which will split into four respective tendons inserting onto digits 2-5.

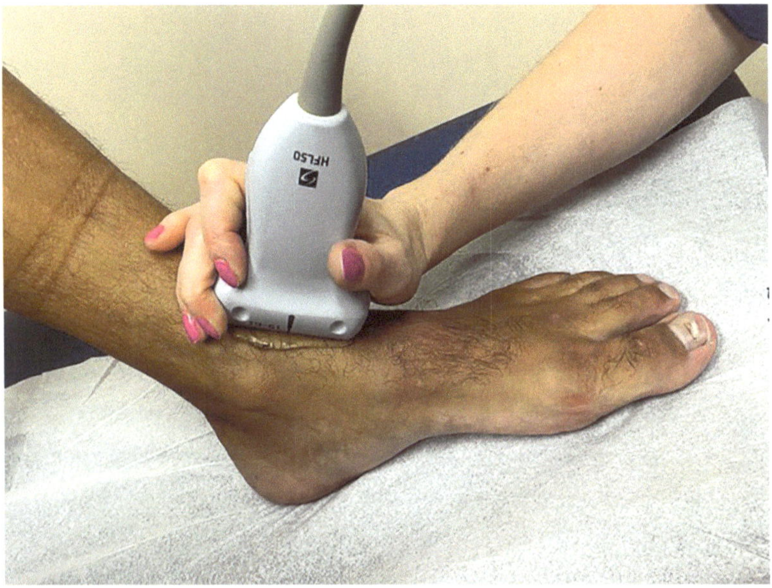

Figure 7-1: Probe positioning in the sagittal plane over the tibiotalar joint.

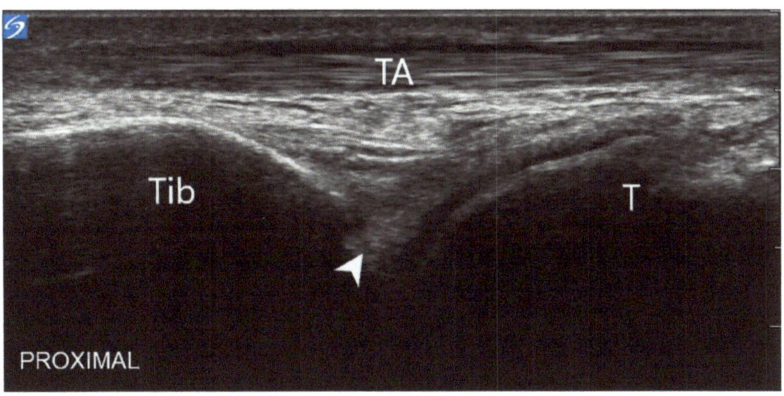

Figure 7-2: Sagittal view over the anterior tibiotalar joint recess between the tibia (Tib) and talus (T) with the hyperechoic anterior fat pad (arrowhead). The fibrillar tibialis anterior (TA) tendon is noted overlying the joint.

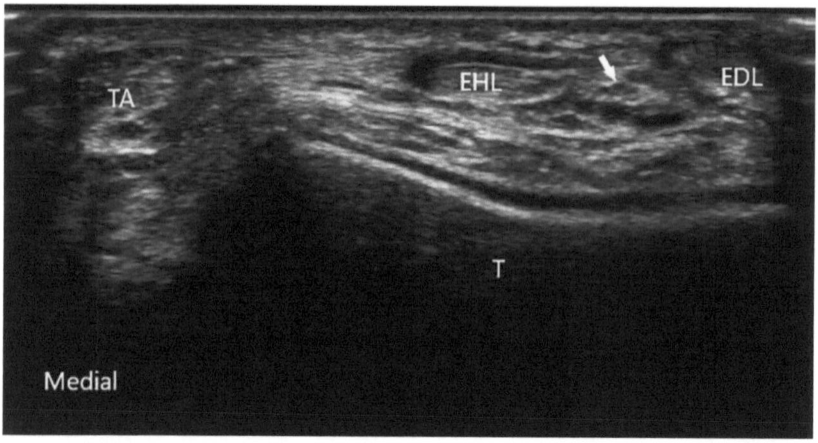

Figure 7-3: Transverse view of the anterior ankle tendons in short axis. The tibialis anterior (TA), extensor hallucis longus (EHL), and extensor digitorum longus (EDL) tendons are seen with the hyperechoic talus (T). The deep peroneal nerve (arrow) is seen running with the anterior tibial artery and vein which are the circular hypoechoic structures between the EHL and EDL tendons.

All structures should then be evaluated in long axis via the sagittal plane from the level of the ankle joint to the bony insertions to evaluate for tenosynovitis, tendon thickening, or tears (Figure 7-2). On ultrasound evaluation of tendinosis, tendons may appear thickened and hypoechogenic with loss of normal fibrillar echotexture. Split longitudinal tendon tears or partial tears will appear as a linear hypoechoic disruption within the tendon[2,4]. Hyperemia secondary to neovascularization can be evident with use of power or color Doppler[2].

b. Medial Ankle:

For evaluation of the medial ankle, the patient will externally rotate the hip while lying supine or lie in a lateral decubitus position. Placing a towel roll under the lateral ankle helps with evaluation of the medial ankle (Figure 7-4). The structures of interest include the elements of the tarsal tunnel, i.e. posterior tibialis tendon (PTT), flexor digitorum longus tendon (FDL), tibial artery and vein, tibial nerve, and flexor hallucis longus tendon (FHL), as well as the deltoid ligament.

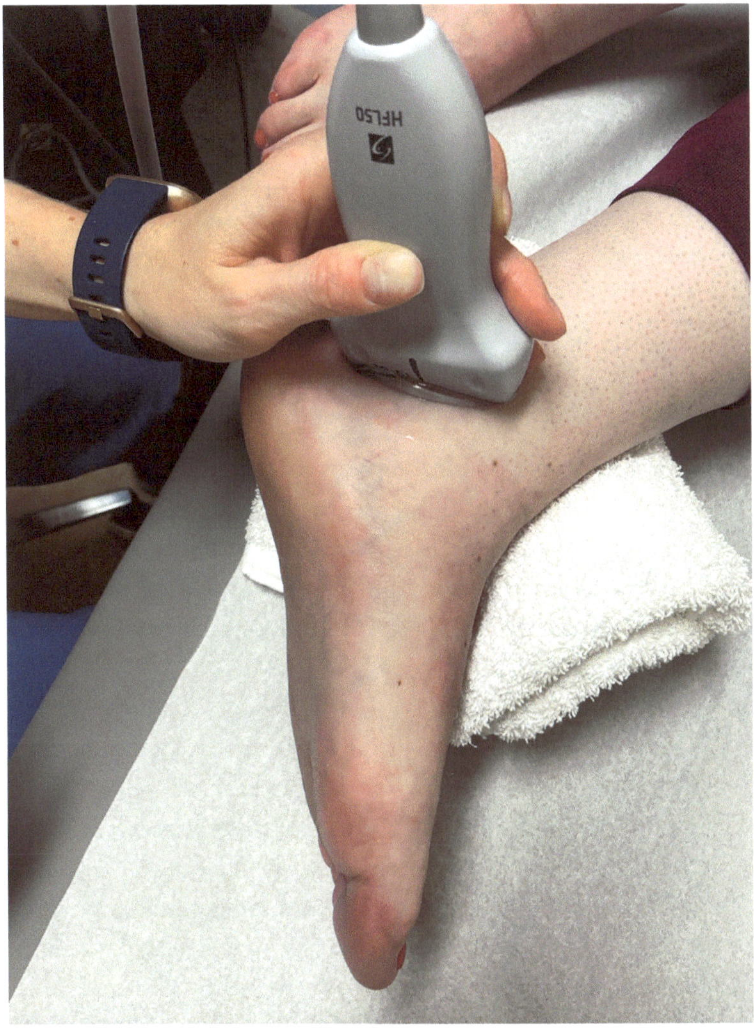

Figure 7-4: Probe positioning in transverse oblique plane over the medial ankle to view the tarsal tunnel elements.

Start with the transducer in transverse plane just proximal and posterior to the medial malleolus. The posterior end of the transducer will be angled slightly inferior to visualize the thin hyperechoic flexor retinaculum connecting the medial malleolus to the calcaneus. The PTT will be twice as large as the adjacent FDL tendon and can demonstrate a small amount of hypoechoic tenosynovial fluid along one side of the tendon in the distal sheath[4] (Figure 7-5).

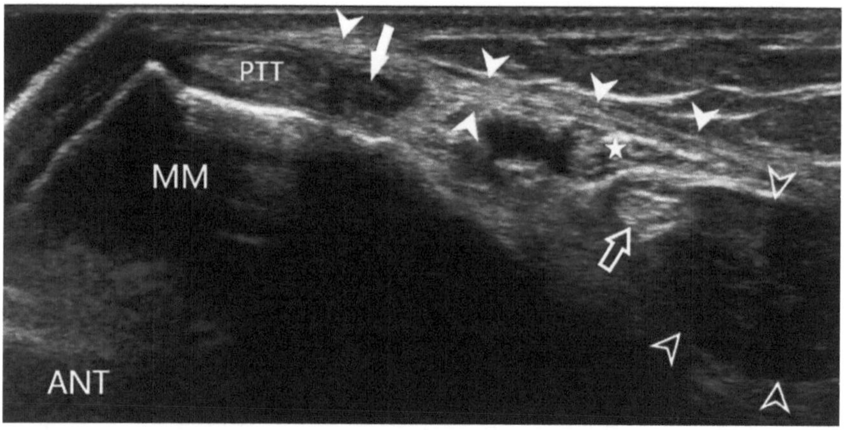

Figure 7-5: Transverse oblique view of tarsal tunnel structures in short axis with the thin hyperechoic flexor retinaculum (solid arrowheads). ANT= anterior, MM= medial malleolus, PTT= posterior tibialis tendon, arrow= flexor digitorum longus, star= tibial nerve, open arrow= flexor hallucis longus tendon, open arrowheads = flexor hallucis longus muscle.

As the PTT is followed distally, the sustentaculum tali, a bony protuberance off the calcaneus, will divide the PTT and FDL and FHL tendons (Figure 7-6). Continue to follow the PTT distally to the insertion on the navicular. To view the tendon in long axis while assessing for pathology, start back at the tarsal tunnel over the PTT and rotate the transducer 90 degrees to the coronal plane. As the tendon is followed, the plane will transition to the transverse plane at the navicular insertion where the tendon may appear less defined, thickened, and hypoechoic secondary to anisotropy and the division of some of the tendon fibers to their insertion on the cuneiforms and metatarsals 2-4[5] (Figure 7-7).

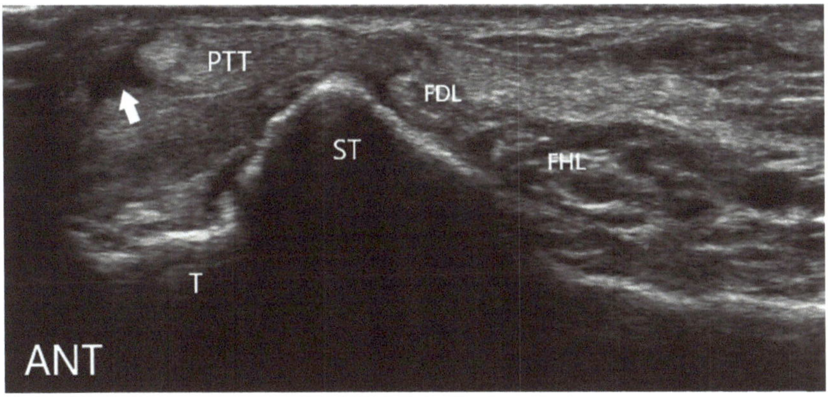

Figure 7-6: Short axis view distal to the medial malleolus. Anterior/ dorsal (ANT) is to the left of the image with the posterior tibialis tendon (PTT) with physiologic fluid (arrow) anterior to the sustentaculum tali (ST) of the calcaneus and the flexor digitorum longus (FDL) and flexor hallucis longus (FHL) posteriorly; T= talus.

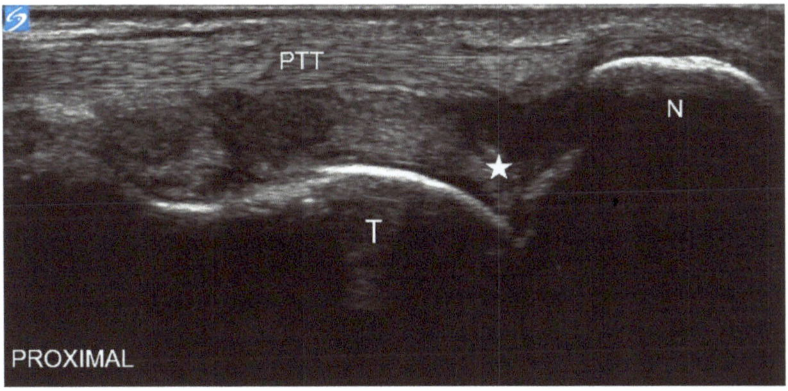

Figure 7-7: Long axis view of the posterior tibialis tendon (PTT) inserting on the Navicular (N). The spring ligament (star) will be deep to the PTT running between the navicular and calcaneus; T= talus.

Ultrasound is typically accurate in diagnosing PTT pathology including tenosynovitis, tendinosis, partial or split tendon tears, or complete tendon tears. Tendinosis is characterized by thickened and heterogenous echotexture while partial tears appear as a linear hypoechoic disruption within the tendon[4] (Figure 7-8). Hypoechoic fluid with or without hyperemia on power Doppler is seen surrounding the tendon when tenosynovitis is present (Figure 7-9). The FDL and FHL tendons can be followed in short and long axis in a similar manner (Figure 7-10). The FHL muscle will extend more inferiorly than the adjacent muscles and appear hypoechoic compared to the tendon. The FDL and FHL tendons can be followed distally to the plantar aspect of the mid foot where they cross at a location termed 'Knot of Henry'. The FDL will cross superficial to the FHL and move from medial to lateral across the plantar aspect of the foot (Figure 7-11).

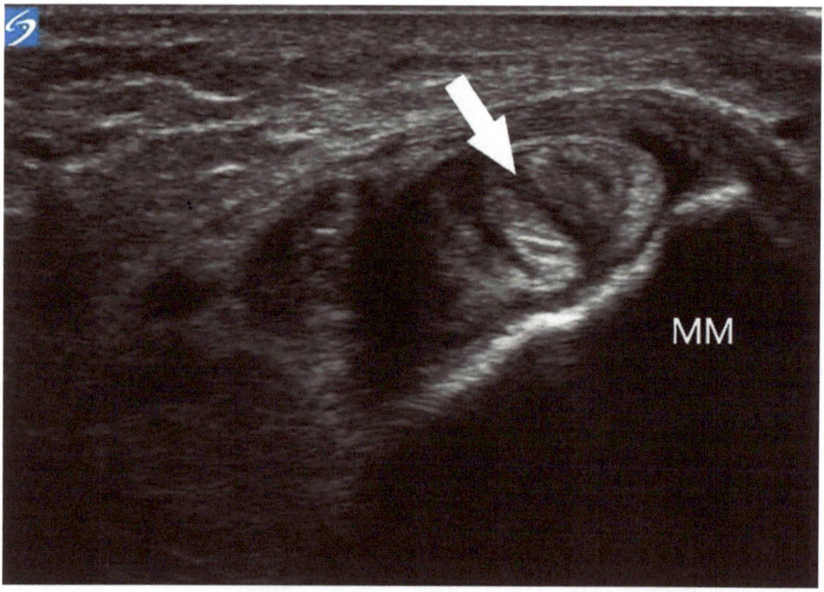

Figure 7-8: Short axis view of the posterior tibialis tendon (PTT) with a hypoechoic line through the tendon and thickening consistent with tendinosis and partial split tendon tear; MM= medial malleolus.

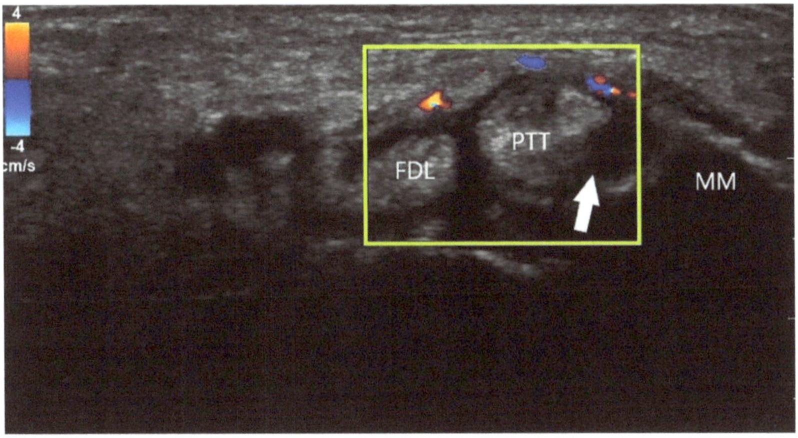

Figure 7-9: Short axis view of the posterior tibialis tendon (PTT) and flexor digitorum longus (FDL) with hypoechoic sheath fluid and hyperemia on power Doppler consistent with tenosynovitis; MM= medial malleolus.

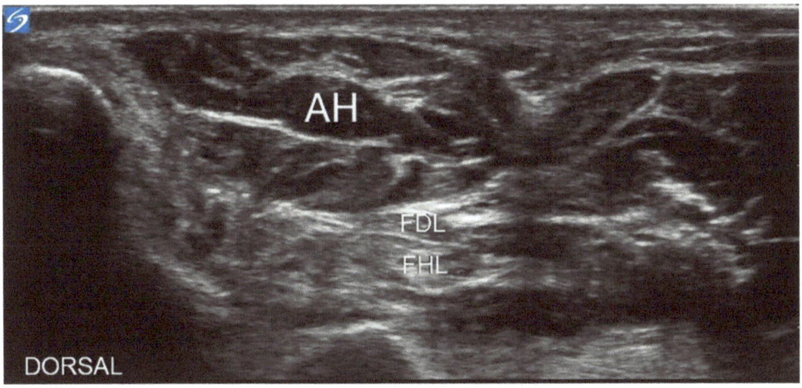

Figure 7-10: Short axis view of the flexor digitorum longus (FDL) crossing over the flexor hallucis longus (FHL) at the 'Knot of Henry'; AH= abductor hallucis muscle in the midfoot.

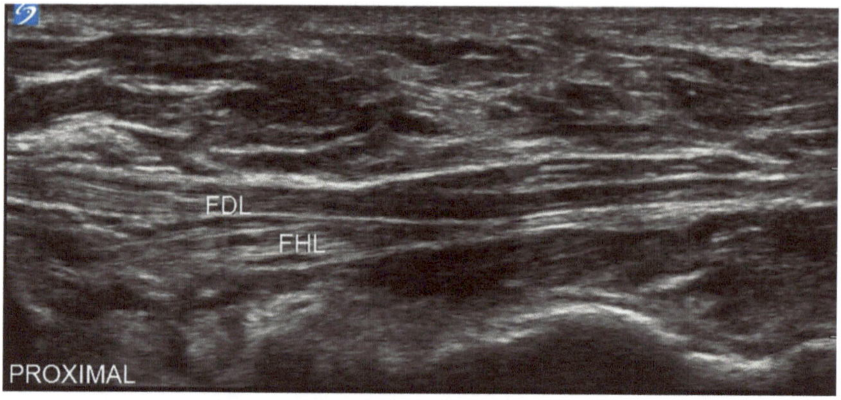

Figure 7-11: Long axis view of the flexor digitorum longus (FDL) crossing over the flexor hallucis longus (FHL) at the 'Knot of Henry' in the midfoot.

In short axis, the tibial nerve demonstrates a honeycomb appearance with hypoechoic nerve fascicles and hyperechoic connective tissue and collagen. In long axis, the nerve will be hypoechoic and coarser compared to the more dense fibrillar tendon structure[6]. A lack of anisotropy will also distinguish nerves from tendons. The tarsal tunnel can be a potential site of entrapment of the tibial nerve secondary to osteophytes, retinacular injury, tendinopathy/ tenosynovitis, or soft tissue masses. Fusiform swelling proximal and distal to the site of entrapment can be seen. Symptoms include paresthesia or pain in the medial ankle radiating to the plantar arch[6]. The tibial nerve will divide distal to the tarsal tunnel into the medial plantar nerve (MPN) and lateral plantar nerve (LPN) which course across the plantar foot (Figure 7-12). The MPN is larger than the LPN and will travel with the medial plantar artery between the flexor hallucis brevis and quadratus plantae muscles. The MPN can be entrapped at the Knot of Henry and is termed 'jogger's foot'. The LPN travels from medial to lateral across the plantar foot alongside the lateral tibial artery. The first branch of the LPN is the inferior calcaneal nerve (Baxter's nerve) which can be compressed between the abductor hallucis longus and quadratus plantae muscles or at a medial calcaneal spur secondary to plantar fasciitis[6]. Baxter's neuropathy can mimic plantar fasciitis. This nerve branch is difficult to visualize due to the small size (1-2 mm) but the abductor digiti minimi can be evaluated for signs of atrophy on ultrasound or MRI.

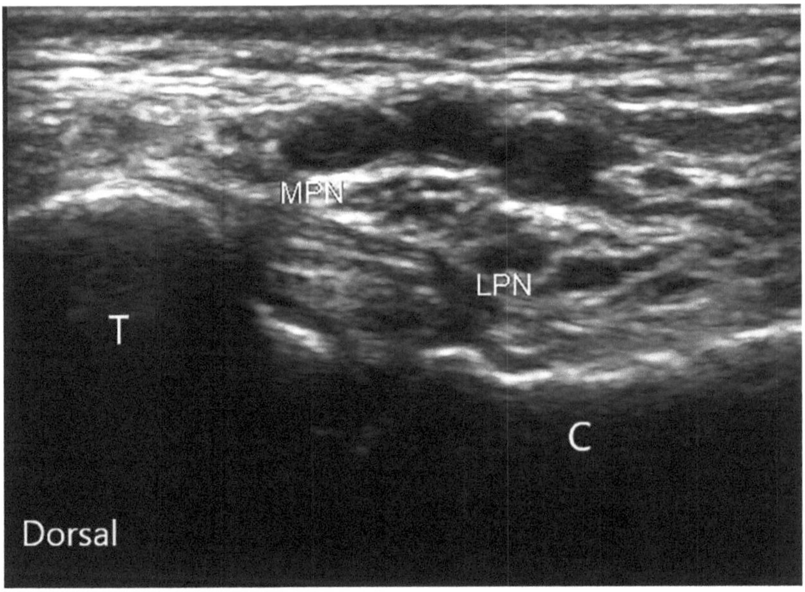

Figure 7-12: Short axis view of the tibial nerve splitting into the medial plantar nerve (MPN) and lateral plantar nerve (LPN) with the characteristic honeycomb appearance. T=talus, C= calcaneus.

After assessing the tarsal tunnel contents, the deltoid and spring ligament complexes should be assessed. The deltoid ligament is composed of deep and superficial portions which are difficult to distinguish. The superficial portion includes the tibiocalcaneal, tibiotalar, and tibionavicular components[4]. To view the tibiocalcaneal portion, the transducer should first be placed in the coronal plane over the medial ankle with the proximal end of the transducer over the distal tibia. The ligament will appear as a thin, superficial, hyperechoic fibrillar band with the bright hyperechoic talus deep (Figure 7-13). The distal end of the transducer can then be fanned anteriorly to view the superficial tibionavicular (Figure 7-14) and deeper anterior tibiotalar components. The posterior tibiotalar component can be viewed by fanning the distal end of the transducer posteriorly to visualize the deep thick fibrillar band running deep to the tibialis posterior tendon[5].

While isolated deltoid ligament tears are rare, hypoechoic thickening and hypoechoic intra-substance tears can be seen with injury[4].

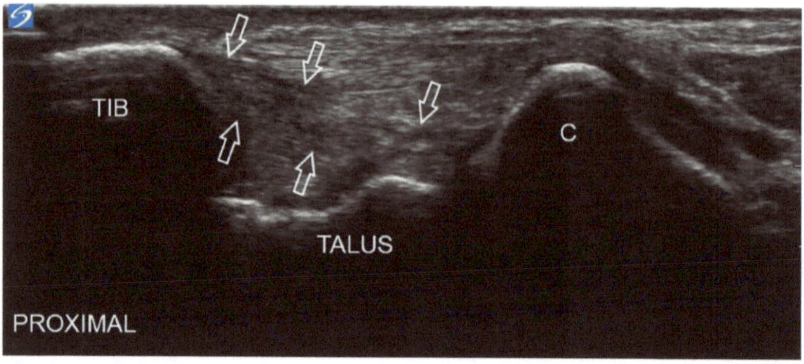

Figure 7-13: Coronal imaging over the tibiocalcaneal component (open arrows) of the deltoid ligament; Tib= tibia, C= calcaneus.

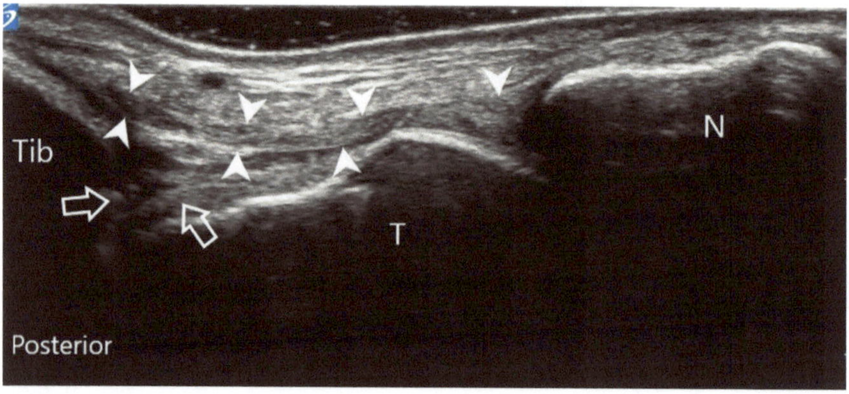

Figure 7-14: Coronal oblique imaging over the tibionavicular (arrowheads) and deeper anterior tibiotalar (open arrows) components of the deltoid ligament; Tib= tibia, T= talus, N= navicular.

Lastly, the spring ligament helps maintain the arch of the foot along with the PTT. The spring ligament connects the calcaneus and navicular bones and is composed of the superomedial, medioplantar, and inferoplantar ligaments. The transducer will be placed in the transverse plane over the sustentaculum tali of the calcaneus and then translated anteriorly and angled slightly superior toward the talus. Here, the superomedial calcaneonavicular ligament will be visualized with the posterior tibialis tendon running superficially and the talus deep (Figure 7-15)[4,5]. Abnormal thickening (>4 mm) of the spring ligament can be noted with intra-substance partial tears and PTT dysfunction. Visualization of the PTT directly contacting the talus in this location is characteristic of a complete spring ligament tears[4].

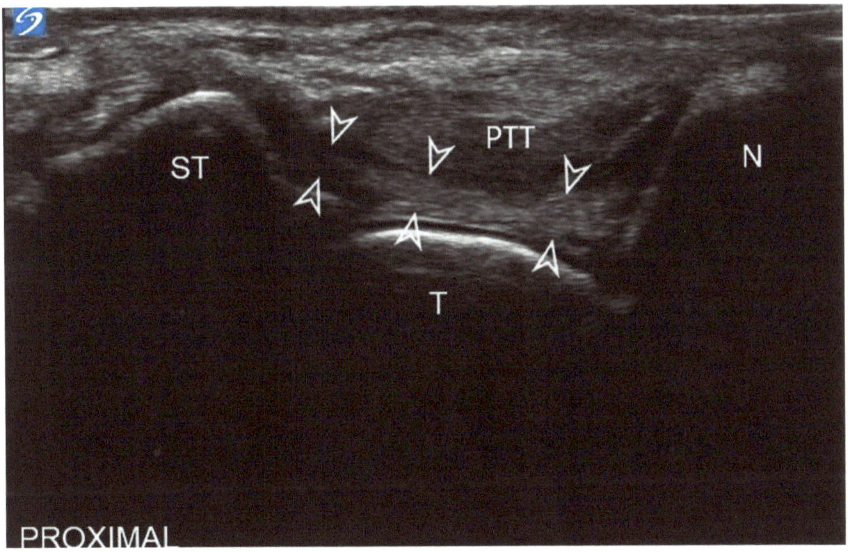

Figure 7-15: Transverse imaging over the plantar arch with the hyperechoic spring (superomedial calcaneonavicular) ligament (open arrowheads) running between the sustentaculum tali (ST) of the calcaneus to the navicular (N) with the talus (T) deep and the posterior tibialis tendon more superficial (PTT).

c. **Lateral ankle:**

For evaluation of the lateral ankle, the patient can internally rotate the hip while lying supine or lie in a lateral decubitus position with the foot in slight plantar flexion. Placing a towel roll under the medial ankle helps with evaluation of the lateral ankle (Figure 7-16). The structures of interest in the lateral ankle include peroneus longus and brevis tendons, superior peroneal retinaculum, anterior talofibular ligament (ATFL), calcaneofibular ligament (CFL), anterior inferior tibiofibular ligament (AITFL), superficial peroneal nerve, and sural nerve.

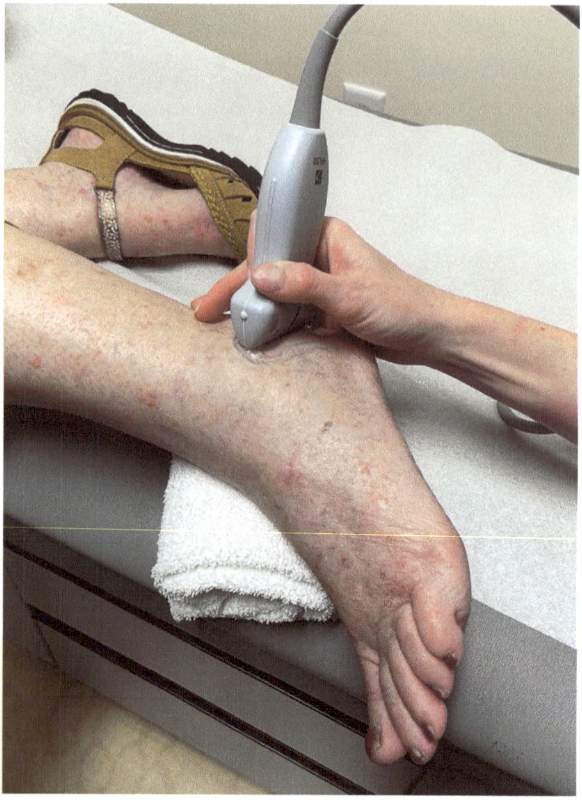

Figure 7-16: Probe positioning in transverse oblique plane over the lateral ankle, posterior to the lateral malleolus.

Evaluation will begin with the transducer in a transverse plane in the retro malleolar groove. A large amount of ultrasound gel is required due to the bony contours of this region. The peroneus longus tendon appears heterogenous in short axis, slightly superficial and anterior to the peroneus brevis, which demonstrates a more hyperechoic tendon and hypoechoic muscle belly at this location. As the transducer is translated inferiorly, the orientation will need to become more oblique to follow the course of the tendon. The peroneus brevis muscle should taper and disappear by the distal lateral malleolar tip. If muscle tissue is seen beyond the lateral malleous, it is considered a low-lying muscle belly which may predispose the tendon to pathology[5]. The peroneus brevis tendon typically lies directly against the bone with the peroneus longus located more posteriorly. The superior peroneal retinaculum will overlie the tendons and appear as a hyperechoic thin fibrillar structure extending from the distal fibula to the posterior calcaneus (Figure 7-17). As the tendons are examined in short axis, frequent toggling will be necessary to minimize anisotropy. Once the tendons course around the lateral malleolus, the transducer should be in an oblique coronal plane and the peroneal tubercle, a bony protuberance on the lateral calcaneus, will be visualized. At this location, the peroneus brevis is anterior (dorsal) to the peroneal tubercle and the peroneus longus is posterior (plantar). Due to the divergent orientation of the tendons, one tendon will typically demonstrate anisotropy and appear falsely hypoechoic while the other tendon is in view (Figure 7-18). Perform gentle toggling and rotating of the transducer to evaluate each tendon individually. Some sonographers use negative anisotropy to outline the peroneal tendons for easier identification due to the echogenic surrounding tissue. The peroneus brevis can be followed to the insertion on the base of the 5th metatarsal and the longus can be followed to the plantar mid foot, through the cuboid tunnel, and to the insertion on the medial cuneiform and base of 1st metatarsal.

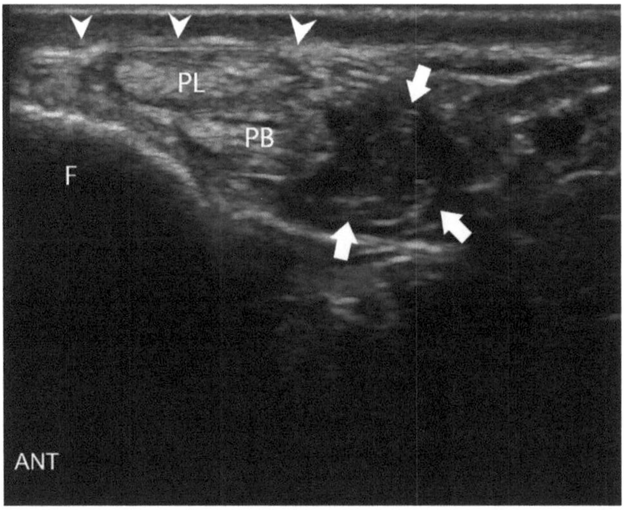

Figure 7-17: Short axis view of the peroneus longus (PL) and peroneus brevis (PB) tendons and hypoechoic peroneus brevis muscle (arrows) with the overlying thin hyperechoic superior peroneal retinaculum (arrowheads); F= fibula; ANT= anterior.

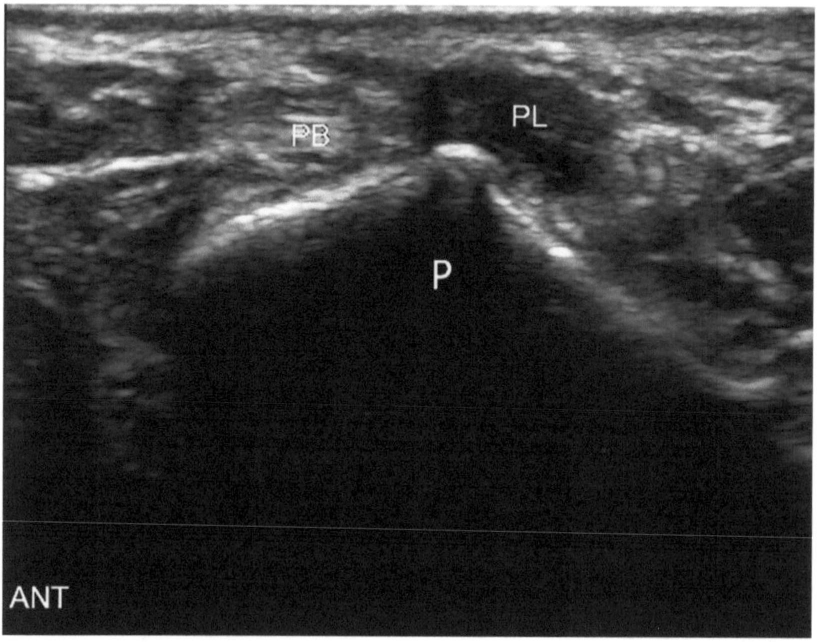

Fig 7-18: Coronal view of the peroneal tendons in short axis at the level of the peroneal tubercle (P) of the calcaneus. The peroneus brevis is anterior (ANT)/dorsal to the tubercle while the peroneus longus (PL) is posterior/plantar with anisotropy demonstrated.

Tendon tears and tendinosis are best evaluated with the tendons in short axis. The most common type of peroneus brevis tear is a longitudinal split tear which generally occurs at the level of the retro malleolar groove and is demonstrated by a horseshoe shape of the tendon wrapping around the peroneus longus tendon (Figure 7-19a) or by observation of a hypoechoic line in the center of the tendon in short axis (Figure 7-19b)[7]. Peroneus longus tendon tears are rarer but can occur at the cuboid tunnel or in association with an os peroneum. An os peroneum is a sesamoid bone within the distal peroneus longus tendon in up to 30% of people and is bilateral in 60% of those individuals. Typically, these are asymptomatic but hypoechoic changes or increased power Doppler flow can signify tendinopathy and inflammation associated with the sesamoid[7].

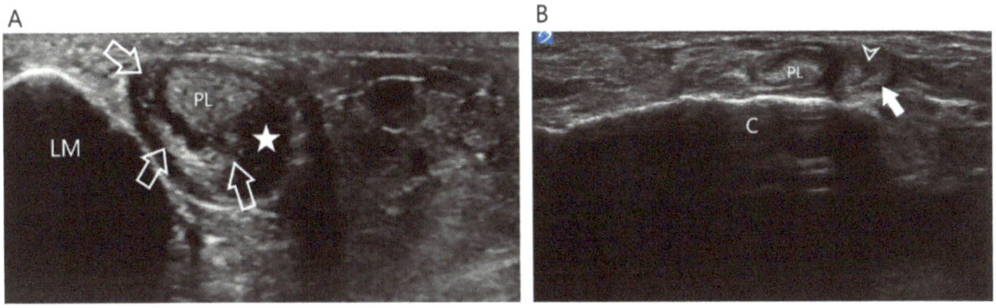

Fig 7-19a: Short axis view of the peroneus longus (PL) and peroneus brevis tendons (open arrows) at the level of the lateral malleolus (LM). There is a split tendon tear of the peroneus brevis which is seen wrapping around the PL. There is also fluid within the sheath (star).

Fig. 7-19b: Short axis view distal to image a., noting the peroneus longus (PL) and peroneus brevis tendons (arrow) with a hypoechoic cleft (open arrowhead) within the peroneus brevis consistent with a partial tear; C= calcaneus.

Dynamic evaluation of the tendons within the retro malleolar groove in short axis should be done to evaluate for instability resulting in subluxation, dislocation, or intra-sheath snapping. The patient should lie supine and perform slow circumduction of their ankle as well as resisted dorsiflexion and eversion during direct visualization. The transducer will be placed in the transverse oblique plane posterior to the fibula. Light transducer pressure is important, as to not artificially stabilize the tendons. With intra-sheath snapping, the tendons will roll over each other and switch anterior and posterior positions[8]. If the tendons are noted to transiently subluxate or dislocate out of the retro malleolar groove, there is likely an injury to the retinaculum. Retinacular injuries appear thickened and heterogeneous on US[7].

For long axis assessment of the tendons, the transducer is rotated 90 degrees to an oblique-coronal plane within the retro malleolar groove and angled toward the posterior aspect of the fibula. Again, the peroneus brevis will lie along the bone with the peroneus longus more superficially. The tendons can be followed distally until they deviate to their respective insertions as they are followed individually (Figure

7-20). Cortical irregularities at the insertion can signify insertional tendinopathy/enthesopathy.

The lateral ankle ligaments are assessed starting with the anterior talofibular ligament (ATFL). The transducer is placed transversely over the distal fibula and then translated anteriorly with the distal end slightly inferior to view the talus. The ATFL appears as a hypoechoic compact structure. Anisotropy can be reduced with a heel-toe maneuver, aiming the ultrasound beam toward the talus (Figure 7-21). An acute ATFL injury is demonstrated by hypoechoic discontinuity within the ligament or will have a heterogenous non-uniform appearance, with possible hyperechoic avulsion fracture fragments; more remote injury shows hypoechoic thickening[5]. Dynamic evaluation can be performed using the anterior drawer physical exam test under ultrasound guidance to assess for instability.

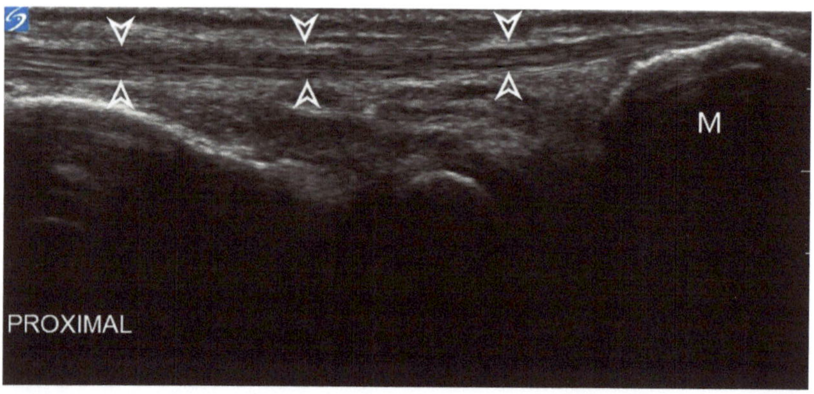

Fig 7-20: Long axis view of the peroneus brevis (open arrowheads) inserting on the base of the 5th metatarsal (M). Proximal end of the image is to the left.

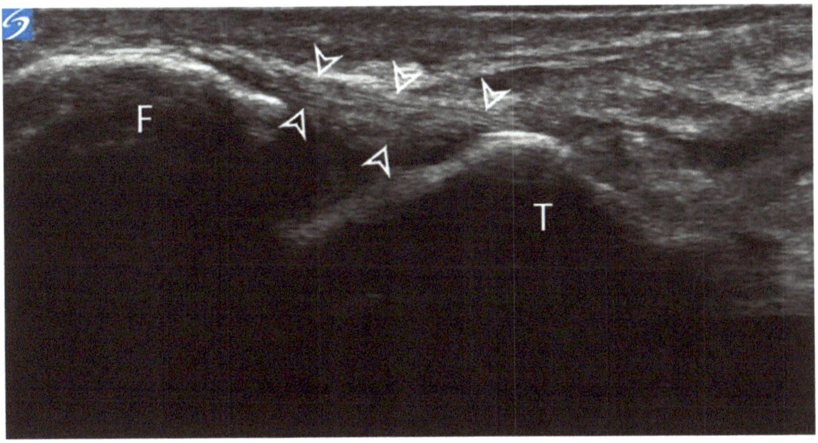

Fig 7-21: Transverse oblique view of the fibrillar anterior talofibular ligament (open arrowheads) extending from the fibula (F) to the talus (T).

To evaluate the calcaneofibular ligament (CFL), the transducer is placed in a coronal oblique plane between the tip of the lateral malleolus and the posteroinferior calcaneus. The peroneal tendons will be viewed in short axis with the fibrillar CFL in long axis deeply (Figure 7-22). Hypoechoic swelling deep to the peroneal tendons is consistent with CFL tear[5]. A complete tear may be suspected if the peroneal tendons do not elevate with dynamic evaluation due to loss of contraction of the CFL.

The anterior inferior tibiofibular ligament (AITFL) is a compact fibrillar structure, identified by starting on the ATFL and rotating the medial aspect of the transducer superiorly from the talus to the tibia, ending in the oblique transverse plane (Figure 7-23). If there is concern for an AITFL injury, the remaining interosseous membrane should be evaluated by translating the transducer superiorly in the transverse plane. The interosseous membrane appears as a thin hyperechoic structure that thickens at the inferior aspect as it approaches the tibiotalar joint[5].

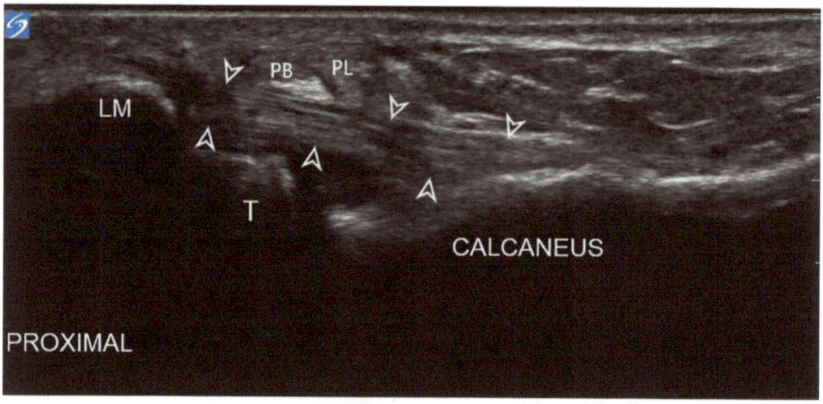

Fig 7-22: Coronal oblique imaging between the lateral malleolus (LM) and calcaneus of the calcaneofibular ligament (open arrowheads) with the peroneus brevis (PB) and peroneus longus (PL) tendons in short axis; T= talus.

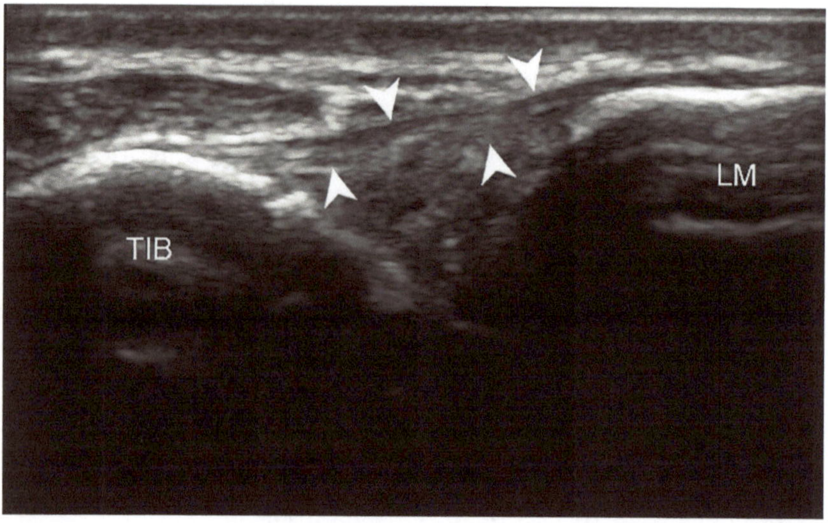

Fig 7-23: Transverse oblique imaging of the thin, compact, anterior inferior tibiofibular ligament (white arrowheads) between the tibia (TIB) and lateral malleolus (LM) of the fibula.

The superficial peroneal nerve (SPN) can be viewed in the transverse plane between the peroneal muscles and extensor digitorum longus in the lateral calf compartment, after it divides from the common peroneal nerve. The nerve will demonstrate the typical honeycomb appearance in short axis. It can be followed distally as it crosses anteriorly to pierce the fascia and course in the subcutaneous fat. The nerve is the easiest to identify in this tissue layer and it is also the most common site of entrapment. The SPN can commonly become stretched during an inversion ankle injury resulting in paresthesia in the lower lateral calf and dorsal foot[6]. If there is entrapment, there may be fusiform swelling of the nerve proximal and distal to the site of entrapment or hyperechoic scar tissue surrounding the nerve.

Lastly, the sural nerve is a pure sensory nerve to the posterolateral leg with innervation from the tibial and common peroneal nerve. The sural nerve travels with the lesser saphenous vein in the midline posterior calf, superficial to the gastrocnemius, and then crosses lateral to the Achilles tendon approximately 3-4 inches proximal to the calcaneus. The transducer should be placed in the transverse plane to view the Achilles tendon in short axis and then follow it to the lateral aspect of the heel where the sural nerve can easily be identified in the subcutaneous fat between the Achilles tendon and lateral malleolus[6] (Figure 7-24).

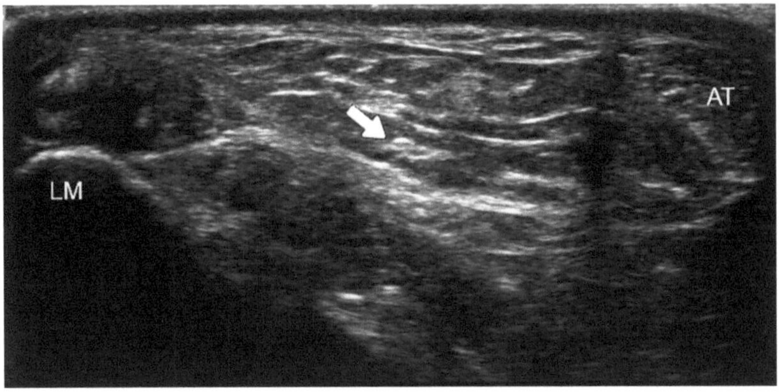

Fig 7-24: Transverse imaging of the sural nerve (arrow) in short axis within the subcutaneous fat between the Achilles tendon (AT) and the lateral malleolus (LM).

d. Posterior ankle/heel/calf:

For sonographic evaluation of the posterior ankle, heel, and calf, the patient should lie prone on the exam table with the foot hanging off the end of the table. The structures of interest in the posterior ankle and heel include the Achilles tendon, retrocalcaneal and retroAchilles bursae, and the plantar fascia. The structures of interest in the calf include the medial and lateral gastrocnemius and plantaris muscles.

First, place the transducer in the sagittal plane over the Achilles tendon to view the tendon in long axis (Figure 7-25). The tendon should appear as a thin, uniform, fibrillar structure spanning from the myotendinous junction of the gastrocnemius/soleus complex to the calcaneus[5] (Figure 7-26). Rotate the transducer 90 degrees to evaluate the tendon in short axis along its course. In short axis, the Achilles will appear relatively flat or slightly concave. The plantaris is a much smaller tendon that can be seen slightly deep and medial to the Achilles and is present in up to 90% of people[9] (Figure 7-27). Thickening of the plantaris tendon has been found to be associated with mid portion Achilles tendinopathy refractory to conservative treatments[10]. The Achilles tendon should be assessed for paratendinitis, tendinosis, and partial or full thickness tears. Paratendinitis is demonstrated by superficial hypoechoic fluid adjacent to the Achilles tendon with or without abnormal power Doppler flow[5]. Midportion Achilles tendinosis is easily identifiable as hypoechoic tendon swelling or thickening without fiber discontinuity but often with evidence of neovascularization on power Doppler (Figure 7-28). Similarly, insertional Achilles tendinosis is demonstrated by thickened hypoechoic tendon, often with hyperechoic enthesophytes off of the calcaneus. Partial Achilles tendon tears appear as focal hypoechoic regions of fiber discontinuity within a swollen tendon while full thickness tears show complete fiber discontinuity with tendon retraction[5] (Figure 7-29).

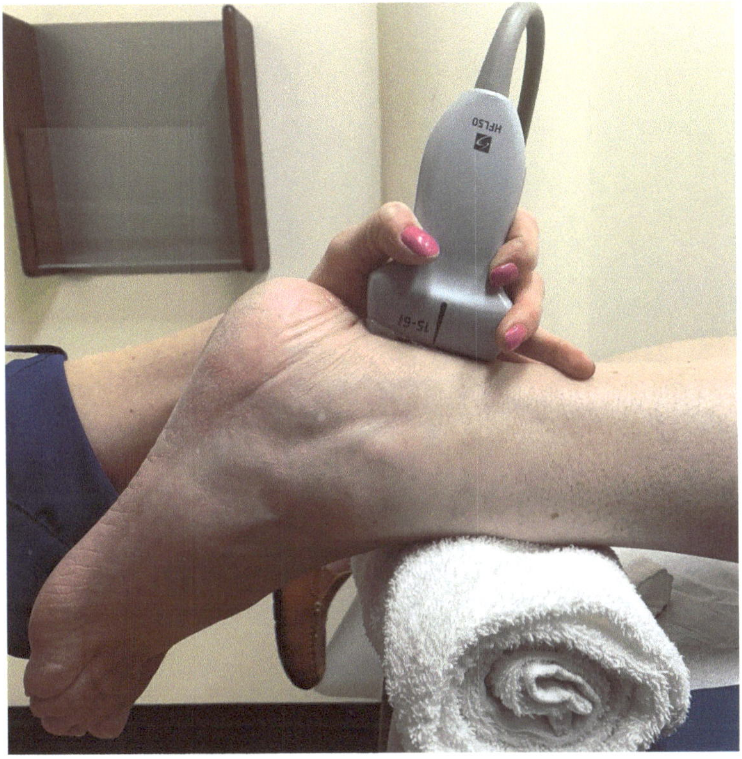

Fig 7-25: Probe positioning in the sagittal plane over the Achilles tendon.

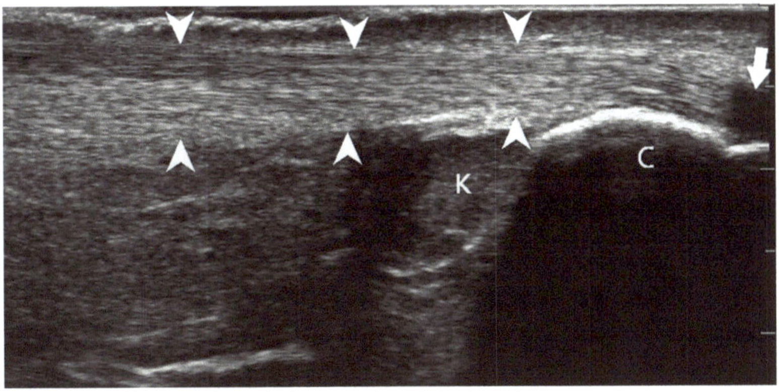

Fig 7-26: Sagittal imaging of the Achilles tendon (arrowheads) in long axis inserting on the calcaneus (C). The Kager fat pad (K) is seen deep to the tendon. The Achilles tendon fibers are anisotropic at the distal most insertion (arrow).

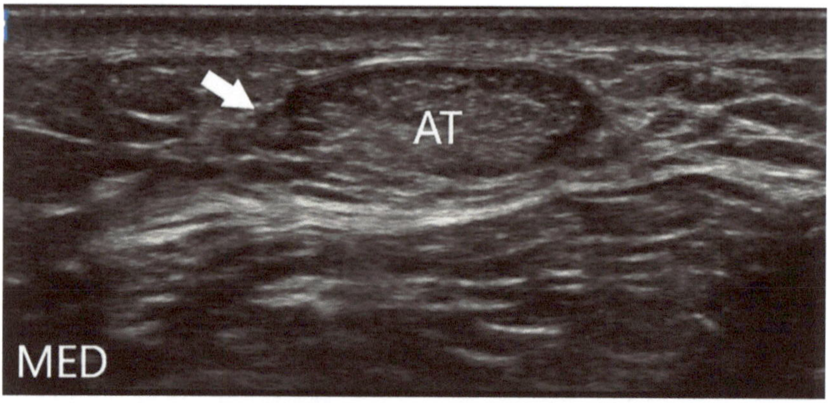

Fig 7-27: Transverse imaging of the Achilles tendon (AT) in short axis with the plantaris tendon (arrow) located medial (MED) to the Achilles.

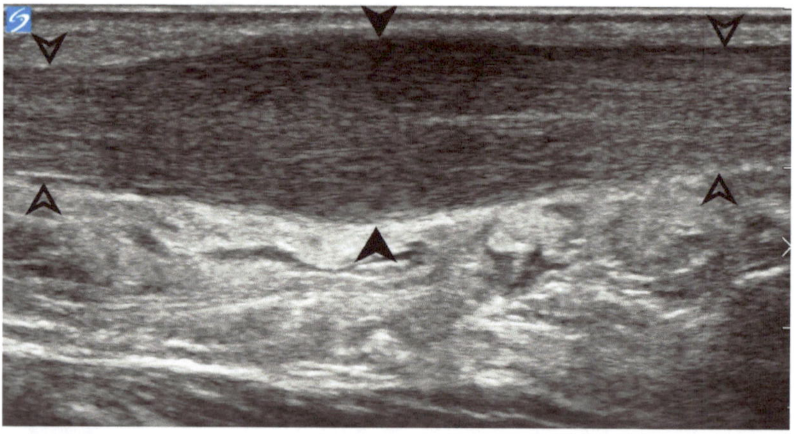

Fig 7-28: Long axis view of the mid portion Achilles tendon with notable fusiform swelling (closed arrowheads) consistent with tendinopathy. Open arrowheads demonstrate normal thickness of the tendon.

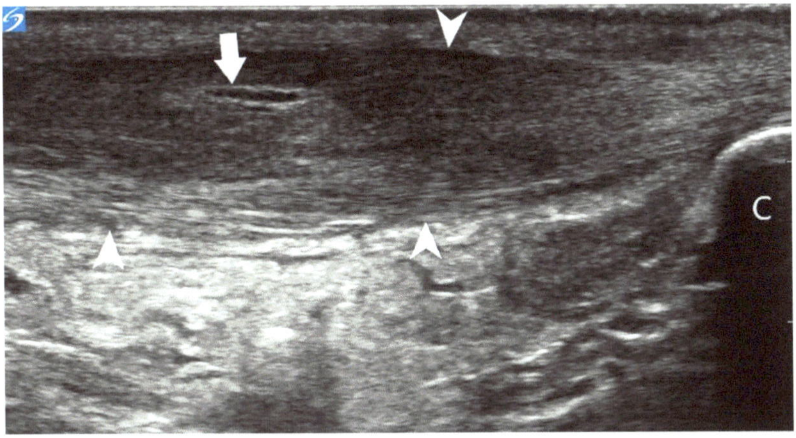

Fig 7-29: Long axis view of the mid portion Achilles tendon with the distal insertion on the calcaneus (C) demonstrating diffuse swelling/ thickening (arrowheads) and a linear hypoechoic intra-substance partial tendon tear (arrow).

The Kager fat pad is a hypoechoic, heterogeneous structure that sits anterior/deep to the Achilles tendon. The retrocalcaneal bursa may ordinarily contain up to 2.5 mm of anechoic fluid sitting at the calcaneal insertion between the Achilles tendon and Kager fat pad. Abnormal distension, or bursitis, can be seen with adjacent tendon tears, inflammation, or enthesopathy[5] (Figure 7-30). The retro-Achilles bursa sits superficial to the distal Achilles tendon and can be inflamed secondary to mechanical effects[5]. To evaluate for retro-Achilles bursitis, one must use a thick layer of ultrasound gel and minimal transducer pressure to avoid compressive obliteration of the bursa. Haglund syndrome signifies the combination of retro-Achilles and retrocalcaneal bursitis with tendinosis of the distal Achilles and enlarged prominence of the posterior superior calcaneus which irritates the Achilles[11].

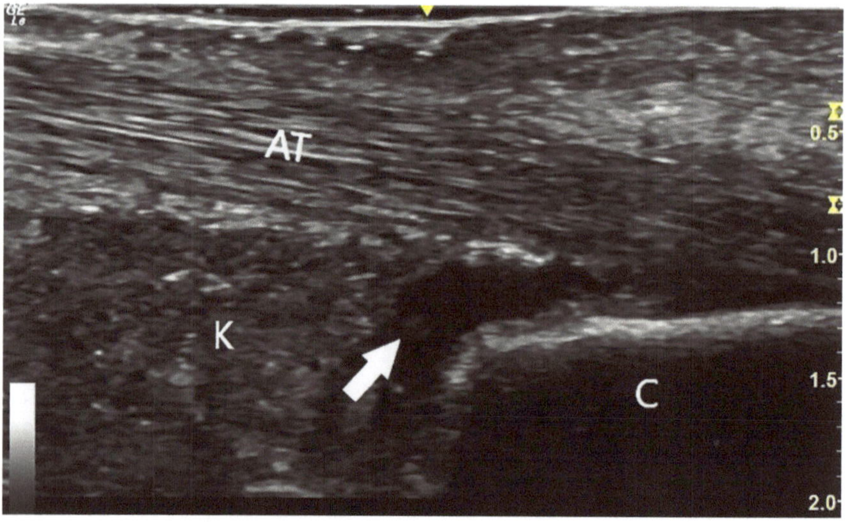

Fig 7-30: Sagittal imaging with long axis view of the Achilles tendon (AT) inserting on the calcaneus (C) with an anechoic retrocalcaneal effusion (arrow) within the bursa between the Achilles tendon and Kager fat pad (K).

The transducer is then moved to the plantar aspect of the heel in the sagittal plane to evaluate the plantar fascia/aponeurosis in long axis (Figure 7-31). With the transducer over the medial calcaneal tubercle, the plantar fascia will appear as a thin, (<4 mm) hyperechoic, linear structure deep to the fat pad of the heel. The gain of the machine typically needs to be turned up to penetrate the more hyperechoic fat pad and bring the plantar fascia into view (Figure 7-32). The transducer should be rotated 90 degrees to view the plantar aponeurosis in short axis as well. Plantar fasciitis is represented by hypoechoic thickening of the fascia > 4mm[5]. Plantar fibromatosis is caused by fibroblastic proliferation of the fascia and can also be evaluated with ultrasound. Plantar fibromatosis appears as multiple hypoechoic masses or thickening of the fascia, often bilateral[5].

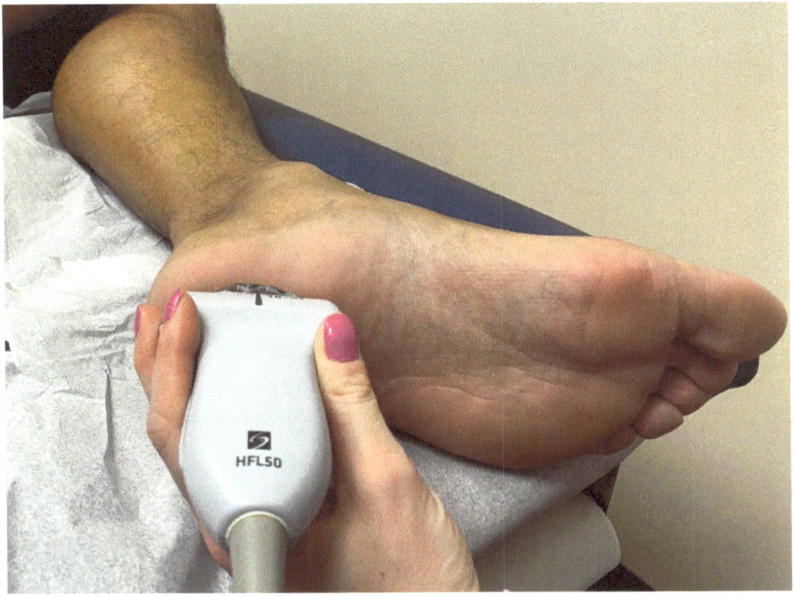

Fig 7-31: Probe positioning over the plantar surface of the heel in the sagittal plane to evaluate the plantar fascia.

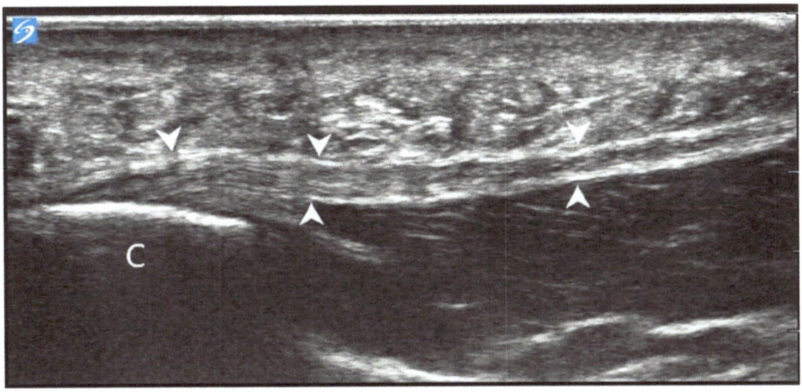

Fig 7-32: Sagittal imaging of the plantar fascia in long axis demonstrated by the thin hyperechoic fibrillar appearance originating from the calcaneus (C). Proximal is to the left of the image.

For evaluation of the calf, place the transducer in transverse plane over the mid posterior calf. Here, the medial and lateral heads of the gastrocnemius muscle and deeper soleus muscle are viewed in short axis (Figure 7-33). The transducer is rotated 90 degrees to evaluate the medial gastrocnemius in long axis as it starts to taper toward the soleus (Figure 7-34). This myotendinous region is a very common site of injury, i.e. 'tennis leg'. Disruption of fibers at this location is noted by hypoechoic or mixed echogenic fluid (often hemorrhage) with surrounding tendon retraction (Figure 7-35). The entire muscle should be followed in both long and short axis. Remote injury is characterized by loss of the normal fibrillar echotexture and hyperechoic scar tissue[5]. The medial and lateral heads of the gastrocnemius and the soleus will combine distally to form the Achilles tendon. The plantaris tendon runs between the medial gastrocnemius and soleus muscles and along the medial aspect of the Achilles tendon to its insertion on the calcaneus[9,10].

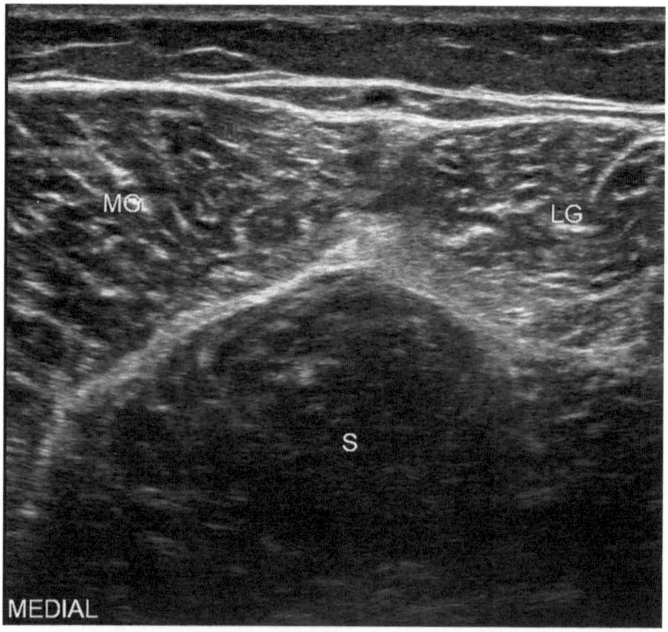

Fig 7-33: Transverse imaging of the posterior calf demonstrating the medial gastrocnemius (MG), lateral gastrocnemius (LG), and soleus (S) muscles in short axis.

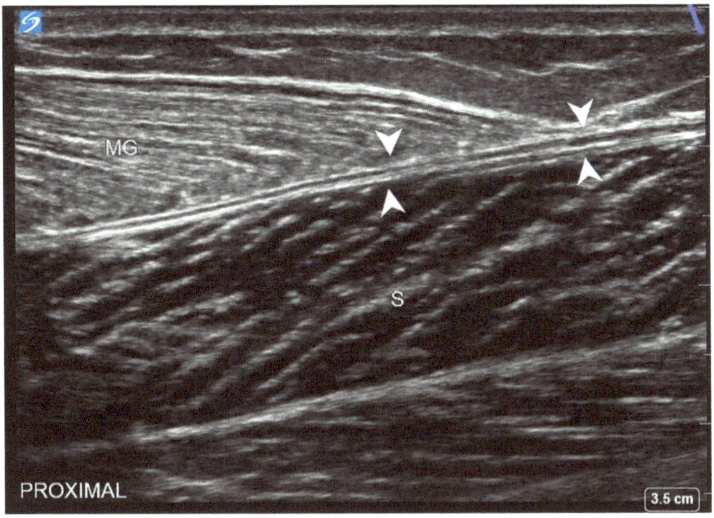

Fig 7-34: Parasagittal imaging of the posterior calf demonstrating the medial gastrocnemius (MG) in long axis tapering toward the soleus (S) muscle with the plantaris noted (arrowheads).

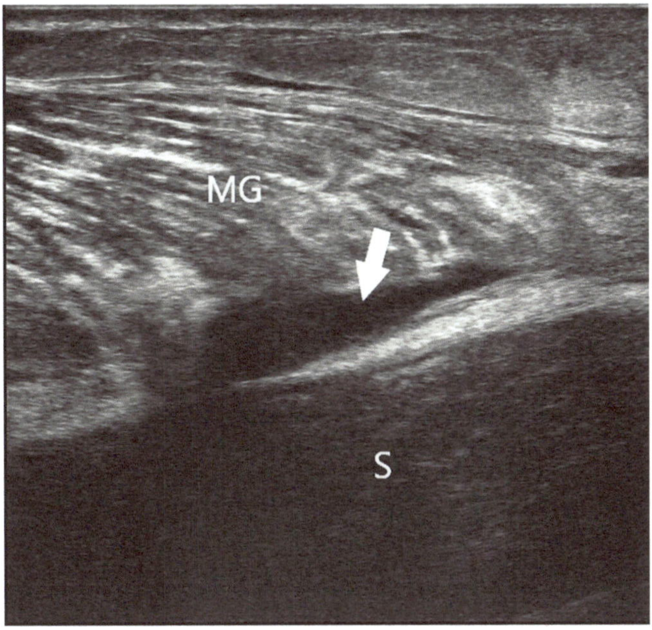

Fig 7-35: Parasagittal imaging of the posterior calf demonstrating a hypoechoic tear of the medial gastrocnemius (MG) at the aponeurosis with the soleus (S) in long axis.

e. **Forefoot:**

The most evaluated structures in the forefoot are Morton's neuromas and the plantar plate. Evaluation for a Morton's neuroma starts with the patient in supine position with the foot dorsiflexed and the transducer in the coronal plane over the plantar aspect of the metatarsal heads (Figure 7-36). The interdigital nerves are prone to compression from tight footwear and repetitive trauma. Swelling of the interdigital nerves occurs most commonly between the 3rd and 4th metatarsals. At the level of the metatarsal heads, a Morton's neuroma will appear as a hypoechoic circular structure that will protrude toward the plantar surface of the foot with dynamic evaluation during metatarsal squeeze (Figure 7-37). This sonographic test is termed 'Mulder's sign'. There may be increased through transmission, or hyperechoic artifact, deep to the hypoechoic neuroma[12]. In long axis, the hyperechoic fibrillar nerve fibers may be seen entering the neuroma as noted by a hypoechoic area of swelling[6].

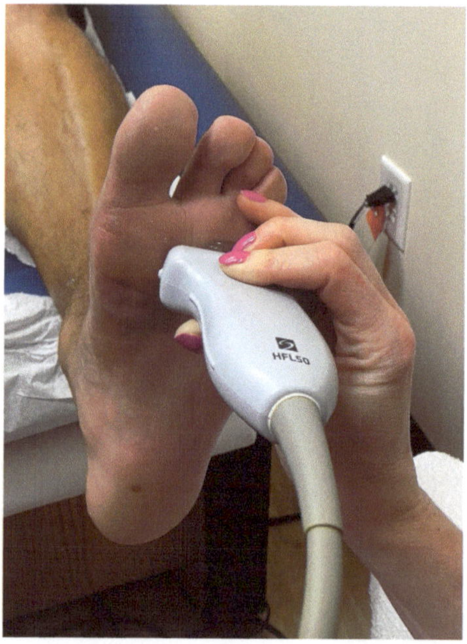

Fig 7-36: Probe positioning in the coronal plane over the plantar aspect of the metatarsal heads.

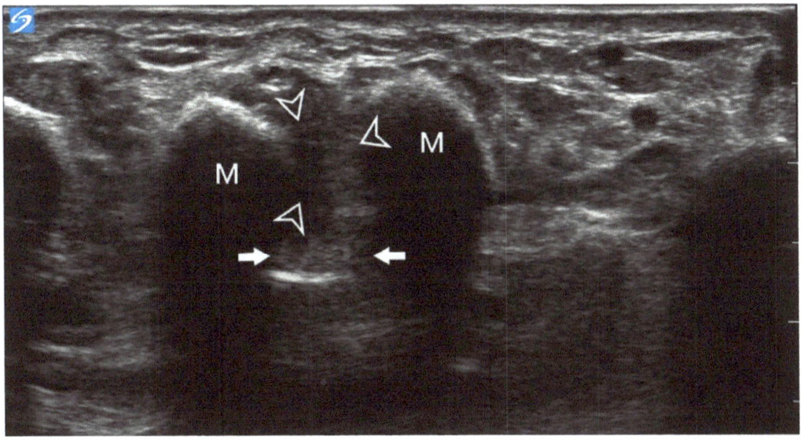

Fig 7-37: Coronal view of the intermetatarsal space with a small hypoechoic Morton's neuroma (open arrowheads) and increased through transmission (arrows); M= metatarsal heads.

The plantar plate is the primary metatarsophalanteal (MTP) joint stabilizer and injury in the first digit is termed 'turf toe'. The plantar plate is reportedly torn in 40% of patients with metatarsalgia of the lesser toes and is typically degenerative in middle-aged patients[13]. For evaluation of the plantar plate, place the transducer in the sagittal plane over the plantar aspect of the MTP joint of interest. Normal appearance of the plantar plate is a mildly hyperechogenic curvilinear structure with a granular texture when compared to the overlying fibrillar flexor digitorum tendons (Figure 7-38). Plantar plate tears appear as a hypoechoic defect (partial or full thickness) or non-visualization of the plantar plate. A hyperechoic curvilinear artifact known as a 'cartilage interface sign' may be seen between the hypoechoic cartilage and hypoechoic fluid in a partial plantar plate tear[12]. A small hyperechoic cortical avulsion from the base of the proximal phalanx may be seen with traumatic full thickness plantar plate tears[13]. In one systematic review, MRI was found to be more accurate than ultrasound in detection of plantar plate tears[14]. Although ultrasound is cheaper and provides the opportunity for dynamic evaluation during a Lachman test, it is highly user dependent. [I'm unfamiliar with this Lachman test]

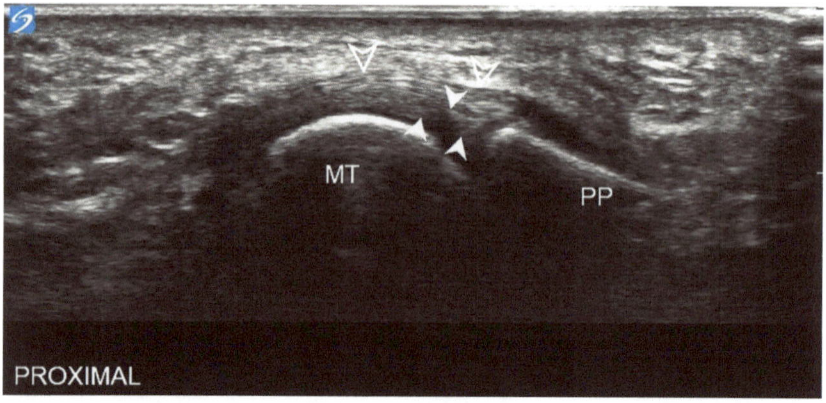

Fig 7-38: Sagittal plane over the plantar metatarsophalangeal joint with the fibrillar flexor digitorum tendon (open arrowheads) with the more granular plantar plate (filled arrowheads), deep to the tendon, connecting the proximal phalanx (PP) and metatarsal (M).

Pathology and Ultrasound-Guided Interventions in the Foot and Ankle

Arthritis

Arthritis of the ankle, hindfoot and midfoot can be due to several causes. In the foot and ankle, most arthritis is post-traumatic. Subtalar arthritis is also often the result of trauma, most commonly as a sequela of calcaneal fractures, but may also be due to inflammatory arthritis, malalignment and congenital factors. Midfoot arthritis is also most commonly seen as a result of trauma. Other causes include rheumatoid arthritis and degeneration due to suboptimal loading due to planovalgus alignment. Regardless of the etiology of foot and ankle arthritis, ultrasound guided injections can be beneficial as a diagnostic and therapeutic tool. While palpation guided tibiotalar joint injections are rather straightforward, ultrasound enhances the ability to visualize joint effusions and assist in aspiration for evaluation of inflammatory arthritis, gout, or infectious etiology[15].

a. Tibiotalar joint injection

i. Injectate: 2-4 mL of local anesthetic with or without 1 mL of corticosteroid.

ii. Technique: The patient may be sitting or lying supine with their knee flexed to 90 degrees and foot flat on the table in approximately 40 degrees of plantar flexion to open the tibiotalar joint space. Using a linear array transducer in the parasagittal plane just medial to the tibialis anterior tendon, the tibiotalar joint is identified. Power Doppler should be utilized to ensure there is no vasculature in the region. The preferred needle trajectory is in plane to the transducer via a distal to proximal approach, just superficial to the talar dome (Fig 7-39). Once the anterior recess is reached, the injectate will be seen distending the anterior joint capsule[16].

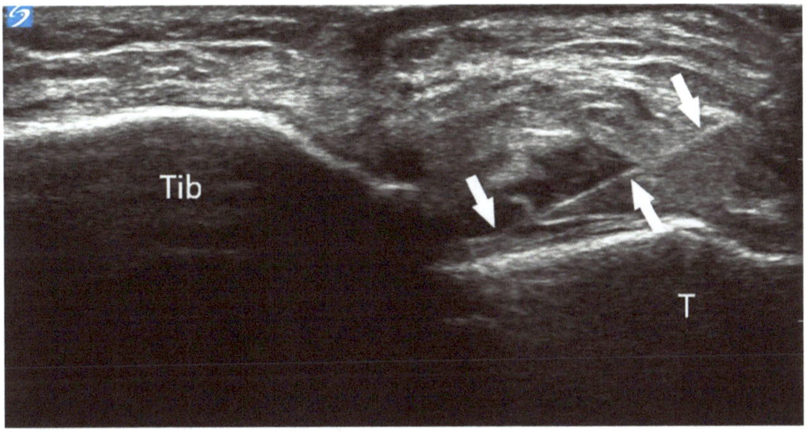

Fig 7-39: Parasagittal view of the tibiotalar joint with the hyperechoic needle (arrows) approaching the joint from distal to proximal trajectory; Tib= tibia, T= talus.

b. Subtalar joint injection

i. Indications: The subtalar joint allows for inversion and eversion of the hindfoot. Instability can result after inversion ankle injuries with CFL ligament rupture. Indications for diagnostic or steroid injection include chronic pain after ankle sprain, posterolateral impingement, osteoarthritis, gout, or other inflammatory arthropathies.

ii. Injectate: 2-4 mL of local anesthetic with or without 1 mL of corticosteroid.

iii. Technique: The subtalar joint can be accessed via the anterolateral, posterolateral, and posteromedial approaches however due the decreased proximity of neurovascular structures, the posterolateral approach is preferred[17]. The patient will lie prone on the exam table with the foot hanging off the edge. Using a linear array transducer along the parasagittal plane just lateral to the Achilles tendon, the subtalar (talocalcaneal) joint space is visualized. The needle will be directed via a steep in plane posterior to anterior approach along the calcaneus to the subtalar joint space (Fig 7-40). Local anesthetic may be given along the planned track. The needle will be difficult to visualize due to the steep trajectory so an inferior angling of the transducer toward the calcaneus can be helpful[16].

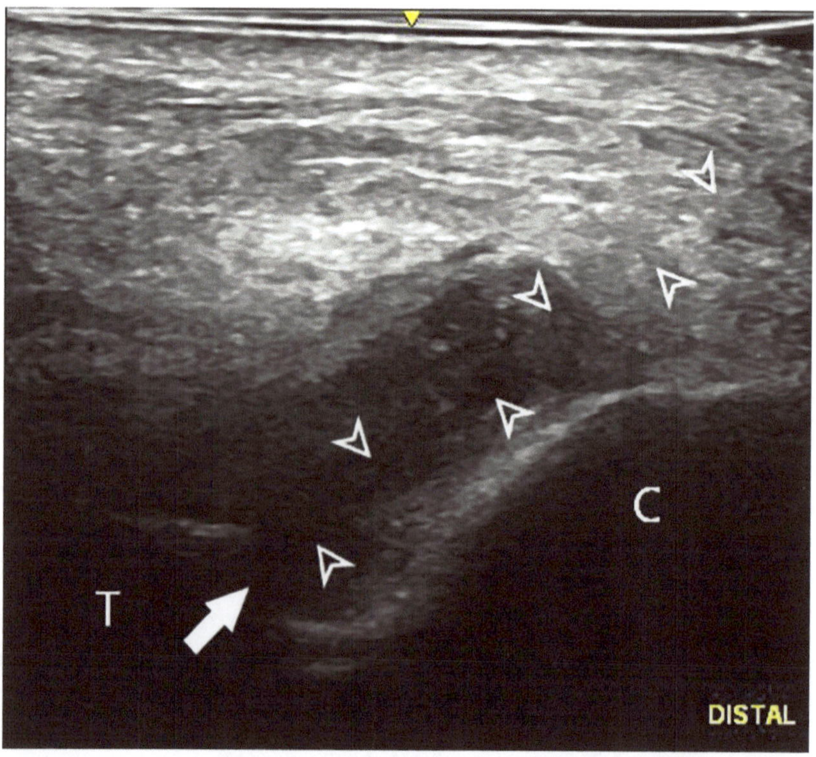

Fig 7-40: Parasagittal view of the posterolateral aspect of the subtalar joint (arrow) with the steep posterior to anterior needle trajectory noted (open arrowheads); T= talus, C= calcaneus.

c. **Mid foot joint injections**

i. Indications: There are many joints of the foot that are prone to pain associated with osteoarthritis or inflammatory arthritis. Each of these joints can be injected via a similar technique but we will specifically discuss tarsometatarsal (TMT) and metatarsophalangeal (MTP) joints. The TMT joint is termed the 'Lisfranc joint' because of the Lisfranc ligament, which acts as an important stabilizer of the 1st and 2nd MTP joints and midfoot. Midfoot sprains often require surgical stabilization. Chronic post injury pain is frequently an indication for injection. Ultrasound guided injection of the TMT joint offers far superior accuracy at 64% compared to palpation guided injections at 24%[15,20]. Khosla et al. also found that the injectate often extended beyond the intended TMT joint after injection so multiple isolated TMT joint injections may not be necessary[20]. The 1st MTP joint is the most common location of gout and ultrasound guided injections and aspirations can aid in diagnosis and treatment[21].

ii. Injectate: 1 mL of local anesthetic and 1 mL of corticosteroid (lesser MTP joints will require smaller volumes).

iii. Technique: The patient will lie supine with the knee flexed to 90 degrees and the foot flat on the table. Using a linear array transducer in the sagittal plane over the dorsal foot, the TMT or MTP joint of interest will be observed. Power Doppler should always be reviewed to assess for the dorsalis pedis artery which runs over the 1st and 2nd TMT joints. We recommend staying over the dorsal foot to avoid the digital neurovascular structures located medially and laterally and the extensor tendons. The needle will enter via an out of plane medial to lateral walk down technique to enter the joint space (Fig 7-41). The joint will distend as the fluid is injected.

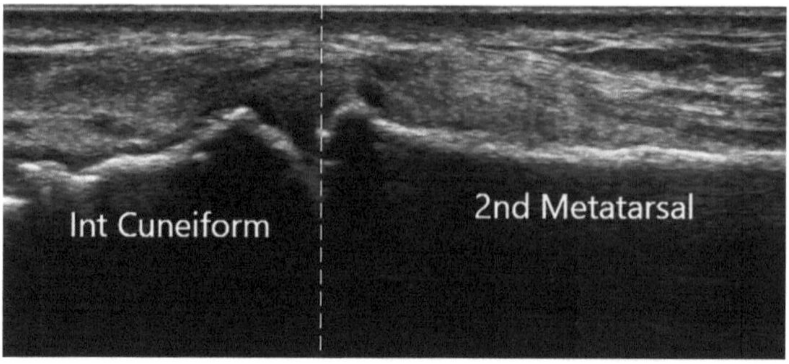

Fig 7-41: Sagittal view of the 2nd tarsometatarsal joint with the out of plane needle trajectory demonstrated by the dashed line between the intermediate cuneiform and 2nd metatarsal.

Ankle impingement

Anterior impingement refers to a syndrome of anterior ankle pain due to soft tissue or bony impingement. Soft tissue impingement is most commonly due to soft tissue proliferation in the setting of chronic ankle instability. Bony impingement is most likely due to early ankle arthritis in the setting of chronic ankle instability. Other causes include post-traumatic bony impingement due to ankle fracture or pilon malunion and post traumatic soft tissue impingement due to a build-up of scar tissue.

Posterior ankle impingement (PAI) can be due to several bony or soft tissue disorders. Regardless of cause, PAI generally leads to posterior ankle pain, worse with plantarflexion activities such as running downhill, en pointe positioning, and kicking. PAI is most commonly caused by edema around an os trigonum or FHL synovitis but can also be a result of acute trauma such as a fracture of the posterior process of the talus. Ultrasound can be used to help localize injections and to assess excursion and triggering of the FHL tendon.

Flexor hallucis longus tendon sheath injection

i. Injectate: 1 mL of local anesthetic with or without 1 mL of corticosteroid or ketorolac.

ii. Technique: Patient will lie prone with a towel roll under the anterior ankle or under the lateral ankle with the foot externally rotated. The transducer will be in the transverse plane over the medial malleolus and tarsal tunnel with a short axis view of the FHL tendon and other tarsal tunnel contents. Needle trajectory will be in plane with a posterior to anterior approach to the FHL sheath starting either medial or lateral to the Achilles tendon (Fig 7-42). The tibial artery, vein, and nerve should be identified and avoided prior to injection.

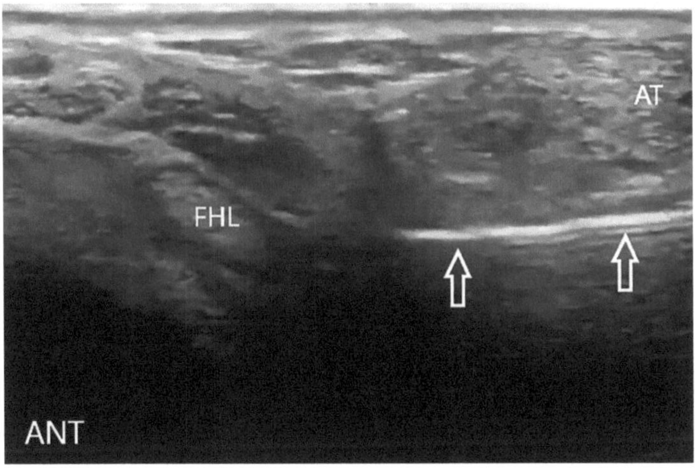

Fig 7-42: Short axis view of the flexor hallucis longus (FHL) tendon with the needle (open arrows) in plane from posterior to anterior (ANT). The needle can be inserted medial or lateral to the Achilles tendon (AT). Initiating the insertion on the lateral side makes the path of the needle less steep with respect to the probe surface.

Sinus tarsi syndrome

i. Indications: The sinus tarsi is a cavity located laterally between the posterior and anterior subtalar joints and contains fat, arterial anastomoses, nerve branches, proprioceptive nerve endings, and five ligamentous structures[18]. Sinus tarsi syndrome (STS) includes multiple possible diagnoses that present with pain localized in the lateral hindfoot near the sinus tarsi. Possible underlying diagnoses include subtalar instability, osteochondral lesion, subtalar arthritis, coalition, interosseous ligament tear, fat and synovial hypertrophy and arthrofibrosis. Regardless of underlying diagnosis, a diagnostic injection can help differentiate STS from peroneal and ankle pathology. If conservative measures fail, and the patient gains relief from a diagnostic injection, subtalar arthroscopy may be considered[22]. Wisniewski et al. found a 35% accuracy rate with palpation guided sinus tarsi injections versus 90% accuracy using ultrasound guidance[19].

ii. Injectate: 1-2 mL of local anesthetic with or without 1 mL of corticosteroid.

iii. Technique: The patient will lie supine with the ankle slightly inverted and plantar flexed or in lateral decubitus position with a towel roll under the medial ankle with slight plantar flexion. The transducer will be placed in a coronal oblique plane between the talus and the calcaneus with the inferior end rotated more anteriorly. The needle trajectory will be an out of plane approach from anterior to posterior using a walk down technique (Fig 7-43). A centerline can be placed on the screen to visualize the target trajectory when the needle is placed at the center marking on the probe. Once the needle passes the edge of the talus and calcaneus, the tip will become more difficult to visualize and the user must monitor for the feeling of the needle dropping into the sinus tarsi[16]. There should not be any resistance when injecting the solution.

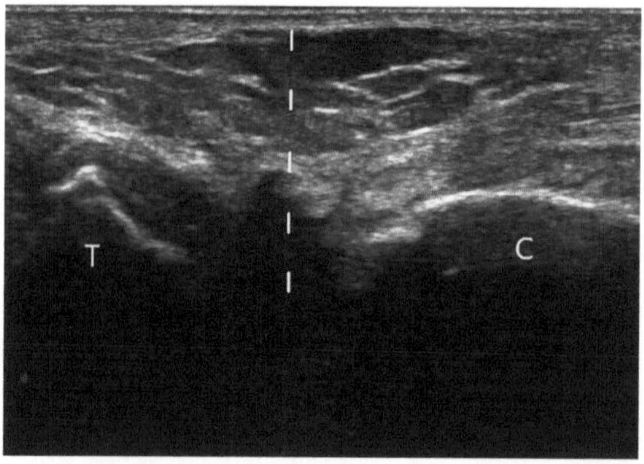

Fig 7-43: Coronal oblique view of the sinus tarsi between the talus (T) and calcaneus (C). The out of plane needle trajectory is noted via the dashed line.

Achilles

Achilles tendon injuries can be broadly classified as acute or chronic. Achilles tendon pathology can also be categorized by severity ranging from mild, overuse-related inflammatory responses to acute, traumatic tendon rupture. Achilles tendon ruptures can also be classified according to the location of the rupture: insertional, midsubstance, and musculotendinous junction. Most acute ruptures can be diagnosed without advanced imaging, but access to office-based ultrasound can help in atypical presentations and exams. Ultrasound can aid in evaluation of chronic Achilles ruptures where there is potential for retraction; Ultrasound can also help approximate the tendon gap.

Achilles hydro-dissection

i. Indications: Chronic tendinopathy is quite common in the mid portion Achilles tendon due to the poor blood supply of this region. Blood vessels grow into the tendon as part of the healing process, however the nerves that travel with the vessels are frequently responsible for the associated pain. Often, fusiform swelling with neovascularization on power Doppler will be noted on ultrasound. Occasionally, Kager's fat pad scarring can be responsible for tendon tethering, resulting in symptomatology[23]. Ultrasound guided hydro-dissection of these tissue layers is a low-risk procedure that can treat the tethering or reduce neovascularization in Achilles tendon problems. Alternatively, platelet rich plasma (PRP) has shown promise for treating refractory Achilles tendinopathy, however more randomized controlled trials are needed[24,25]. Corticosteroid injections around the Achilles tendon are controversial and have been loosely associated with tendon rupture in some studies[26,27].

ii. Injectate: 9 mL of D5W and 1 mL of local anesthetic for hydro-dissection.

iii. Technique: Patient will lie prone with the foot hanging over the edge of the table. The Achilles tendon should be viewed in both short and long axis to identify the region of tendon thickening and possible hyperemia signifying neovascularization. The transducer will be in transverse plane with the tendon in short axis at the region of interest. The needle trajectory will be in plane, lateral to medial to target the tissue plane between the tendon and the Kager fat pad (Fig 7-44). Identify the sural nerve and saphenous vein which sit lateral to the Achilles tendon prior to injection to avoid injury. As the solution is injected, the fat pad should be seen peeling away from the tendon. Switch the transducer between short and long axis views of the tendon during the procedure to ensure the needle tip is in the intended tissue plane. Post injection, power Doppler can be utilized to ensure the neovascular tendon infiltration has been decreased. There are no major activity restrictions after this procedure since the tendon was not injected.

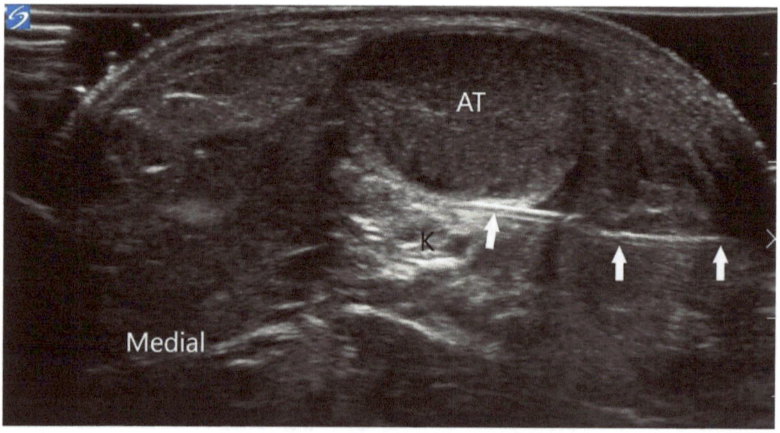

Fig 7-44: Short axis view of the Achilles tendon (AT) with the needle (arrows) entering via an in-plane lateral to medial approach to the plane between the Achilles and Kager fat pad (K) for fluid deposition during an Achilles hydro-dissection injection.

Posterior tibial tendon

Posterior tibial tendon dysfunction has long been seen as the most common cause of adult acquired flatfoot deformity (AAFD). The tibialis posterior muscle originates from the posterior tibia, fibula and interosseous membrane of the deep posterior compartment of the leg. The muscle becomes tendinous in distal 1/3 of the leg. The posterior tibial tendon (PTT) travels posterior to the medial malleolus and inserts on the navicular tuberosity. The PTT is prone to injury due to its anatomical orientation and repetitive loading. Early stages of AAFD involve tenosynovitis of the PTT with flexible deformities. Ultrasound guided injection of the PTT sheath can provide pain relief and is a useful adjunct to physical therapy for tenosynovitis. As always, caution should be advised when administering corticosteroids, especially in the presence of partial tendon tears.

Posterior tibialis tendon sheath injection

i. Injectate: 1-2 mL of local anesthetic with or without 1 mL of corticosteroid or ketorolac.

ii. Technique: Patient will lie in a lateral decubitus position with the affected medial ankle facing upward and a towel roll under the lateral ankle. The transducer will be in the transverse oblique plane over the medial malleolus and tarsal tunnel with a short axis view of the PTT tendon. Needle trajectory will be in plane with an anterior to posterior or posterior to anterior approach to the PTT sheath (Fig 7-45). The tibial artery, vein, and nerve should be identified and avoided prior to injection. The anterior approach allows for the shortest distance and avoidance of the neurovascular structures; however, it can be difficult to pass over the medial malleolus and enter the tendon sheath. The gel standoff technique can be helpful with the anterior approach[16].

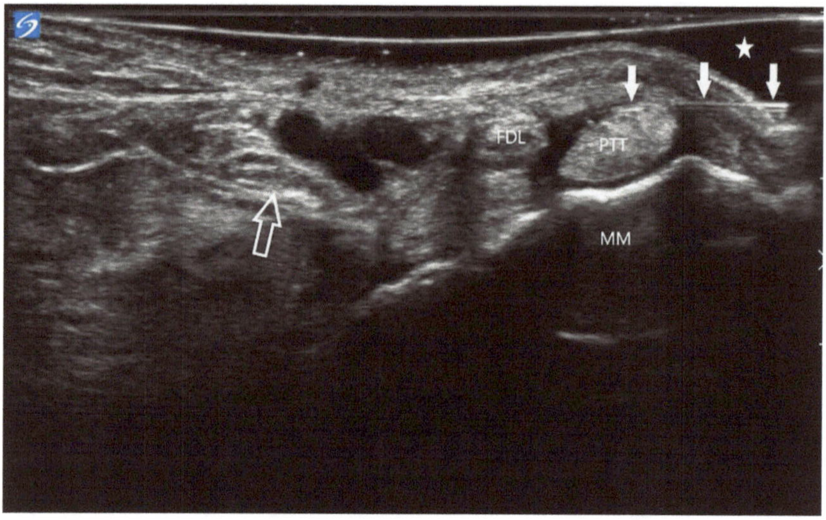

Fig 7-45: Short axis view of the posterior tibialis tendon (PTT) with the needle (arrows) seen entering the tendon sheath via an anterior to posterior approach. Note the gel standoff assisting with needle entry (star); FDL= flexor digitorum longus tendon; MM= medial malleolus; open arrow= tibial nerve.

Peroneal tendon injury

Peroneal tendon injury is typically classified as tenosynovitis with or without subluxation, chronic peroneal tendinopathy, and peroneal tendon tears. The peroneal muscles lie in the lateral compartment of the leg and become tendinous in the distal aspect as they traverse through the fibro-osseous peroneal tunnel. The tunnel lies posterior to the fibula and is composed of retro-fibular surface anteriorly, the superior peroneal retinaculum (SPR) laterally and the calcaneofibular and posterior talofibular ligaments medially. The peroneus longus runs posteriorly to the peroneus brevis tendon through this tunnel and both make obtuse turns around the distal fibula and then reflect along the lateral calcaneus. The brevis then inserts on the proximal aspect of the fifth metatarsal while the longus tendon traverses beneath the cuboid where it takes another sharp turn as it travels to its insertion on the plantar aspect of the first metatarsal bone. The peroneus brevis and longus tendons function to evert the foot and plantar flex the first ray, respectively. Ultrasound may be used to visualize soft tissue structures. It permits dynamic imaging of the tendons as well. For chronic peroneal tendinopathy, ultrasound may be particularly useful as it can demonstrate tendon excursion, or the lack thereof, which is a key factor in operative decision making as noted below.

Peroneal tendon sheath injection

i. Indications: Peroneal tendinopathy, tenosynovitis, and partial tears are common etiologies for which diagnostic anesthetic or ketorolac injections may be useful. Caution should be used when administering corticosteroid around the peroneal tendons and a relative contraindication exists for corticosteroid injection in the setting of partial tendon tear due to the potential side effects of tendon rupture. Ultrasound guided peroneal tendon sheath injections were found to be 100% accurate versus 60% accurate for palpation guided injections in one study[28].

ii. Injectate: 0.5-1 mL of local anesthetic with or without 1 mL of corticosteroid or ketorolac.

iii. Technique: Patient will lie in a lateral decubitus position with the affected lateral ankle facing upward and a towel roll under the medial ankle. The transducer will be in the transverse oblique plane over the lateral malleolus and retro malleolar groove with a short axis view of the tendons. Needle trajectory will be in plane with a posterior to anterior approach to the common peroneal tendon sheath (Fig 7-46). A gel standoff technique can assist with needle entry.

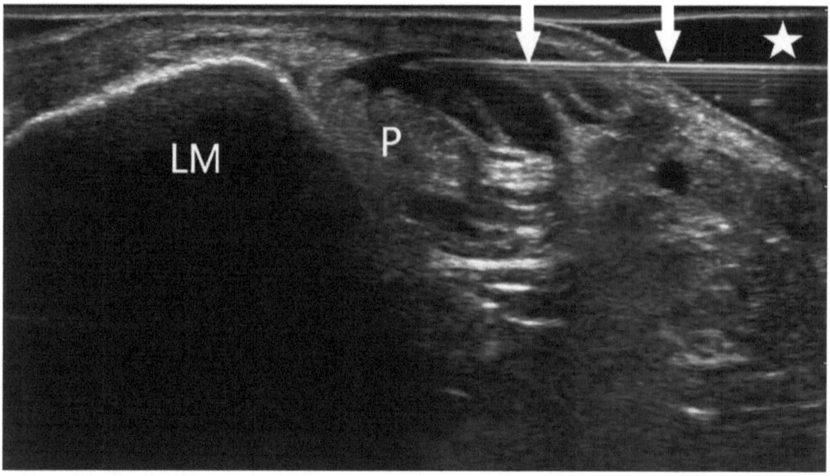

Fig 7-46: Short axis view of the peroneal tendons (P) with the needle seen entering the tendon sheath via a posterior to anterior approach (arrows). Note the gel standoff assisting with needle entry (star); LM= lateral malleolus.

Knot of Henry

The FDL tendon crosses over the FHL tendon distal to the sustentaculum tali at the 'knot of Henry'. There is substantial variation in the numbers of interconnections between the FHL and FDL tendons at the knot of Henry[29]. Adhesions or friction between the tendons and interconnections can lead to pain on the plantar medial foot secondary to tenosynovitis or an intersection syndrome[16]. Patients may also feel popping or snapping with motion of the toes and ankle. Due to the infrequency of the diagnosis, a diagnostic injection can be helpful prior to a planned surgery'.

Knot of Henry injection

i. Injectate: 1 mL of local anesthetic and 1 mL of corticosteroid.

ii. Technique: Patient will lie in a lateral decubitus position with the affected medial ankle/foot facing upward and a towel roll under the lateral ankle. The transducer will be in a sagittal oblique plane in the medial arch of the foot distal to the sustentaculum tali to view the tendons in short axis as they cross.

The needle trajectory will be in an in plane medial to lateral approach to the crossing point between the two tendons. Local anesthetic can be used for a skin wheel and needle entry. Check power Doppler flow prior to injection to ensure adjacent vessels and the medial plantar nerve are not injected. The tendons can also be viewed in long axis with an out of plane medial to lateral needle trajectory toward the tendons (Fig 7-47).

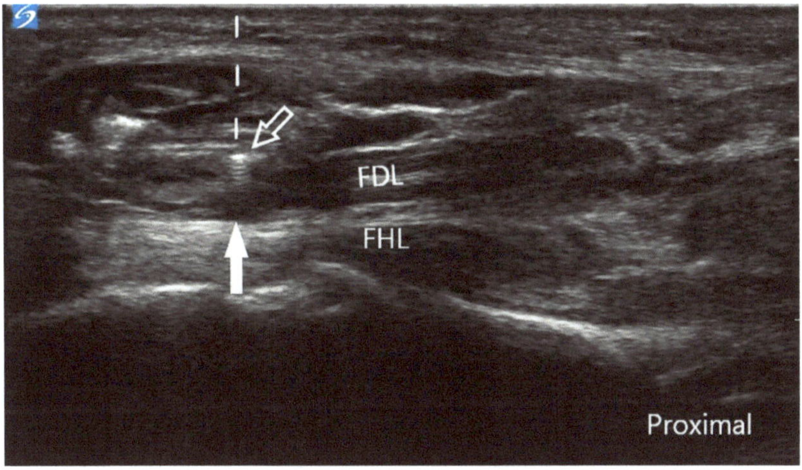

Fig 7-47: Long axis view of the intersection of the flexor hallucis longus (FHL) and flexor digitorum longus (FDL) tendons at the Knot of Henry (arrow) with the out of plane needle trajectory (dashed line) and needle tip (open arrow) noted.

Plantar fascia injection

i. Indications: Plantar fasciopathy is one of the most common complaints in a foot and ankle clinical setting. Peri-plantar fascia steroid injections can be indicated for patients with recalcitrant plantar fasciitis despite all conservative treatments. Long term benefit has been shown for intra-fascial dextrose prolotherapy or PRP injections for chronic pain associated with chronic plantar fasciitis, fascial thickening, or partial plantar fascia tear[25,30,31].

ii. Injectate: 1 mL of local anesthetic and 1 mL of corticosteroid or 1-2 mL of 25% dextrose solution or PRP for intrafascial injections.

iii. Technique: Patient will lie in a lateral decubitus position with the medial heel facing upwards and a towel roll under the lateral foot/ankle. The transducer will be in a transverse plane over the plantar aspect of the heel with the plantar fascia in short axis. The target is at the origin of the plantar fascia on the medial calcaneal tubercle between the calcaneus and plantar fascia for peri-fascial injections and directly into the plantar fascia for intra-fascial injections. Injecting corticosteroid deep to the plantar fascia reduces the risk of fat pad atrophy[16]. The needle trajectory is an in plane medial to lateral approach (Fig 7-48). For peri-plantar fascia injections, the soft tissue should be anesthetized with local anesthetic prior to transitioning to a 22-gauge needle for the corticosteroid mixture administration. For intra-fasical dextrose prolotherapy or PRP injections, a posterior tibial nerve block with local anesthetic is first recommended to decrease pain and increase procedure tolerance (See tibial nerve injection below). After the tibial nerve block, local tissue anesthetic is not likely needed but can be given to ensure proper anesthesia of the region. The plantar fascia should then be fenestrated multiple times with peppering of the solution throughout. Typically, after intra-fascial injections, the patient will be protected with weight bearing as tolerated in walking boot for 1-2 weeks.

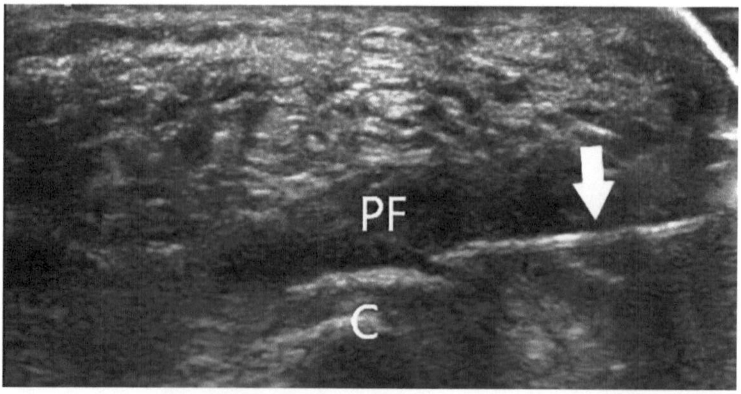

Fig 7-48: Short axis view of the plantar fascia (PF) with the needle (arrow) entering from medial to lateral to the target between the plantar fascia and calcaneus (C).

Interdigital Neuromas

The 1st, 2nd and 3rd web spaces are innervated by the medial plantar nerve by way of the common digital nerve branches. The lateral plantar nerve provides a common digital nerve to the 4th webspace as well as a communicating branch to the 3rd webspace. Interdigital neuromas are most common in the third webspace. Patients most commonly complain of neuritic-type pain along the plantar foot and toes in the affected webspace. Symptoms are generally worsened by conditions that overload or compress the forefoot such as shoes with a raised heel and tight fitting footwear[32]. Injections to the affected webspace plantar to the transverse metatarsal ligament can be both diagnostic and therapeutic for interdigital neuromas. Ultrasound has similar sensitivity to MRI but higher specificity in identification of a Morton's neuroma[14]. Ultrasound guided Morton's neuroma steroid injection provides better short-term pain relief than palpation guided injections[33]. If a neuroma injection is helpful in the acute period, it can aid in diagnostic confidence. If a patient has good relief of symptoms from an Ultrasound guided neuroma injection, but the effect wanes, the injection can be repeated if adequate time has passed or offered surgical excision of the neuroma.

Morton's neuroma injection

i. Injectate: 0.5 mL of local anesthetic and 0.5-1 mL of corticosteroid.

ii. Technique: Injection can be performed through the plantar foot which is closer to the neuroma or through the dorsal foot. The dorsal approach tends to be less painful and better tolerated so we will review that approach. The patient will lie supine on the table with the knee flexed and foot flat on the table. The transducer will be in transverse axis over the dorsal metatarsal heads. The needle trajectory will be an out of plane distal to proximal approach with a walk down technique to the targeted deep inter-metatarsal space (Fig 7-49). Local anesthetic can be used prior to steroid injection if preferred. Always check power Doppler prior to injection to avoid the interdigital neuro-vasculature.

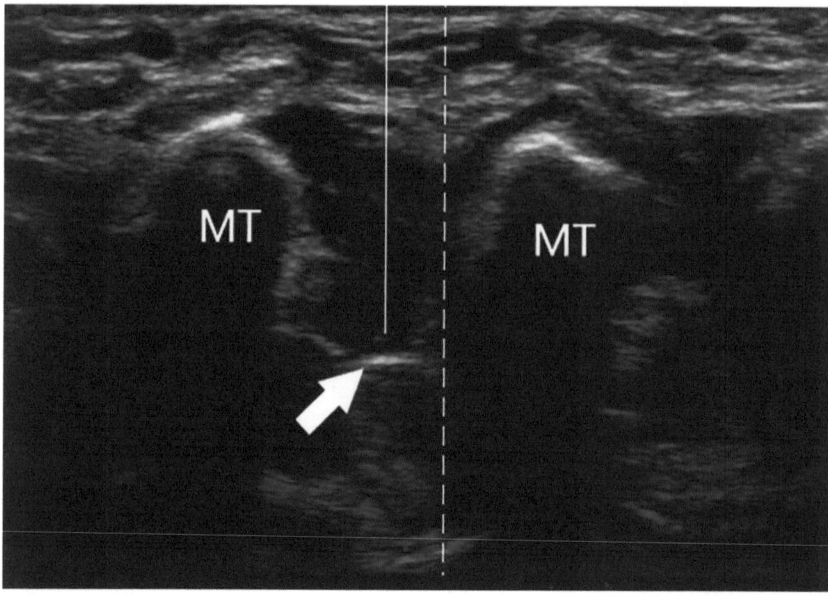

Fig 7-49: Transverse plane over the dorsal aspect of the metatarsal heads (MT). Out of plane distal to proximal needle trajectory (solid white line) will be parallel to the centerline (white dashed line) utilizing walk down technique between the metatarsal heads with the needle tip demonstrated (arrow) in the inter-metatarsal space.

Foreign bodies

Puncture wounds are common to the plantar aspect of the foot. Many of the most common penetrating substances are not detected on radiographs. Without removal, patients are at risk for infections ranging from mild cellulitis to chronic osteomyelitis. Ultrasound can aid in foreign body removal in the operating room or in office-based procedures[34].

Tarsal Tunnel

The tarsal tunnel is the distal continuation of the deep posterior compartment of the leg. In over 90% of the population, the tibial nerve divides into the medial and lateral plantar nerves within the tarsal tunnel. The most common variant is a proximal bifurcation of the tibial nerve. Etiologies of tarsal tunnel include varicosities, ganglion cysts, bony exostoses, hypertrophic and/or accessory muscles, hypertrophic ligaments bordering the tunnel, and trauma. Ultrasound can be useful to identify ganglia and other space occupying lesions. Ultrasound-guided tarsal tunnel injection can also provide another diagnostic tool when MRI and nerve conduction exams are inconclusive. Rarely, patients may have compression of individual branches of the nerves such as the medial and lateral plantar nerves, or Baxter's nerve which is the first branch of the lateral plantar nerve. Diagnostic blocks of these nerves can help guide surgical planning.

a. Tarsal tunnel/tibial nerve injection

i. Indications: Injection of local anesthetic around the tibial nerve within the tarsal tunnel can be done prior to distal foot procedures such as a plantar fascia fenestration as discussed above or prior to surgery. This injection can also be done for tarsal tunnel syndrome in which tibial nerve entrapment is suspected within the tarsal tunnel. Infiltration of anesthetic around the nerve can mechanically free the nerve from surrounding scar tissue and aid in diagnosis.

ii. Injectate: 2-5 mL of local anesthetic.

iii. Technique: Patient will lie in a lateral decubitus position with the affected medial ankle facing upward and a towel roll under the lateral ankle. The transducer will be in the transverse oblique plane over the medial malleolus and tarsal tunnel with a short axis view of the tarsal tunnel contents. Needle trajectory will be in plane with a posterior to anterior approach to the tibial nerve (Fig 7-50). The tibial vasculature should be identified and avoided prior to injection using power Doppler flow. The nerve will be slightly deep and posterior to the vasculature. Make sure to inject around the nerve and not directly into the nerve or surrounding vasculature. Allow 5 minutes for the block to take effect prior to proceeding with any subsequent procedures.

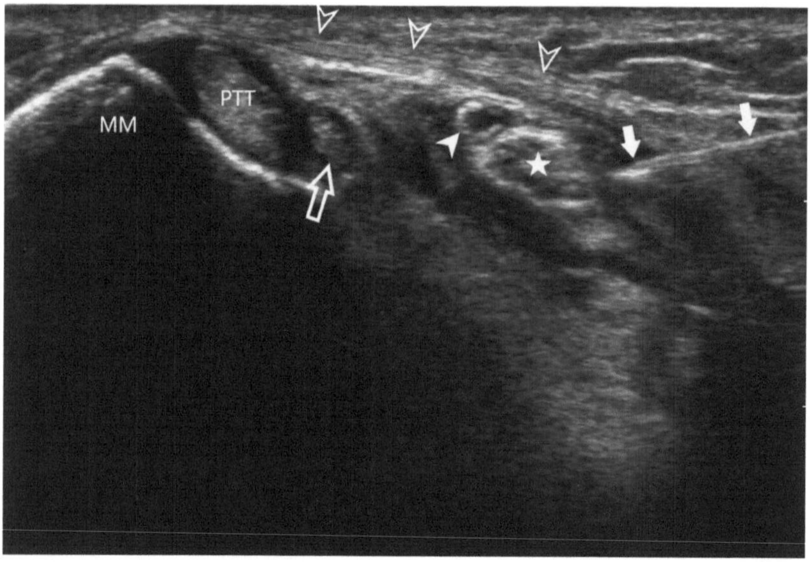

Fig 7-50: Transverse oblique plane posterior to the medial malleolus (MM) over the tarsal tunnel. The needle (arrows) enters via a posterior to anterior approach to the tibial nerve (star) to inject the surrounding tissue. Make sure to avoid the tibial artery and vein (arrowhead); MM= medial malleolus, PTT= posterior tibialis tendon; open arrow= flexor digitorum longus tendon, open arrowheads= flexor retinaculum.

Superficial Peroneal Nerve (SPN) and Sural Nerve

SPN entrapment is a relatively uncommon cause of anterolateral leg pain. Entrapment most commonly occurs as the nerve emerges from the deep fascia and begins to cross from the lateral to anterior compartments. It tends to occur in a younger, athletic population. Reported anatomic variations include nerve origination from the anterior compartment, adherence to the lateral compartment fascial near the anterior intermuscular septum, a proximal split into the two terminal branches, and muscle herniation through the fascial opening for the SPN. Compression or stretch neuropathy of the sural nerve is common in lateral ankle sprains or chronic instability. Extrinsic compression from ganglion cysts, hypertrophic muscles, or tenosynovitis can also cause symptoms. While the sural nerve may be injured in surgical approaches, it is uncommon to see true entrapment. If prior surgery leads to significant scarring, the nerve can become locally entrapped in scar tissue. Occasionally, compression or stretch neuropathy of the sural nerve can occur after lateral ankle sprains or chronic instability. Extrinsic compression from ganglion cysts, hypertrophic muscles, or tenosynovitis can also cause symptoms. Anesthetic, steroid, or larger volume hydro-dissection injection can be considered for patients with pain along the posterolateral lower leg and foot. Hydro-dissection involves mechanical separation of surrounding tissue from the nerve. Some studies demonstrate a direct analgesic effect of 5% dextrose solution on neuropathic pain, so D5W is the preferred solution for hydro-dissection[35].

Sural nerve and SPN injection

i. Injectate: 3-4 mL of local anesthetic and 1 mL of corticosteroid or 1 mL of local anesthetic and 9 mL of D5W for hydro-dissection.

ii. Technique: The patient will lie in a contralateral decubitus position with the affected lateral ankle facing upward and a towel roll under the medial ankle. The transducer will be in transverse axis with the SPN and sural nerve in short axis in the region of interest. For the sural nerve, this will typically be between the lateral malleolus and Achilles tendon while the SPN target will be more proximal and anterior in the distal calf subcutaneous tissue. The needle trajectory is an in-plane posterior to anterior approach (Fig 7-51) targeting the perineural tissue superficial and deep to the indicated nerve, attempting to create a neurogram of hypoechoic fluid surrounding the nerve (Fig 7-52). Check power Doppler prior to injection to avoid the saphenous vein running with the sural nerve and the anterior tibial vein running anterior to the SPN.

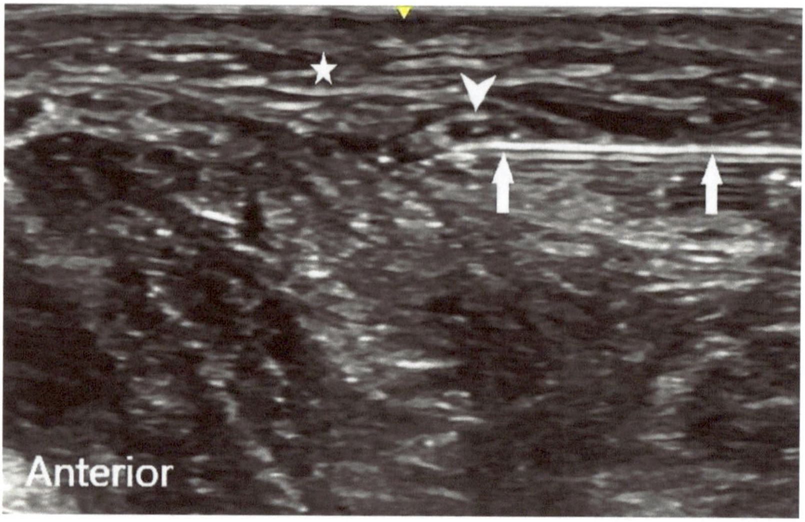

Fig 7-51: Short axis view of the superficial peroneal nerve (arrowhead) within the subcutaneous tissue (star) of the lateral calf with the needle (arrows) entering deep to the nerve via an in-plane posterior to anterior approach.

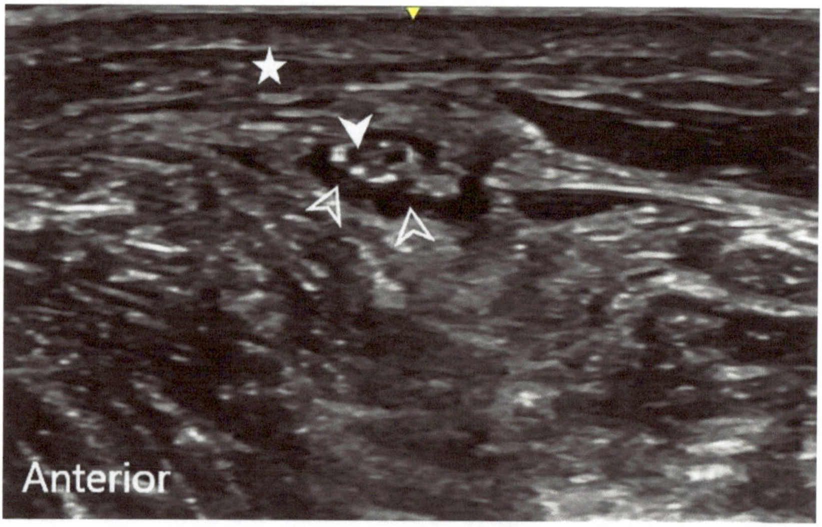

Fig 7-52: Short axis view of the superficial peroneal nerve (arrowhead) within the subcutaneous tissue (star) of the lateral calf after hyro-dissection with the anechoic fluid neurogram noted (open arrowhead).

Summary

While most clinicians are less familiar with ultrasound as compared to other advanced imaging modalities, knowledge of ultrasound techniques can be invaluable. This chapter shows the vast breadth of uses for ultrasound for the foot and ankle alone. In the senior authors' practices, ultrasound is used daily to perform diagnostic and therapeutic injections, as well as in the perioperative setting to guide peripheral nerve blocks by the anesthesia team. Knowledge of these techniques along with others mentioned in the chapter have greatly aided diagnosis and treatment for many different foot and ankle pathologies.

References

1. Jain Nm Omar I, Kelikian A, van Holsbeeck L, Grant T. Prevalence of and factors associated with posterior tibial tendon pathology on sonographic assessment. *PMR* 2011; 3(11): 998-1004.

2. Neustadter J, Raikin S, Nazarian L, Dynamic sonographic evaluation of peroneal tendon subluxation. *Am J Roentgenol* 2004; 183 (4): 985-988.

3. Chang A, Miller TT. Imaging of tendons. *Sports Health.* 2009; 1(4):293-300. doi:10.1177/1941738109338361

4. Connolly DJ, Berman L, McNally EG. The use of beam angulation to overcome anisotropy when viewing human tendon with high frequency linear array ultrasound. *Br J Radiol.* 2001; 74(878):183-185. doi:10.1259/bjr.74.878.740183

5. Kotnis N, Harish S, Popowich T. Medial ankle and heel: ultrasound evaluation and sonographic appearances of conditions causing symptoms. *Semin Ultrasound CT MR.* 2011; 32(2):125-141. doi:10.1053/j.sult.2010.11.001

6. Jacobson JA. Ankle, foot, and lower leg ultrasound. In: *Fundamentals of musculoskeletal ultrasound.* Elsevier; 2007:264-331. doi:10.1016/B978-1-4160-3593-0.50013-1

7. Yablon CM, Hammer MR, Morag Y, Brandon CJ, Fessell DP, Jacobson JA. US of the peripheral nerves of the lower extremity: A landmark approach. *Radiographics.* 2016; 36(2):464-478. doi:10.1148/rg.2016150120

8. Taljanovic MS, Alcala JN, Gimber LH, Rieke JD, Chilvers MM, Latt LD. High-resolution US and MR imaging of

peroneal tendon injuries. *Radiographics*. 2015; 35(1):179-199. doi:10.1148/rg.351130062

9. Draghi F, Bortolotto C, Draghi AG, Gitto S. Intrasheath instability of the peroneal tendons: dynamic ultrasound imaging. *J Ultrasound Med*. 2018; 37(12):2753-2758. doi:10.1002/jum.14633

10. Olewnik Ł, Wysiadecki G, Podgórski M, Polguj M, Topol M. The plantaris muscle tendon and its relationship with the Achilles tendinopathy. *Biomed Res Int*. 2018; 2018:9623579. doi:10.1155/2018/9623579

11. Spang C, Alfredson H, Docking SI, Masci L, Andersson G. The plantaris tendon: a narrative review focusing on anatomical features and clinical importance. *Bone Joint J*. 2016; 98-B(10):1312-1319. doi:10.1302/0301-620X.98b10.37939

12. Vaishya R, Agarwal AK, Azizi AT, Vijay V. Haglund's syndrome: A commonly seen mysterious condition. *Cureus*. 2016; 8(10):e820. doi:10.7759/cureus.820

13. Feldman MK, Katyal S, Blackwood MS. US artifacts. *Radiographics*. 2009; 29(4):1179-1189. doi:10.1148/rg.294085199

14. McCarthy CL, Thompson GV. Ultrasound findings of plantar plate tears of the lesser metatarsophalangeal joints. *Skeletal Radiol*. 2021; 50(8):1513-1525. doi:10.1007/s00256-020-03708-1

15. Duan X, Li L, Wei D-Q, et al. Role of magnetic resonance imaging versus ultrasound for detection of plantar plate tear. *J Orthop Surg Res*. 2017; 12(1):14. doi:10.1186/s13018-016-0507-6

16. Daniels EW, Cole D, Jacobs B, Phillips SF. Existing evidence on ultrasound-guided injections in sports medicine.

Orthop J Sports Med. 2018; 6(2):2325967118756576. doi:10.1177/2325967118756576

17. Malanga GA, Mautner KR, eds. Foot & ankle. In: *Atlas of Ultrasound-Guided Musculoskeletal Injections.* McGraw-Hill Education; 2014:325-418.

18. Henning T, Finnoff JT, Smith J. Sonographically guided posterior subtalar joint injections: anatomic study and validation of 3 approaches. *PM R.* 2009; 1(10):925-931. doi:10.1016/j.pmrj.2009.09.006

19. Taillard W, Meyer JM, Garcia J, Blanc Y. The sinus tarsi syndrome. *Int Orthop.* 1981; 5(2):117-130. doi:10.1007/BF00267842

20. Wisniewski SJ, Smith J, Patterson DG, Carmichael SW, Pawlina W. Ultrasound-guided versus nonguided tibiotalar joint and sinus tarsi injections: a cadaveric study. *PM R.* 2010; 2(4):277-281. doi:10.1016/j.pmrj.2010.03.013

21. Khosla S, Thiele R, Baumhauer JF. Ultrasound guidance for intra-articular injections of the foot and ankle. *Foot Ankle Int.* 2009; 30(9):886-890. doi:10.3113/FAI.2009.0886

22. Kang MH, Moon KW, Jeon YH, Cho SW. Sonography of the first metatarsophalangeal joint and sonographically guided intraarticular injection of corticosteroid in acute gout attack. *J Clin Ultrasound.* 2015; 43(3):179-186. doi:10.1002/jcu.22206

23. Frey C, Feder KS, DiGiovanni C. Arthroscopic evaluation of the subtalar joint: does sinus tarsi syndrome exist? *Foot Ankle Int.* 1999 Mar; 20(3):185-91. doi: 10.1177/107110079902000309. PMID: 10195298.

24. He L, Genin J, Delzell P. Ultrasound diagnosis and percutaneous treatment of Achilles tendon tethering: a case series. *Skeletal Radiol.* 2016; 45(9):1293-1298. doi:10.1007/s00256-016-2416-5

25. Mautner K, Colberg RE, Malanga G, et al. Outcomes after ultrasound-guided platelet-rich plasma injections for chronic tendinopathy: a multicenter, retrospective review. *PM R.* 2013; 5(3):169-175. doi:10.1016/j.pmrj.2012.12.010

26. Filardo G, Kon E, Di Matteo B, et al. Platelet-rich plasma injections for the treatment of refractory Achilles tendinopathy: results at 4 years. *Blood Transfus.* 2014; 12(4):533-540. doi:10.2450/2014.0289-13

27. Boone SL, Uzor R, Walter E, et al. Safety and efficacy of image-guided retrocalcaneal bursa corticosteroid injection for the treatment of retrocalcaneal bursitis. *Skeletal Radiol.* May 2021. doi:10.1007/s00256-021-03783-y

28. Speed CA. Fortnightly review: Corticosteroid injections in tendon lesions. *BMJ.* 2001; 323(7309):382-386. doi:10.1136/bmj.323.7309.382

29. Muir JJ, Curtiss HM, Hollman J, Smith J, Finnoff JT. The accuracy of ultrasound-guided and palpation-guided peroneal tendon sheath injections. *Am J Phys Med Rehabil.* 2011; 90(7):564-571. doi:10.1097/PHM.0b013e31821f6e63

30. Vasudha TK, Vani PC, Sankaranarayanan G, Rajasekhar SSSN, Dinesh Kumar V. Communications between the tendons of flexor hallucis longus and flexor digitorum longus: a cadaveric study. *Surg Radiol Anat.* 2019 Dec; 41(12):1411-1419. doi: 10.1007/s00276-019-02311-x. Epub 2019 Sep 20. PMID: 31541272.

31. Raissi G, Arbabi A, Rafiei M, et al. Ultrasound-guided injection of dextrose versus corticosteroid in chronic plantar fasciitis management: a randomized, double-blind clinical trial. *Foot Ankle Spec.* January 2021:1938640020980924. doi:10.1177/1938640020980924

32. Kalia RB, Singh V, Chowdhury N, Jain A, Singh SK, Das L. Role of platelet rich plasma in chronic plantar fasciitis: a prospective study. *Indian J Orthop.* 2021; 55(Suppl 1):142-148. doi:10.1007/s43465-020-00261-w

33. Mak MS, Chowdhury R, Johnson R. Morton's neuroma: review of anatomy, pathomechanism, and imaging. *Clin Radiol.* 2021; 76(3):235.e15-235.e23. doi:10.1016/j.crad.2020.10.006

34. Ruiz Santiago F, Prados Olleta N, Tomás Muñoz P, Guzmán Álvarez L, Martínez Martínez A. Short term comparison between blind and ultrasound guided injection in morton neuroma. *Eur Radiol.* 2019; 29(2):620-627. doi:10.1007/s00330-018-5670-1

35. Banerjee B, Das RK. Sonographic detection of foreign bodies of the extremities. *Br J Radiol.* 1991 Feb; 64(758):107-12. doi: 10.1259/0007-1285-64-758-107. PMID: 2004200.

36. Lam KHS, Hung C-Y, Chiang Y-P, et al. Ultrasound-guided nerve hydrodissection for pain management: rationale, methods, current literature, and theoretical mechanisms. *J Pain Res.* 2020; 13:1957-1968. doi:10.2147/JPR.S247208

References (alphabetical)

Banerjee B, Das RK. Sonographic detection of foreign bodies of the extremities. Br J Radiol. 1991 Feb;64(758):107-12. doi: 10.1259/0007-1285-64-758-107. PMID: 2004200.

Boone SL, Uzor R, Walter E, et al. Safety and efficacy of image-guided retrocalcaneal bursa corticosteroid injection for the treatment of retrocalcaneal bursitis. Skeletal Radiol. May 2021. doi:10.1007/s00256-021-03783-y

Chang A, Miller TT. Imaging of tendons. Sports Health. 2009;1(4):293-300. doi:10.1177/1941738109338361

Connolly DJ, Berman L, McNally EG. The use of beam angulation to overcome anisotropy when viewing human tendon with high frequency linear array ultrasound. Br J Radiol. 2001;74(878):183-185. doi:10.1259/bjr.74.878.740183

Daniels EW, Cole D, Jacobs B, Phillips SF. Existing Evidence on Ultrasound-Guided Injections in Sports Medicine. Orthop J Sports Med. 2018;6(2):2325967118756576. doi:10.1177/2325967118756576

Draghi F, Bortolotto C, Draghi AG, Gitto S. Intrasheath instability of the peroneal tendons: dynamic ultrasound imaging. J Ultrasound Med. 2018;37(12):2753-2758. doi:10.1002/jum.14633

Duan X, Li L, Wei D-Q, et al. Role of magnetic resonance imaging versus ultrasound for detection of plantar plate tear. J Orthop Surg Res. 2017;12(1):14. doi:10.1186/s13018-016-0507-6

Feldman MK, Katyal S, Blackwood MS. US artifacts. Radiographics. 2009;29(4):1179-1189. doi:10.1148/rg.294085199

Filardo G, Kon E, Di Matteo B, et al. Platelet-rich plasma injections for the treatment of refractory Achilles tendinopathy: results at 4 years. Blood Transfus. 2014;12(4):533-540. doi:10.2450/2014.0289-13

Frey C, Feder KS, DiGiovanni C. Arthroscopic evaluation of the subtalar joint: does sinus tarsi syndrome exist? Foot Ankle Int. 1999 Mar;20(3):185-91. doi: 10.1177/107110079902000309. PMID: 10195298.

He L, Genin J, Delzell P. Ultrasound diagnosis and percutaneous treatment of Achilles tendon tethering: a case series. Skeletal Radiol. 2016;45(9):1293-1298. doi:10.1007/s00256-016-2416-5

Henning T, Finnoff JT, Smith J. Sonographically guided posterior subtalar joint injections: anatomic study and validation of 3 approaches. PM R. 2009;1(10):925-931. doi:10.1016/j.pmrj.2009.09.006

Jacobson JA. Ankle, foot, and lower leg ultrasound. In: Fundamentals of musculoskeletal ultrasound. Elsevier; 2007:264-331. doi:10.1016/B978-1-4160-3593-0.50013-1

Jain Nm Omar I, Kelikian A, van Holsbeeck L, Grant T. Prevalence of and Factors Associated with posterior tibial tendon pathology on sonographic assessment. PMR 2011; 3(11): 998-1004.) (Neustadter J, Raikin S, Nazarian L, Dynamic sonographic evaluation of peroneal tendon subluxation. Am J Roentgenol 2004; 183 (4): 985-988.

Kalia RB, Singh V, Chowdhury N, Jain A, Singh SK, Das L. Role of platelet rich plasma in chronic plantar fasciitis: A prospective study. Indian J Orthop. 2021;55(Suppl 1):142-148. doi:10.1007/s43465-020-00261-w

Kang MH, Moon KW, Jeon YH, Cho SW. Sonography of the first metatarsophalangeal joint and sonographically guided intraarticular injection of corticosteroid in acute gout attack. J Clin Ultrasound. 2015;43(3):179-186. doi:10.1002/jcu.22206

Khosla S, Thiele R, Baumhauer JF. Ultrasound guidance for intra-articular injections of the foot and ankle. Foot Ankle Int. 2009;30(9):886-890. doi:10.3113/FAI.2009.0886

Kotnis N, Harish S, Popowich T. Medial ankle and heel: ultrasound evaluation and sonographic appearances of conditions causing symptoms. Semin Ultrasound CT MR. 2011;32(2):125-141. doi:10.1053/j.sult.2010.11.001

Lam KHS, Hung C-Y, Chiang Y-P, et al. Ultrasound-Guided Nerve Hydrodissection for Pain Management: Rationale, Methods, Current Literature, and Theoretical Mechanisms. J Pain Res. 2020;13:1957-1968. doi:10.2147/JPR.S247208

Mak MS, Chowdhury R, Johnson R. Morton's neuroma: review of anatomy, pathomechanism, and imaging. Clin Radiol. 2021;76(3):235.e15-235.e23. doi:10.1016/j.crad.2020.10.006

Malanga GA, Mautner KR, eds. Foot & Ankle. In: Atlas of Ultrasound-Guided Musculoskeletal Injections. McGraw-Hill Education; 2014:325-418.

Mautner K, Colberg RE, Malanga G, et al. Outcomes after ultrasound-guided platelet-rich plasma injections for chronic tendinopathy: a multicenter, retrospective review. PM R. 2013;5(3):169-175. doi:10.1016/j.pmrj.2012.12.010

McCarthy CL, Thompson GV. Ultrasound findings of plantar plate tears of the lesser metatarsophalangeal joints. Skeletal Radiol. 2021;50(8):1513-1525. doi:10.1007/s00256-020-03708-1

Muir JJ, Curtiss HM, Hollman J, Smith J, Finnoff JT. The accuracy of ultrasound-guided and palpation-guided peroneal tendon sheath injections. Am J Phys Med Rehabil. 2011;90(7):564-571. doi:10.1097/PHM.0b013e31821f6e63

Olewnik Ł, Wysiadecki G, Podgórski M, Polguj M, Topol M. The Plantaris Muscle Tendon and Its Relationship with the Achilles Tendinopathy. Biomed Res Int. 2018;2018:9623579. doi:10.1155/2018/9623579

Raissi G, Arbabi A, Rafiei M, et al. Ultrasound-Guided Injection of Dextrose Versus Corticosteroid in Chronic Plantar Fasciitis Management: A Randomized, Double-Blind Clinical Trial. Foot Ankle Spec. January 2021:1938640020980924. doi:10.1177/1938640020980924

Ruiz Santiago F, Prados Olleta N, Tomás Muñoz P, Guzmán Álvarez L, Martínez Martínez A. Short term comparison between blind and ultrasound guided injection in morton neuroma. Eur Radiol. 2019;29(2):620-627. doi:10.1007/s00330-018-5670-1

Spang C, Alfredson H, Docking SI, Masci L, Andersson G. The plantaris tendon: a narrative review focusing on anatomical features and clinical importance. Bone Joint J. 2016;98-B(10):1312-1319. doi:10.1302/0301-620X.98b10.37939

Speed CA. Fortnightly review: Corticosteroid injections in tendon lesions. BMJ. 2001;323(7309):382-386. doi:10.1136/bmj.323.7309.382

Taillard W, Meyer JM, Garcia J, Blanc Y. The sinus tarsi syndrome. Int Orthop. 1981;5(2):117-130. doi:10.1007/BF00267842

Taljanovic MS, Alcala JN, Gimber LH, Rieke JD, Chilvers MM, Latt LD. High-resolution US and MR imaging of peroneal tendon injuries. Radiographics. 2015;35(1):179-199. doi:10.1148/rg.351130062

Vaishya R, Agarwal AK, Azizi AT, Vijay V. Haglund's syndrome: A commonly seen mysterious condition. Cureus. 2016;8(10):e820. doi:10.7759/cureus.820

Vasudha TK, Vani PC, Sankaranarayanan G, Rajasekhar SSSN, Dinesh Kumar V. Communications between the tendons of flexor hallucis longus and flexor digitorum longus: a cadaveric study. Surg Radiol Anat. 2019 Dec;41(12):1411-1419. doi: 10.1007/s00276-019-02311-x. Epub 2019 Sep 20. PMID: 31541272.

Wisniewski SJ, Smith J, Patterson DG, Carmichael SW, Pawlina W. Ultrasound-guided versus nonguided tibiotalar joint and sinus tarsi injections: a cadaveric study. PM R. 2010;2(4):277-281. doi:10.1016/j.pmrj.2010.03.013

Yablon CM, Hammer MR, Morag Y, Brandon CJ, Fessell DP, Jacobson JA. US of the peripheral nerves of the lower extremity: A landmark approach. Radiographics. 2016;36(2):464-478. doi:10.1148/rg.2016150120

Chapter 8 Pediatrics and Spine surgery

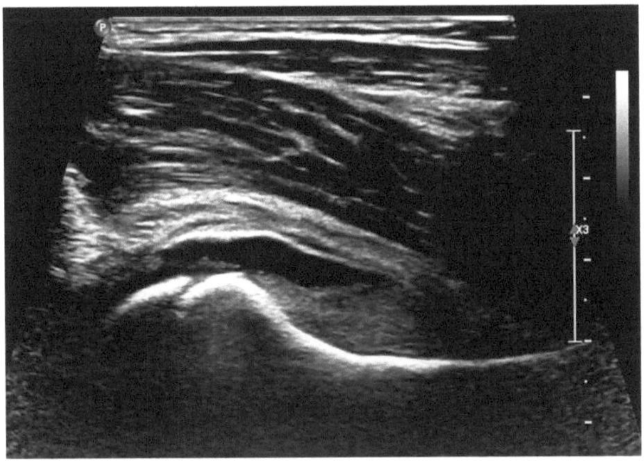

- Edward P. Southern, MD, MBA[1]
- Manaf H. Younis, MD, MPH[2]
- Alvin Camacho, MD[3]

[1]Department of Orthopaedic Surgery and Rehabilitation, The University of Texas Medical Branch at Galveston

[2]Children's Hospital of New Orleans, Louisiana State University Health Science Center

[3]Department of Radiology, The University of Texas Medical Branch at Galveston

Author Note

No grant support or other funding was received for this project.

Novel Uses of Ultrasound in Pediatric Orthopaedic Surgery

Ultrasound in Pediatric Orthopaedics

Ultrasonography is an important imaging modality that can be used by pediatric orthopaedic surgeons to acquire quick, real-time information without exposing the patient to radiation, and has advantages over other imaging modalities in terms of availability, comfort, safety, and diagnostic potential. It is a safe, noninvasive tool that can be used for diagnostic and therapeutic purposes in many orthopaedic conditions. In contrast to computed tomography (CT) and X rays, it does not emit ionizing radiation. Ultrasonography is typically readily accessible in most medical centers and, unlike many imaging tools, can be performed at the bedside through portable devices. Operating costs are low compared to both CT and magnetic resonance imaging (MRI), but the use and interpretation of ultrasonography requires adequate training and experience.

A Brief History of Ultrasound in Pediatric Orthopaedics

Ultrasonic energy was first applied to the human body for medical purposes by Dr. George Ludwig at the Naval Medical Research Institute, Bethesda, Maryland, in the late 1940s. It wasn't until the late 1970s that ultrasound in pediatric orthopaedics became widely used, when Reinhard Graf from Austria introduced the use of hip ultrasonography for the early radiological diagnosis of developmental dysplasia.[1] There have been multiple techniques for ultrasound of the hip; the earliest and most used is the Graf technique, followed by the Harcke technique, which was developed in the late 1980s.[2] Reports of the use of ultrasound in the diagnosis of hip effusions and aspiration date back to the 1980s, in studies to recognize septic hips and transient synovitis.[3,4]

In 1978, Reid first reported the use of focused ultrasound to preoperatively evaluate the spinal cord in a patient with cystic astrocytoma of the cervical cord by asking the patient to flex his neck and looking into the spinal canal with ultrasound via an "interlaminar window."[5] Spinal ultrasound was used in the early 1980s to assess the level of conus medullaris and diagnose congenital spine anomalies.[6] Subsequently, in 1982, Dohrmann and Rubin reported using ultrasound intraoperatively during spinal surgery on 10 patients with varying diagnoses including syringomyelia, spinal cord cysts, and intramedullary and extramedullary tumors.[7]

Ever since the first studies were compiled on the ultrasound imaging of fractures by Gerlanc et al. in 1975, the method has been repeatedly published in the literature.[8] The first report on the use of ultrasound in the evaluation of rib fractures was published in 1990 by Smeets et al. and was proposed as a new sonographic sign in the radiological spectrum of child abuse.[9] According to Griffith et al., X rays revealed only 12% of rib fractures, whereas ultrasound revealed 78%.[10] Wide clinical use of ultrasonography in the pediatric hand and trigger thumb has not been established, other than its use in revealing masses and fluid collections. In 2013 Verma et al. used ultrasound on a wider scale to analyze the etiology of pediatric trigger thumb.[11]

Ultrasound is very often useful in evaluation of soft-tissue masses or suspected infectious etiologies during assessment of a myriad of lesions which may be found in the body, extremities, and around the joints in children.[12] Ultrasound can assess bone infections, and can also readily identify the convex subperiosteal abscesses accompanying osteomyelitis. Its role in confirming effusions of infected or injured joints is well recognized, particularly when also used to obtain joint fluid specimens. The use of ultrasound should continue to play a prominent role in early assessment of lesions in soft tissue and joints, as it readily differentiates more benign cystic lesions from solid lesions, and it often may be diagnostic. At the same time, it can also assist in the evaluation and work-up of solid lesions and malignancies to localize and avoid sampling errors during biopsies.[12] In recent years, ultrasonography has also often been utilized in vascular mapping pre- and intraoperatively for perforator flaps, which has revolutionized modern reconstructive plastic surgery.[13]

Ultrasound for Hip Dysplasia

There are a large number of textbooks and articles documenting the proper evaluation of the hip with ultrasound, and we will briefly review its well-known utility in this setting, to focus on more esoteric uses of ultrasound in children.[14] In addition to the femoral head physis, both the cartilaginous labrum and the bony acetabulum are well visualized on ultrasound. A normal infant hip ultrasound shows a femoral head covered by the bony acetabulum and the cartilaginous component and the labrum (i.e., a "centered" hip according to Graf). To be reproducible, a consistent coronal sonographic section through the hip joint must be defined by three points: (1) The lower limb of the bony ilium in the bottom of the acetabular fossa, (2) the mid portion of the bony acetabular roof, and (3) the acetabular cartilaginous labrum. Graf described 4 major hip types based on the alpha angle, each with subtypes characterized by the beta angles. He pointed out that the alpha angle and the radiographic center edge angle, when combined, have an approximate relationship of 90 degrees. For ultrasound of the hip, the lower limb of the ilium is the center of the acetabulum, and if this landmark is not seen, the study is non-diagnostic. The landmarks of a line bisecting the bony and cartilaginous acetabulum through the center of the joint and a line tangent to the bony roof of the acetabulum defines the alpha angle, which defines the Graf types; the bisecting line through the center of the joint and a line tangent to the cartilaginous, labral acetabular wall defines the beta angle, which further refines the characterization of the hip (Figure 1). In unstable hip joints, the imaging should also document the resting position and displacement caused by manually applied joint stresses. According to Graf, a full description of a child's hip ultrasound must start with the child's age, the preliminary hip type, the given alpha angle measurement, the subtype primarily determined by the beta angle measurement, and a description of any pathological instability changes caused by a manual stressing of the joint (Figure 2).

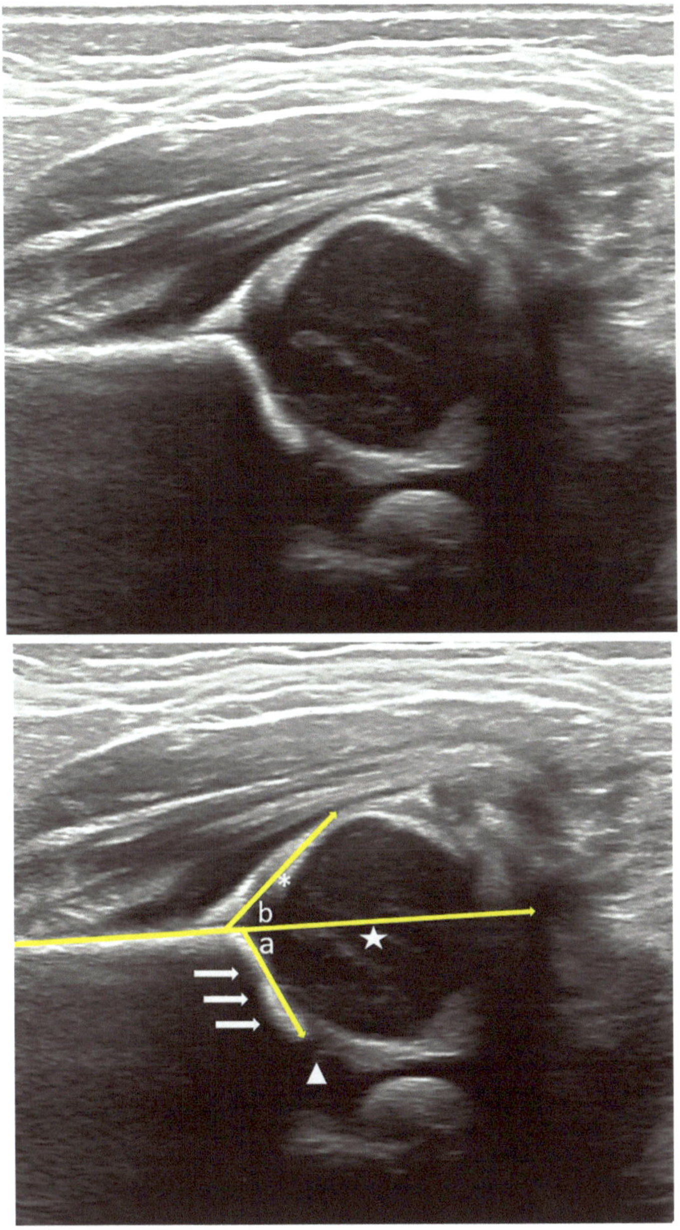

Figure 8-1. Six-week old infant, born breech. Coronal sonogram of the left hip shows a normal, mature hip with adequate coverage of the femoral head and alpha angle of 60 degrees (A). Acetabular roof (white arrows), femoral head (star), triradiate cartilage (arrowhead), labrum (*), alpha angle (a) and beta angle (b).

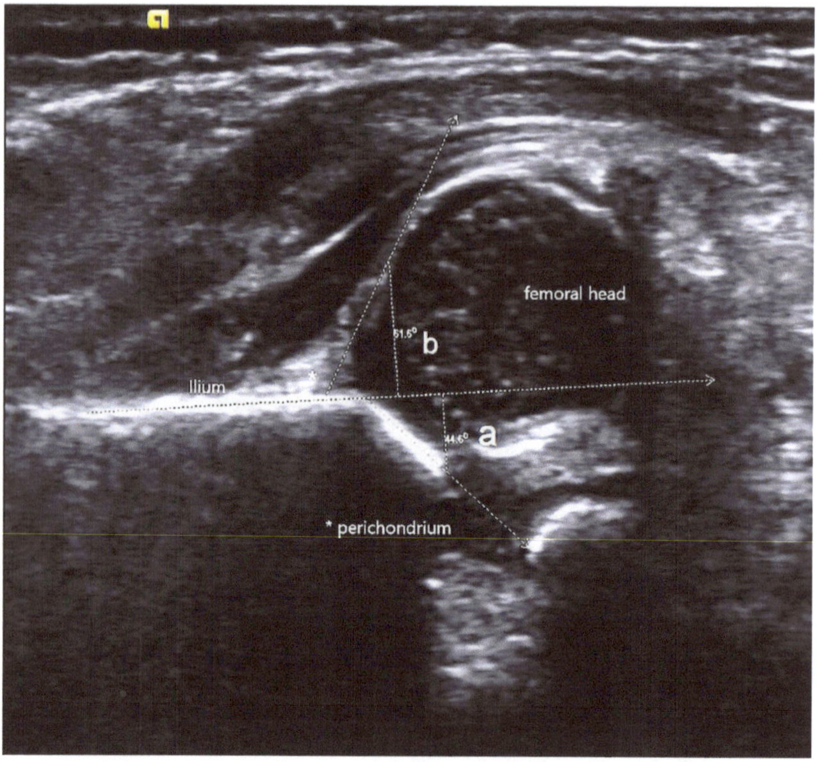

Figure 8-2. Four-week old infant with developmental dysplasia with a Type IIc hip. Coronal sonographic image demonstrates a shallow acetabulum with an alpha angle of 45 degrees. The femoral head is laterally subluxed with poor coverage. The bony acetabular roof is severely deficient with an alpha angle of 44.6 degrees (a). The superior bony rim is flattened but the cartilaginous roof still covers the femoral head with a beta angle of 61.6 degrees (b).

A synopsis of the sonographic hip types is adapted from his textbook on hip ultrasonography and presented in Table 1.[14] The prognosis and treatment of these different types are distinctly different and gestational age must also take into account; a dysplastic appearing hip in a four-month old may demand active treatment, but the same appearance might be perfectly normal in a six-week old child and require observation alone.

Table 1. Synopsis of the sonographic hip types, adapted from Graf, R. *Hip sonography: Diagnosis and management of infant hip dysplasia.* 2nd ed. New York: Springer Berlin Heidelberg; 2006.

Graf Type	Bony Roof: α angle	Perichondrium at Edge of Ilium	Cartilaginous Roof: α angle	Age
I	Well-formed bony roof	Angular or slightly rounded	Well centered with $\beta \geq 60°$	Any age
Ia	Well-formed bony roof	Angular or slightly rounded	Hip centered and cartilage roof extends farther than bony roof with $\beta \leq 55°$	Any age
Ib	Well-formed bony roof	Angular or slightly rounded	Hip is centered and cartilage roof extends farther than bony roof with $\beta > 55°$	Any age
IIa+	Adequate (based upon age) bony roof with α between 50-59°	Rounded	Hip centered and femoral head covered	0-12 weeks
IIa-	Deficient (based upon age) bony roof with α between 50-59°	Rounded	Hip centered and femoral head covered	6-12 weeks

IIb	Deficient (based upon age) with α between 50-59°	Rounded	Hip centered and femoral head covered	>12 weeks
IIc	Highly deficient with α between 43-49°	Rounded to flat	Hip centered and femoral head covered with β ≤ 77°	Any age
IId	Highly deficient with α between 43-49°	Rounded to flat	Hip "about to decenter" with β > 77°	Any age
IIIa	Poorly formed bony roof with α < 43°	Flat	Hip decentered and roof with normal echogenicity and shifted superiorly	Any age
IIIb	Poorly formed bony roof with α < 43°	Flat	Hip is decentered and roof is hyperechoic and shifted superiorly	Any age
IV	Poorly formed bony roof with α < 43°	Flat	Dislocated and roof is shifted inferiorly	Any age

Ultrasound Beyond Hip Dysplasia

Older children with or without hip dysplasia may also be assessed with ultrasound for defining hip anatomy which otherwise might require an MRI; we have diagnosed a large, symptomatic paralabral cyst in a child using ultrasound as an outpatient, facilitating the work-up (Figure 3).

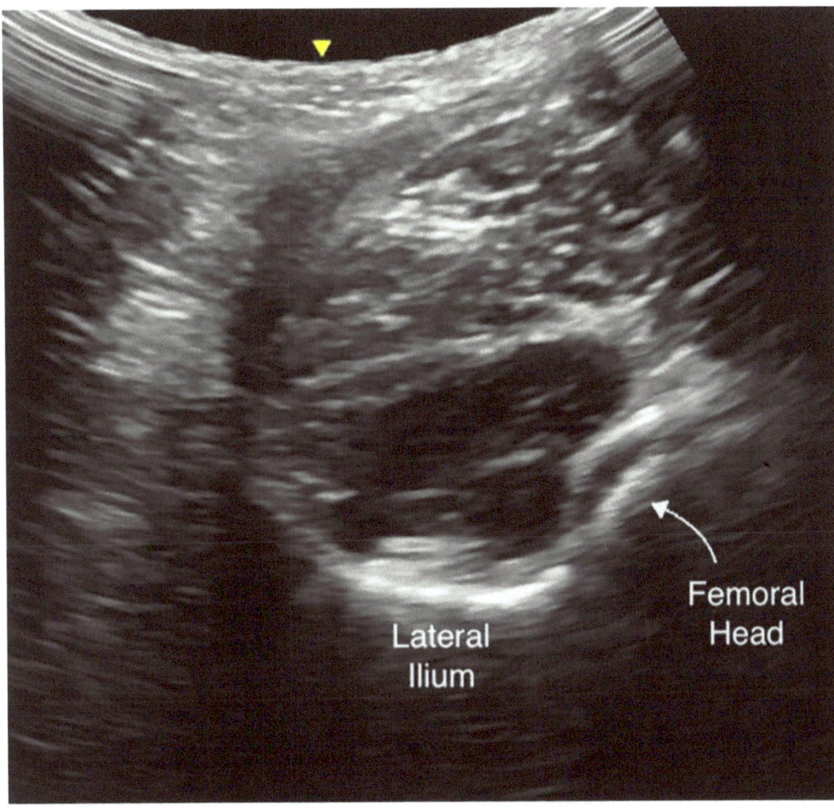

Figure 8-3. Large paralabral cyst hip in a child. *(Courtesy of Christopher Jobe, MD*

Musculoskeletal infections

The investigation of a child with a suspected musculoskeletal infection can present a diagnostic challenge, as radiographs are easily available and inexpensive, but insensitive for joint effusion and the early stages of bone infection.[15] Due to its excellent soft-tissue contrast, its ability to show bone edema early, and its high sensitivity and specificity, MRI is generally regarded as the imaging modality of choice.[16] However, it is expensive, not universally available, and often requires general anesthesia or sedation in young children. Increasing concerns about high radiation exposure has limited the use of scintigraphy and CT in recent years, and sonography offers a cheap, easily available, and radiation-free alternative.[17]

Septic arthritis

The incidence of septic arthritis in children varies in different regions, but ranges between five and 12 per 100,000 per year.[18] Septic arthritis is usually monoarticular, with the hip and knee most commonly affected.[19] It may be associated with osteomyelitis due to direct extension of infection from bone into the joint, which occurs more frequently in joints where the metaphysis is intra-articular, such as in the hip or shoulder.[18] A quick diagnosis and early treatment is important, as joint damage occurs due to bacterial endotoxins, the body's own inflammatory response, and avascular necrosis related to tamponade of nutrient vessels by large-joint effusions.[20,21]

Sonography can usually be performed as the first-line imaging investigation in a young, limping child to exclude a hip-joint effusion, or to investigate any swollen or painful joint; it is frequently used for diagnosis of hip sepsis and has been proven to be quite useful in showing intra-articular fluid and debris (Figure 4).[22] Ultrasound can detect joint effusions as small as 1-2 ml, but it cannot distinguish an infected from a non-infected effusion, regardless of the size or echogenicity of the fluid.[21] While the absence of a joint effusion excludes a diagnosis of septic arthritis, ultrasound may be negative in the first 24 hours after onset of symptoms, when a sufficient effusion has not yet accumulated; thus, it does not take the place of clinical acumen or additional laboratory studies.[23]

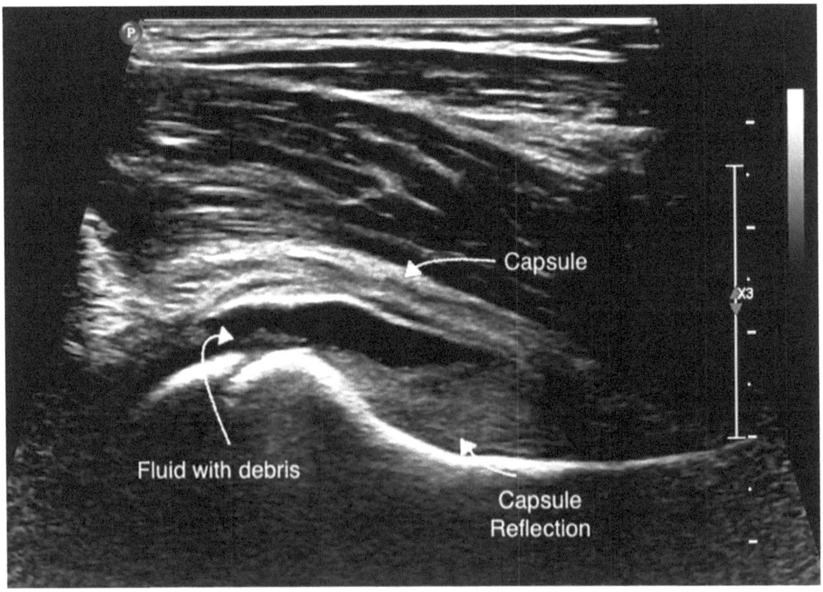

Figure 8-4a

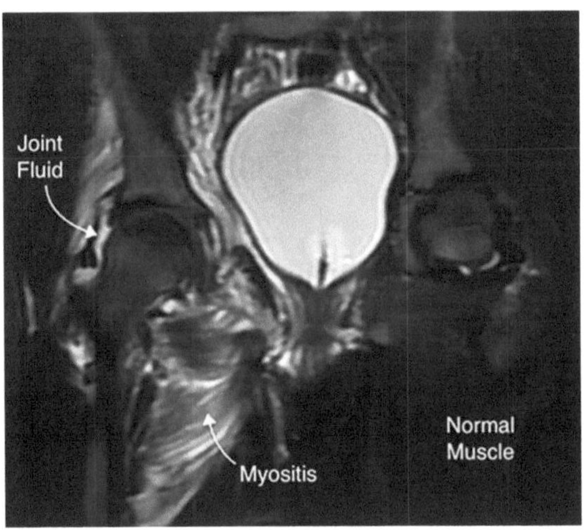

Figure 8-4b

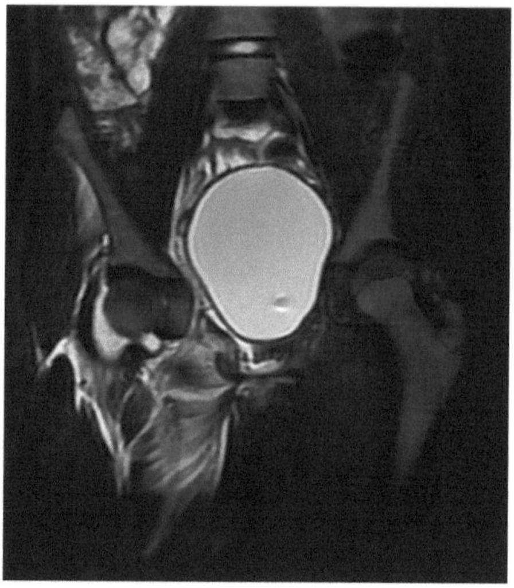

Figure 8-4c

Figure 8-4. A 4-year-old child presented with right hip pain and inability to bear weight. (a) Ultrasound images show a large right-hip effusion with debris. (b, c) Coronal T2 magnetic resonance imaging was performed without contrast, showing the right hip effusion with myositis, but no signs of underlying osteomyelitis. The child was taken to the operating room and underwent incision and drainage for an isolated septic hip joint.

Several authors have described the various clinical decision algorithms evaluating fever, raised C-reactive protein (CRP), erythrocyte sedimentation rate, white blood cell count (WBC), and non-weight-bearing status to differentiate septic arthritis from transient synovitis, a self-limiting benign process.[24,25] However, there is no single investigation or blood test to reliably distinguish the two entities. Many authors regard joint aspiration and culture of the fluid as the definitive investigation if the clinical algorithms point toward septic arthritis or the diagnosis remains unclear, and ultrasound facilitates both the identification of the effusion and its aspiration.[26]

Osteomyelitis

Infection of the bone and bone marrow may occur either from direct or hematogenous spread. The long bones most frequently affected include the femur, tibia, and humerus. Other bones affected include the pelvis and calcaneus.[27] In young children, the periosteum is not firmly attached to the cortex, leading to prominent subperiosteal collections. In older age groups, vascular supply between the epiphysis and metaphysis is separated by the avascular growth plate; it is therefore rare for hematogenous osteomyelitis to spread from the metaphysis to the epiphysis without mechanical disruption of the growth plate.[15,28]

Sonography demonstrates a range of findings as early as one to three days after the onset of symptoms, with juxtacortical deep soft-tissue swelling being the earliest finding visible on ultrasound.[29] This is followed by periosteal thickening or elevation, with a thin layer of fluid and subperiosteal abscess formation.[30] These findings are usually seen on ultrasound before any change is apparent on the radiographs, up to two weeks later.[15] Subperiosteal collections are characterized by a hypoechoic or anechoic lenticular-shaped fluid collection extending along the cortex of the bone. Anechoic collections in continuity with the bone are highly suggestive of osteomyelitis.[31] If soft tissue can be identified between the fluid collection and the bone, the collection is likely of non-osseous origin. Cortical erosions and perforations may be demonstrated, but are not usually apparent until seven to 10 days after onset of symptoms.[31] Reactive or infectious joint effusions may also be identified, and sonography can again be used to guide aspirations.[30] Figure 5 is an example case of primary osteomyelitis of the clavicle diagnosed in a 22-month-old child on her third clinical evaluation after four days of symptoms. The diagnosis was confirmed through clinical, laboratory, and imaging studies, including ultrasound.

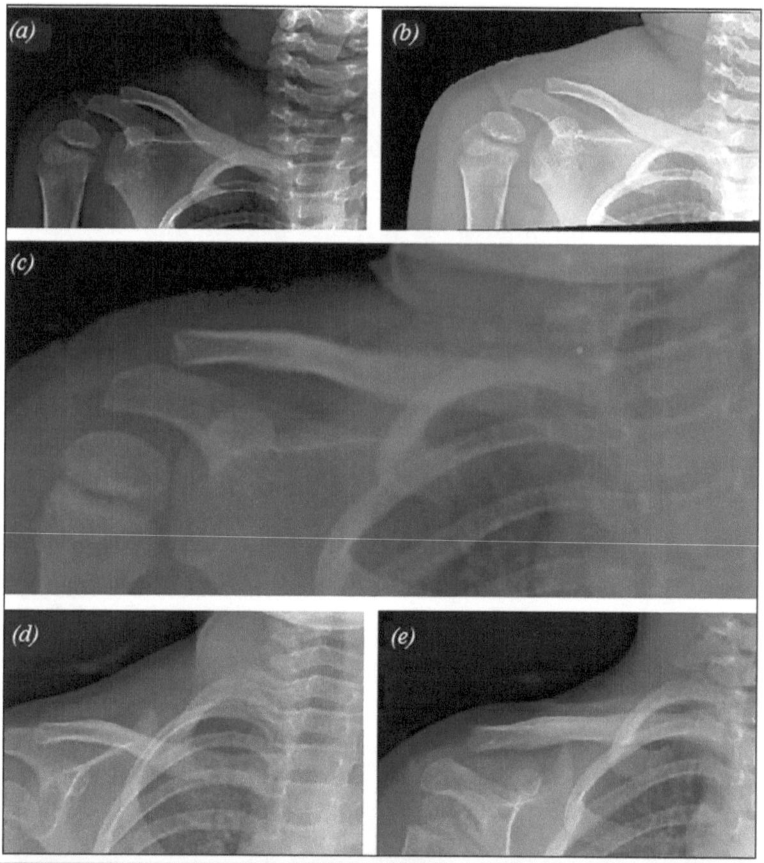
(a)
(b)
(c)
(d)
(e)

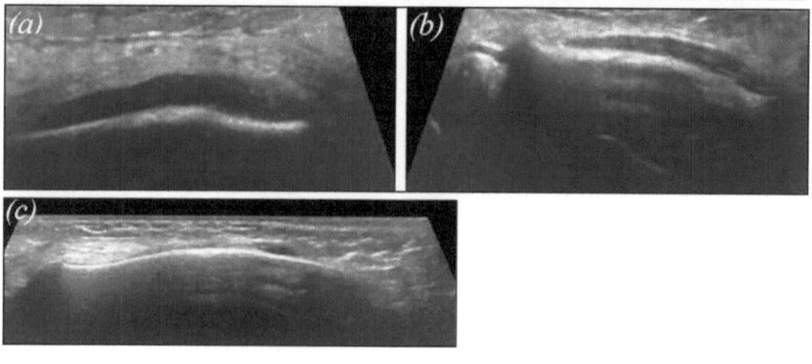
(a)
(b)
(c)

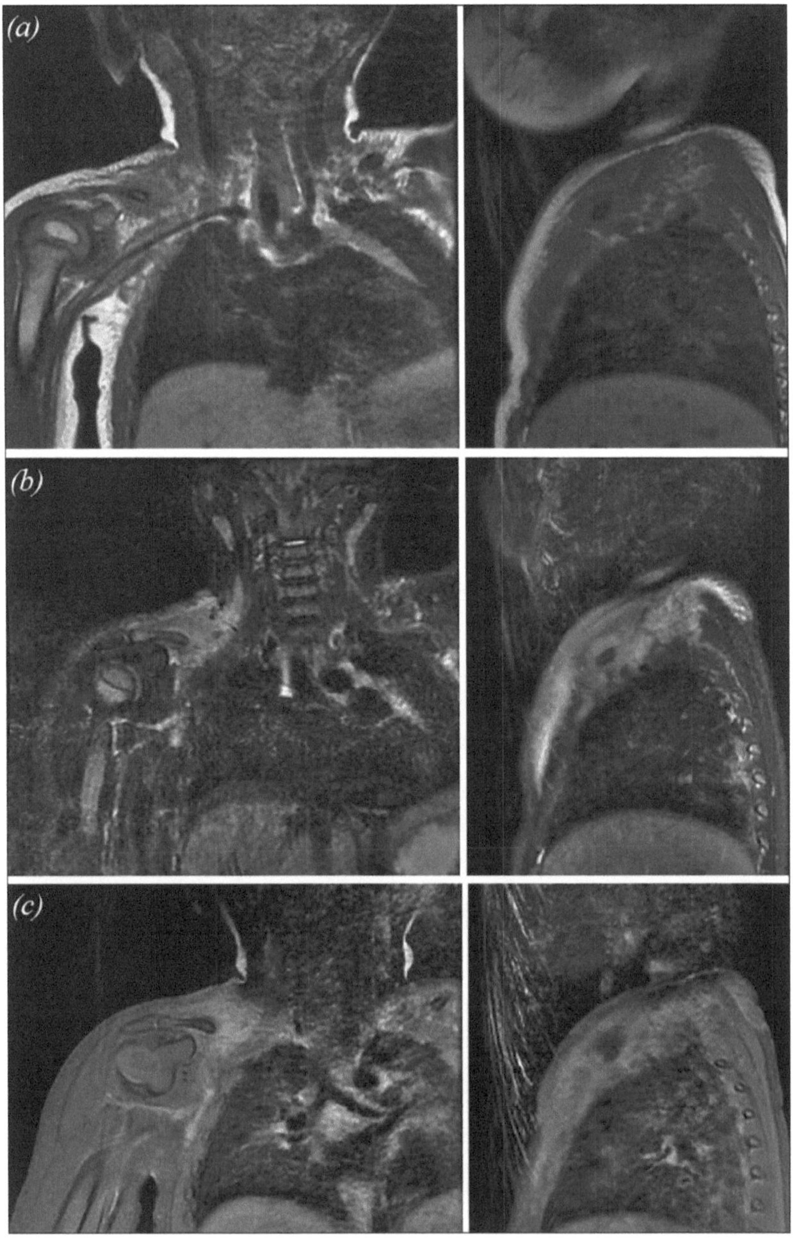

Figure 8-5. A 22-month-old child presented to the pediatric tertiary care emergency department after two outside hospital visits for similar complaints of fever, acute-onset pain, and swelling of her right shoulder and arm. (a) Plain anteroposterior radiographs of the right shoulder on presentation with enhanced bony contrast (top

left) and soft-tissue contrast (top right) show minimal resorption and mild sclerosis of the medial two-thirds of the clavicle. (b) Diagnostic ultrasound revealed a very large subperiosteal abscess as the result of a delay in diagnosis. The right upper chest and shoulder showed soft-tissue swelling near the medial metaphysis of the clavicle (top left). Ultrasound of the left clavicle was normal (bottom). (c) Magnetic resonance imaging: anteroposterior and lateral T1-weighted coronal and sagittal images (top), T2-weighted coronal and sagittal (center), and T1-weighted postcontrast coronal and sagittal (bottom) magnetic resonance imaging show periosteal thickening of the right clavicle subperiosteal fluid with soft-tissue edema and peripheral enhancement, respectively in the negative of inflammatory changes highly suspicious for infection. The patient was treated initially with intravenous antibiotics and underwent therapeutic and diagnostic needle-guided tissue aspiration under ultrasound guidance, which ruled out malignancy, but was not curative. Subperiosteal abscess recurred within 24 hours (b, top right), prompting formal operative irrigation and debridement with excellent localization directed by intraoperative ultrasound, minimizing surgical soft-tissue trauma. Anteroposterior radiographs of the right shoulder at 5 weeks (a, center) and at 5 months, showing resolution of the bony lysis and mild sclerosis is present at 5 months (a, bottom left). The patient was seen for her 12-month postoperative follow-up without complications or evidence of infection recurrence on anteroposterior radiographs (a, bottom right) and resolution of all signs of infection.

Color or power Doppler can demonstrate increased vascularity in the periosteum and surrounding tissues or synovitis in the adjacent joint consistent with an inflammatory response.[31,32] Chao et al. reported that the increased flow on Doppler around the periosteum corresponds to advanced aggressive disease in patients with higher CRP levels, and Ezzat et al. have shown that increased flow on Doppler around the periosteum early in the disease process is likely to progress into a subperiosteal collection, which can be demonstrated on follow-up sonography.[32,33] Therefore, Doppler imaging may identify the patients who require more aggressive management or surgical intervention.

Ultrasound is most sensitive in suspected acute osteomyelitis of the long bones, where there is the greatest tendency to develop periosteal reactions or subperiosteal collections.[30] However, it cannot assess the bone marrow, and therefore may underestimate the degree of bone involvement, and can also miss purulent fluid collections within the bone.[30] Assessment of the pelvis, especially in older children with suspected osteomyelitis, is also often difficult with ultrasound.[34] In these patients, early MRI may be required because the presentations can be non-specific, the pelvic bony anatomy is complex, and the findings of soft-tissue edema and deep pelvic fluid collections can be subtle on ultrasound.[29]

In children with sickle cell disease, acute pain may be due to a vaso-occlusive crisis related to bone infarction or osteomyelitis, and clinical differentiation can be difficult, especially if blood cultures are negative.[35] Ultrasound can help differentiate osteomyelitis from a vaso-occlusive crisis if there are large subperiosteal collections (> 4 mm in depth) detected, especially when seen in conjunction with high CRP and WBC values.[35,36] William et al. suggest that patients with pain and subperiosteal collections of > 4 mm require aspiration of the fluid to diagnose osteomyelitis.[36]

Deep vein thrombosis (DVT) is also a recognized serious complication of osteomyelitis. The localized endothelial damage mediated by surrounding inflammation and release of cytokines that activate the coagulation cascade, are thought to play a role, compounded by the local tissue edema compromising the venous return. Clinically, these patients will complain of rapid onset of intense pain, a greater severity of clinical symptoms, loss of function in the affected extremity, and extensive soft-tissue edema.[37] Ultrasound is an ideal study for assessing the extent of osseous involvement and abscess formation, while at the same time assessing for the presence of DVT.

Pyomyositis

Pyomyositis is an infection of striated skeletal muscle. Although pyomyositis may affect any muscle, there is a predilection for the larger muscles of the pelvis and lower extremity, often with osteomyelitis and septic arthritis concomitantly present in up to two-thirds of cases.[38] Psoas abscesses are a frequent site of pyomyositis, although multiple areas may be affected.[39]

In the early phlegmonous stage of pyomyositis, sonography may identify an increase in muscle volume and edema, with disruption of the hyperechoic muscle fibers with hypoechoic septa and generalized hyperemia.[39] In the later, suppurative stage, a more discrete, complex fluid collection or abscess can be seen, surrounded by a thick hyperechoic and hyperemic wall on color Doppler imaging.[40,41] Gas within the abscess is characteristic of infection and manifests as tiny hyperechoic foci with reverberation artifacts known as "dirty shadowing."[42] Dynamic compression aids in the visualization of an echogenic, liquefied component within the abscess, which can be aspirated with ultrasound guidance.[43] An enlarged proximal psoas muscle and a focal walled-off collection is best evaluated posterior to the kidneys, from the flank or the lower abdomen, where aspiration is also a distinct and safe possibility.[40] Sonography may still underestimate the extent of muscle inflammation in the early stages, where subtle disruption of muscle fibers and changes in echogenicity are the only signs; therefore, concerns for pyomyositis in the deep pelvic muscles, with possible coexistent osteomyelitis and spondylodiscitis, are better evaluated with MRI.[34,39]

Cellulitis and soft-tissue abscess

Cellulitis remains a clinical diagnosis, but ultrasound findings will progress over time, and these correlate well with the clinical findings and the serum CRP levels.[44] In the early stages, thickening and increased echogenicity of the skin and subcutaneous tissues are seen, and as early as 1 to 2 days after the onset of symptoms, an advanced stage with distortion of the tissues and layering of fluid between hyperechoic fatty lobules can be observed as a "cobblestone" appearance (Figure 6).[44]

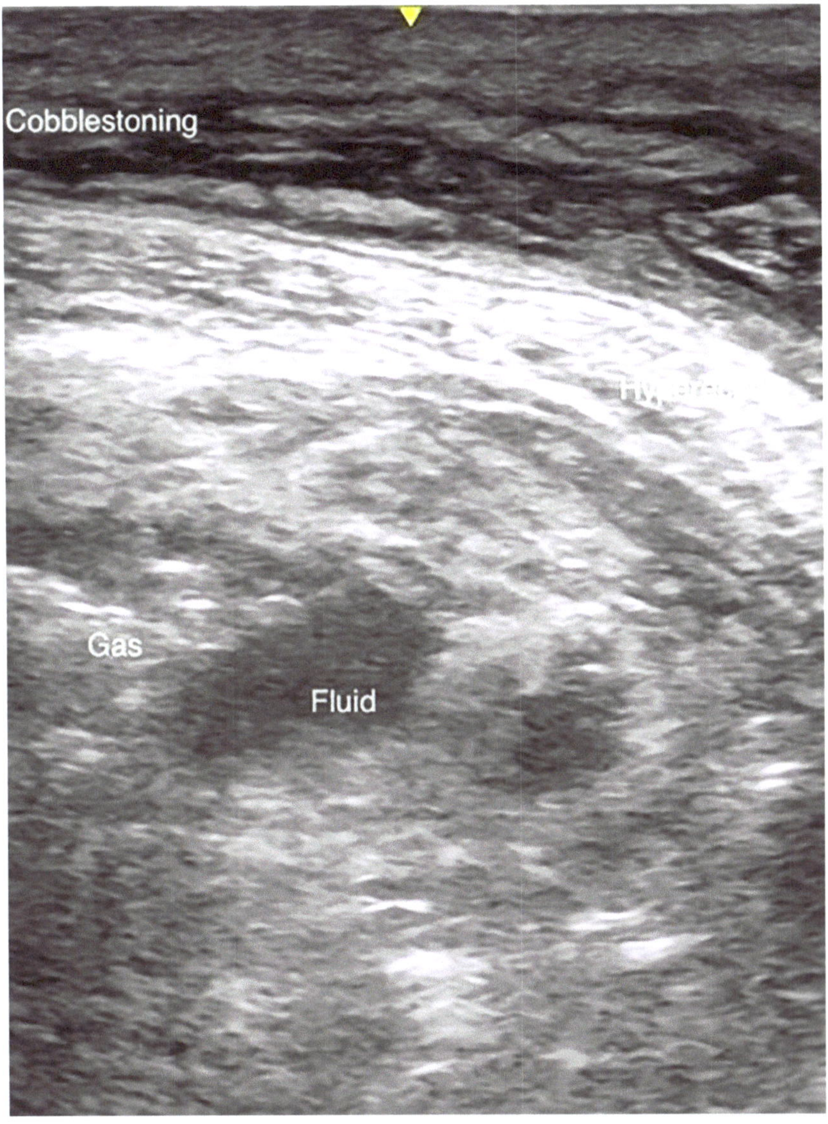

Figure 8-6. Thigh swelling and interstitial gas formation in cellulitis of the thigh. The cobblestone appearance of the superficial fat is created by edema between fat globules The deep fluid is better seen on a dynamic view as the fluid moves. *(Courtesy of Christopher Jobe, MD)*

These findings are nonspecific, and similar appearances may be seen with non-infected subcutaneous edema.[30] Localized abscess formation can be readily identified with sonography and indicates the late stage.[44] Abscesses can demonstrate a hypo- or hyperechoic center. An abscess with a hyperechoic center may be mistaken for a solid lesion, but dynamic assessment will show movement of material within it to aid in its diagnosis, and this will help to assess the need for aspiration. Increased flow on power Doppler within the wall of an abscess, but not in the center, also supports the diagnosis.[41]

Necrotizing fasciitis, a severe soft-tissue infection, may be difficult to diagnose in its early stages, when similar findings to cellulitis are seen; in advanced stages, ultrasound will demonstrate thickening of the fascia with surrounding layered fluid collections and perhaps gas formation.[45] If necrotizing fasciitis is suspected clinically, advanced cross-sectional imaging may be needed to guide acute intervention.

Infective tenosynovitis

Ultrasound findings of infective tenosynovitis include thickening of the tendon and tendon sheath. Color Doppler can demonstrate increased vascularity of the tendon sheath and, less commonly, within the tendon itself. Care should be taken in applying transducer pressure during color Doppler studies, as excessive pressure may eliminate the visualization of neovascularity, a supporting feature seen in infectious tenosynovitis.[46] The use of color Doppler can therefore help distinguish tendon sheath thickening from a synovial sheath effusion, which may benefit from or require drainage while under ultrasound guidance. More pronounced tendon sheath fluid collections are a feature of severe suppurative tenosynovitis, while thickening, edema, and hyperemia of the adjacent subcutaneous tissues indicate peritendinous spread of the infection.[30]

Fracture Diagnosis and Care

Since Roentgen's late-19th century discovery of his eponymous, invisible rays, fracture care has revolved around the use of radiographs, but modern ultrasound has changed everything. Traditionally, fracture diagnosis and confirmation of reduction was performed with the use of radiographic imaging; to further enhance reduction accuracy, some practitioners use fluoroscopy during the reduction maneuvers and splint or cast applications. Recent studies have found that sonographic imaging is also an effective diagnostic test that can be used to identify fractures without exposing the patient to radiation.[47,48] Upper extremity ultrasound for fractures in children has been reviewed extensively, and a review of 32 studies found it was significantly more sensitive to elbow fractures (P < 0.01); overall sensitivity was 95%, but went down to 80% in some studies.[49] Because it is operator-dependent, and intraosseous pathology, like tumors, may be missed if radiographs are not obtained, it may be very useful as a screening tool for fractures, but cannot substitute for radiologic evaluation when fractures are identified.

Distal forearm fractures

This is the most common indication for fracture ultrasound. The data supporting this is very good, with a meta-analysis recently confirming the safety of the method.[50] A study by Chen et al. evaluated 48 patients between the ages of 2 and 21 years in the pediatric emergency department with forearm fractures.[51] For each patient, four views were obtained using ultrasonography and radiographs, and ultrasonography had a 97% sensitivity and 100% specificity in detecting pediatric forearm fractures. Ultrasonography was able to correctly identify the fracture location for 46 of the 48 patients; in the remaining two patients, ultrasonography correctly identified fractures of the metaphysis of the radius, but failed to diagnose the associated ulnar styloid fractures. Ultrasonography can, therefore, be used as a rapid screening tool to quickly identify patients with fractures that may warrant further radiographic imaging. Patients with negative ultrasonography examinations may be reassured that a fracture is quite unlikely and spared the radiation associated with radiographs.

In addition to the diagnosis, ultrasonography can be used as a tool to assist in fracture reduction. Fluoroscopy is often used to aid in accurately reducing and immobilizing forearm fractures. The use of fluoroscopy increases the chance that the initial reduction attempt is adequate, thereby limiting the possibility of repeated reduction attempts and subsequent number of trips to the radiology suite.[52] However, using fluoroscopy during reduction has disadvantages as well, and stand-alone emergency departments and smaller facilities may not have access to a C-arm. Fluoroscopy also exposes both the patient and the practitioner to additional radiation; therefore, using ultrasonography to assist with reductions can be a useful alternative to fluoroscopy.[53]

For a forearm fracture, the patient is positioned supine with the fingers suspended using finger traps, and ultrasonography is used to obtain a baseline understanding of the fracture pattern in two planes, with cross-sectional and longitudinal anatomy views similar to those obtainable with CT scanning.[54] Ultrasonography can then be used in a dynamic fashion to visualize the reduction obtained during the reduction maneuver, but a disadvantage of using ultrasonography for fracture reduction is that it cannot be used during splint or cast application. However, it has been found that ultrasonography obtained after reduction, but before cast application, corresponds well to the post-casting radiographs. Patel et al. have reported a 92.3% agreement between the ultrasonography and the post-reduction radiographs for confirming the adequacy of their reductions.[47,54]

Screening of elbow injuries

The diagnostic value of ultrasound evaluation of pediatric elbow injuries is currently limited to primary evaluation for purely qualitative evidence of a fracture being present, as part of screening, or to otherwise rule out a fracture, such as presents in children with a nursemaid's elbow or a low-energy fall and elbow pain.

Studies have provided evidence on the role of the dorsal fat pad sign as tantamount to an articular effusion in the olecranon fossa. In 90% of patients with a fat pad sign, a fracture is present.[55] In a similar vein, in 98.2% of cases where there is no fat pad sign, there is no fracture (negative predictive value).[56-58] As early as 1998, De Maesener demonstrated that the sensitivity of ultrasound for detection of the fat pad sign is greater than that of X rays, and this was surpassed only by MRI.[59] Using ultrasound on a dorsomedian longitudinal section along the elbow joint, an elbow fracture can quickly be confirmed or ruled out, and a positive sonographic fat pad sign represents a further indication for X-ray examination.

Proximal humerus fractures

Separation of the proximal humeral epiphysis (SPHE) is a well-known occurrence and may occur secondary to trauma, infection, and non-accidental trauma. Since most newborns do not have the proximal humeral epiphysis ossified at birth, the diagnosis may be difficult to make on routine radiographs. Widening of the glenohumeral distance may be a clue on plain film, but it is not always accurate.[60] Ultrasonography of the shoulder in the newborn is a rapid, noninvasive, and non-ionizing imaging technique which can diagnose SPHE. Additionally, it can be performed at the bedside. To the best of our knowledge, there have been few reports in the literature demonstrating SPHE in the newborn period with sonography.[61-64]

Clavicular fractures

Clavicle fractures are also successfully diagnosed with ultrasonography. A study by Cross et al. evaluated 100 pediatric patients in the emergency department presenting with pain around the shoulder or clavicle pain, who would be obtaining a radiograph as part of his or her clinical workup.[48] They observed a 95% sensitivity and 96% specificity for diagnosing clavicle fractures in pediatric patients with ultrasonography. Ultrasonography was unable to identify fractures in two patients, and both had non-displaced fractures of the clavicle visible on the radiograph. The proximity to the head and neck area, however, may result in the examination being more difficult to carry out in small and lively children. Additionally, the highly curved shape of the bone may pose a certain challenge, which may result in the investigation being time-consuming.

Screening examination in cases of suspected long bone fracture

In cases of young children, pinpointing pain can be difficult due to poor cooperation. This can be important, for example, in cases of "toddler's fracture" or a potential case of child abuse,[65,66] often resulting in the entire extremity being X rayed in order to rule out any fractures. When using ultrasound, on the other hand, fractures of the long bones can be identified in children and adolescents in almost 100% of cases.[67] Compared to X ray, ultrasound sensitivity in these cases is 73% to 95.3%, and the specificity is 85.5% to 92%.[68] In these cases, ultrasound can be used at least to establish the location of the fracture, so that X-ray diagnosis does not need to be carried out at all, or only a few additional X-ray images are required to obtain a definitive diagnosis. The decisive factor here is not the exact classification or stability assessment of the fracture, but rather only the identification of evidence of a bone anomaly; this is a form of diagnosis of exclusion. The increased time requirement can be justified by the significantly reduced exposure to radiation, especially in the proximal limbs. Ultrasound also has an advantage over X rays in the neonatal age groups, when the epiphyses of the long bones may still be radiolucent, yet separated from the metaphyses, which are easily seen on ultrasound.

In the newborn, especially a premature infant, ossification centers may not be readily visible, and in such cases, ultrasound can be extremely useful.[69] We used ultrasound for diagnosis and treatment in a newborn premature child with what initially appeared to be a congenital knee dislocation (Figure 7a-c). Using bedside ultrasound requiring no sedation, this was ultimately diagnosed as a Salter I distal femoral physeal birth fracture. The fracture was then reduced under ultrasound guidance and sedation, then followed to healing with subsequent radiographs (Figure 7d-i). Even much older children can be diagnosed with ease using ultrasound, although it may be more of a screening tool in children with trauma and pain about a major joint, such as the knee (Figure 8). Most practitioners of the art will want to also obtain full-length X rays of the extremity, including one joint above and one joint below the injury, as is customary.

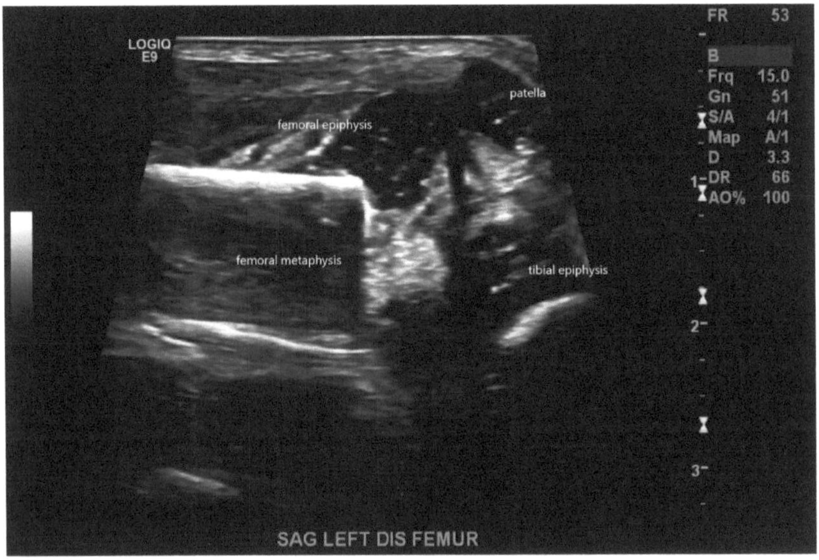

Figure 8-7a

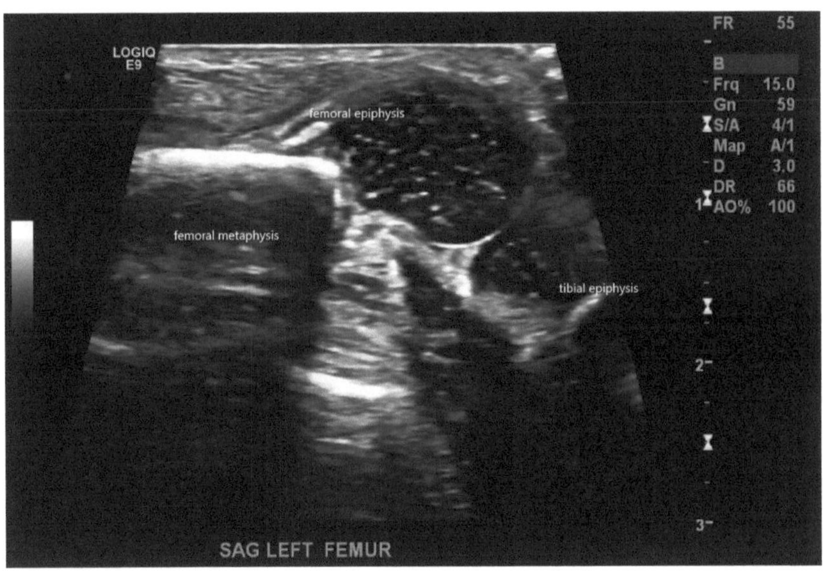

Figure 8-7b

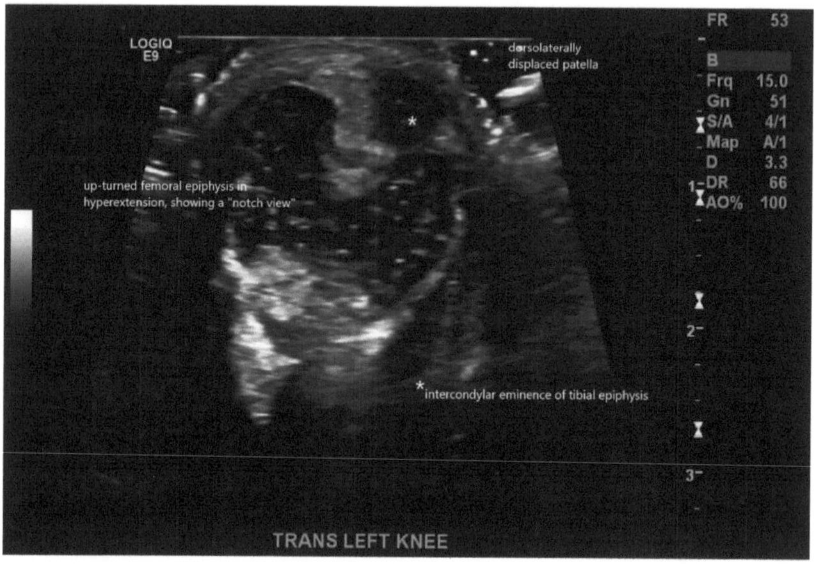

Figure 8-7c

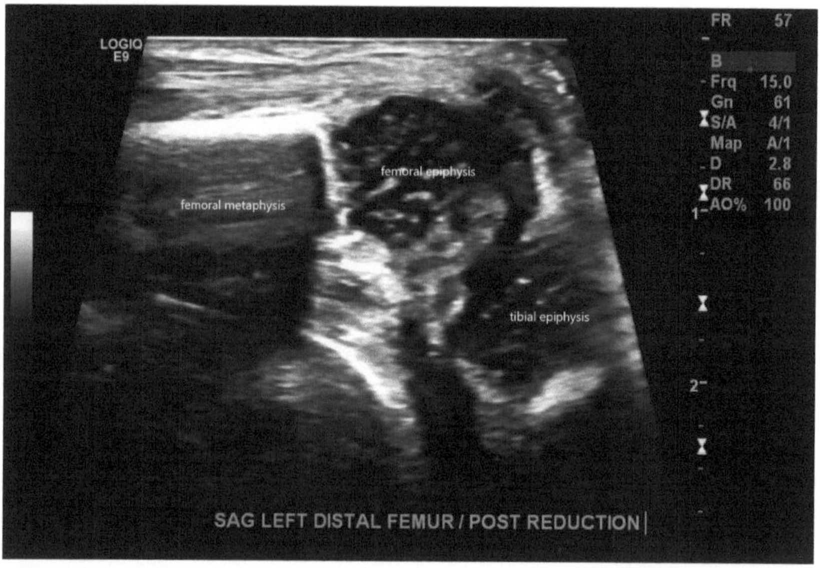

Figure 8-7d

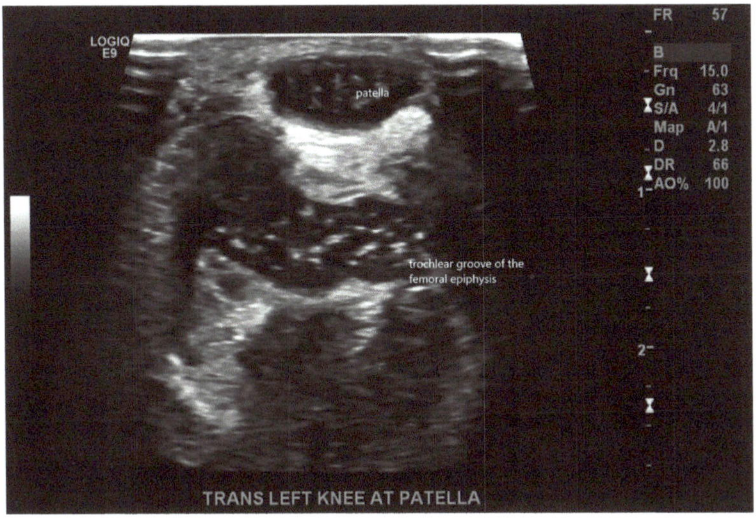

Figure 8-7e

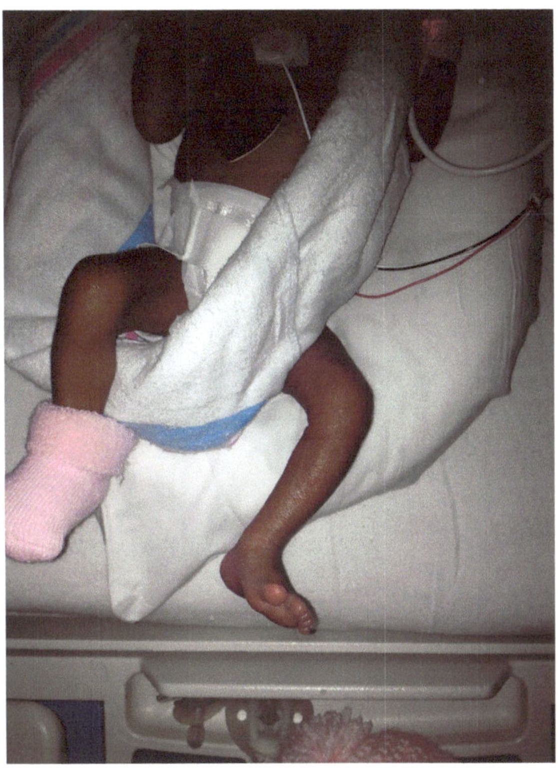

Figure 8-7f

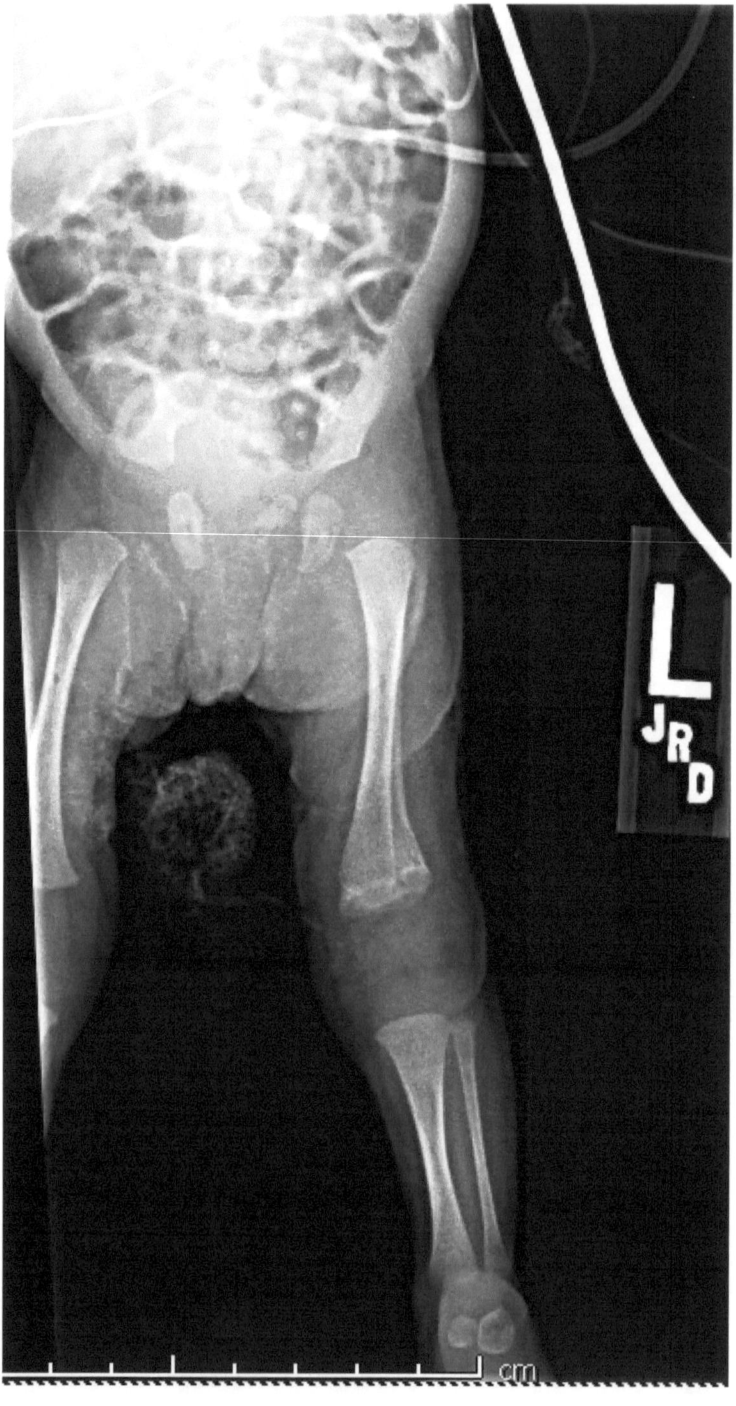

Figure 8-7g

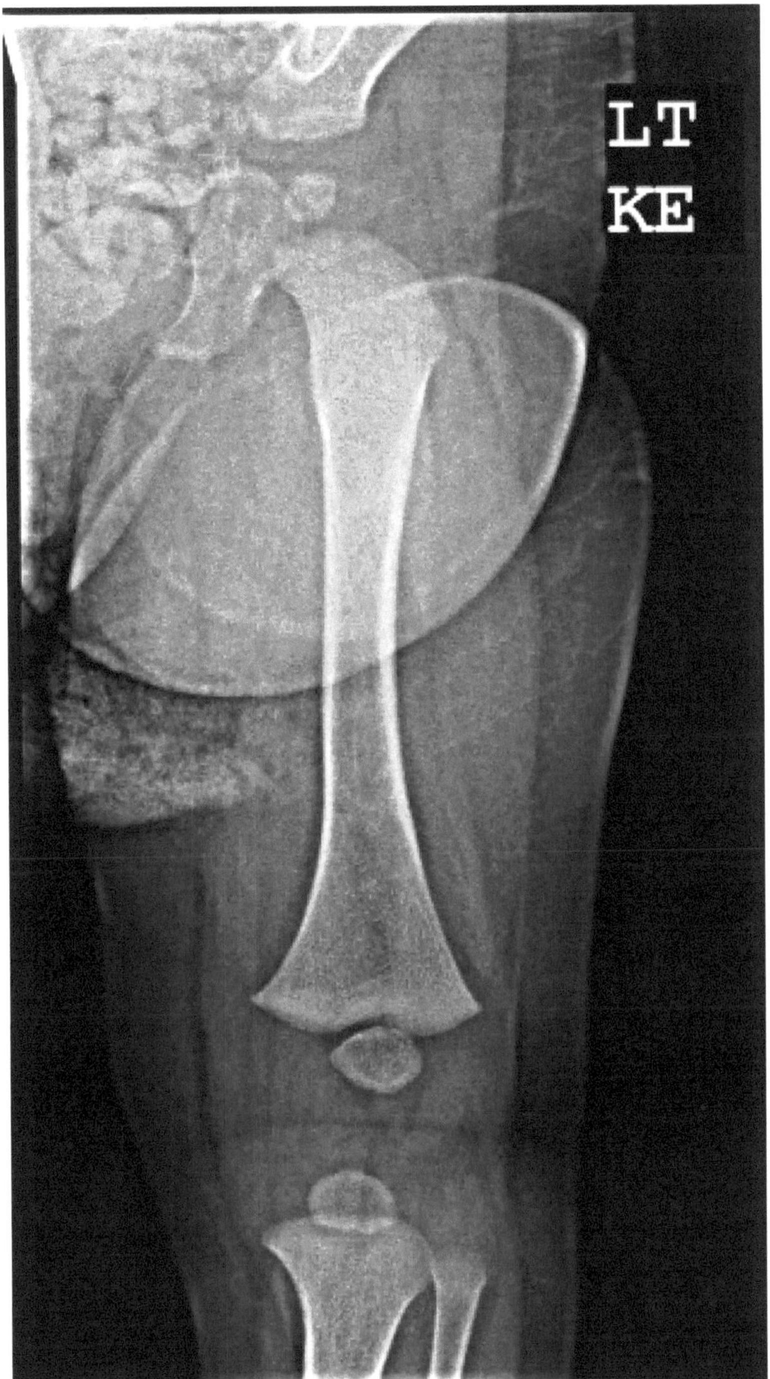

Figure 8-7h

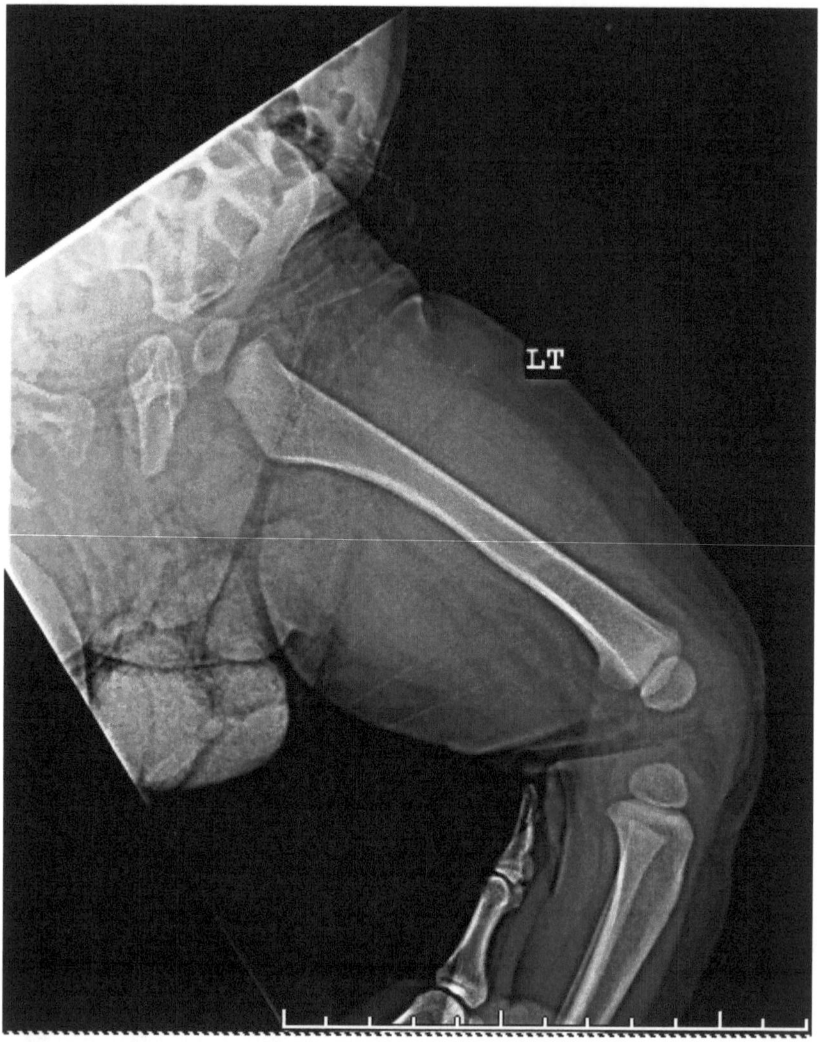

Figure 8-7i

Figure 8-7. A newborn, premature infant was seen in the neonatal intensive care unit after emergency delivery with a left knee deformity initially thought to be a congenital knee dislocation. She had a hyperextended knee deformity in left lower extremity which was evaluated at the bedside with ultrasound. (a) Sagittal and (b) parasagittal left femur ultrasounds show a dorsolaterally located patellar epiphysis above a dorsally displaced and femoral epiphysis rotated in the sagittal plan, with the tibial epiphysis still in continuity.

The stippling seen within the epiphyses are hyperechoic cellular regions within the low ultrasound signal cartilage matrix, typical of an immature physis on ultrasound imaging. (c) Transverse ultrasound view across the distal left femur at the physis showing the patella lying over an axial view of the femoral notch of the displaced, flipped-up distal femoral physis. Closed reduction in the neonatal intensive care unit was performed with sedation using ultrasound guidance, showing restoration of the anatomy. (d) Sagittal ultrasound view of the left femur shows an anatomically repositioned epiphysis with the tibial epiphysis in continuity. (e) Transverse view of the left femur across the physis showing the patella overlying the patellar groove in the physis, now with a large effusion-hemarthrosis. (f) Clinical appearance of the child at 3-week follow-up. (g) Follow-up radiograph at three weeks, showing the initial brisk subperiosteal new bone formation. This was followed by a rapid return to a normal bony appearance with normal physeal ossification and growth on long-term follow-up (h, i).

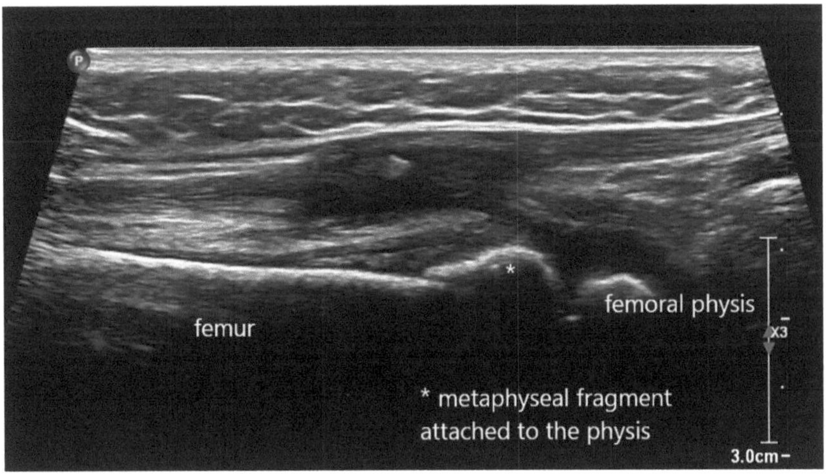

Figure 8-8a

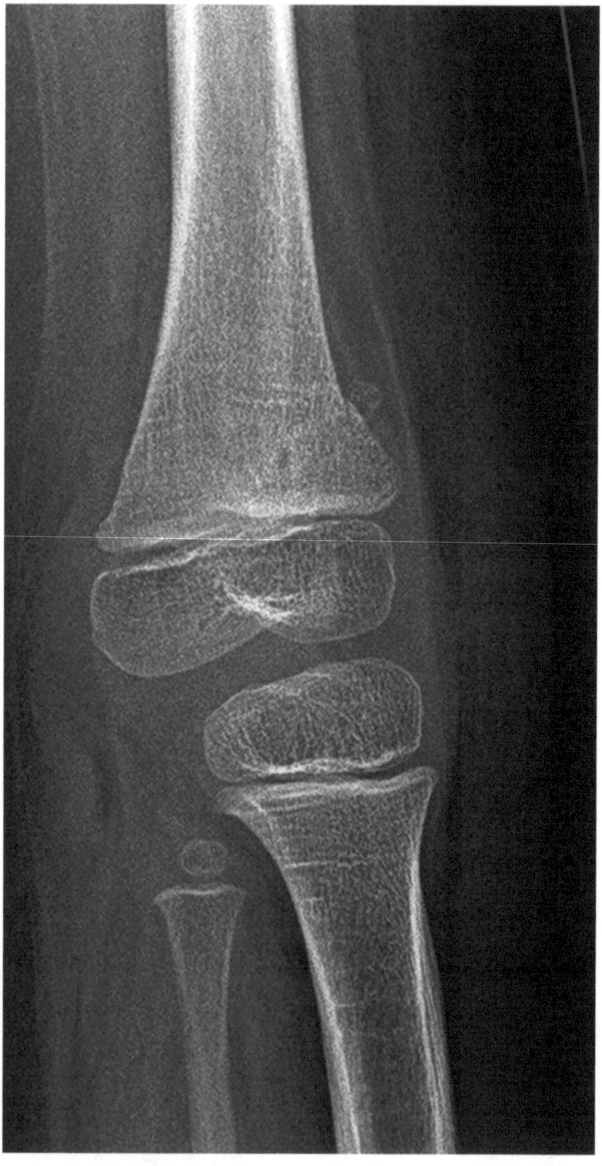

Figure 8-8b

Figure 8-8. (a) An otherwise-healthy 5-year-old presented with post-traumatic right knee pain. Ultrasound images show the cortical discontinuity and the large effusion, representing the fracture and fracture hematoma. (b) X-ray images show a non-displaced Salter-Harris type II distal femoral fracture.

Dislocations of joints other than the hip

Dislocation of joints other than the hip in children is rare, but does occur, especially around the elbow. Ultrasound can differentiate the anatomy of a thickened or torn annular ligament in the nursemaid's elbow, and can readily identify otherwise almost-invisible fractures, such as a transphyseal separation of the distal humerus in a neonate, from true elbow dislocations. The characteristic typical partially calcific fragmentation of the epiphysis in Osgood Schlatter's disease can be demonstrated well on ultrasound. Congenital knee dislocation is an uncommon problem, and often can be diagnosed on clinical exam alone, but ultrasound is useful as an adjunct to X rays in evaluating the abnormal position of the often-unossified and minute patella, its muscle insertions, and the status of the ligamentous structures, bursa, and dynamic aspects of patellar stability.[54] Litrenta et al. have also recommended ultrasound to monitor treatment at the bedside, especially for recalcitrant dislocations.[54] As previously mentioned, we also used ultrasound to differentiate a fracture deformity from a congenital knee dislocation and to treat it at the bedside in a premature infant in the neonatal intensive care unit.

Other uses of ultrasound in pediatric joint evaluation should include shoulder soft-tissue anatomy and evaluation for instability in young patients, which can be readily assessed with ultrasound (Figure 9). Congenital malformations also can be assessed with ultrasound in the shoulder; Figure 10 shows a case of trapezial agenesis treated with scapulothoracic fusion. Three weeks post-operatively she was thought to have an elevated diaphragm on x-ray. On ultrasound this proved to be a loculated pulmonary effusion which was also assessed easily and followed with ultrasound. We also have a case of middle trapezius atrophy whose pain was coming from a dislocating biceps tendon. The segmental trapezius wasting was noted on ultrasound, perhaps a result of a mild brachial plexus palsy (trapezius is eleventh nerve) (Figure 11). The hip can also be assessed with ultrasound for issues other than dysplasia, and we have used it in the diagnosis and evaluation of an acute slipped capital femoral epiphysis (Figure 12).

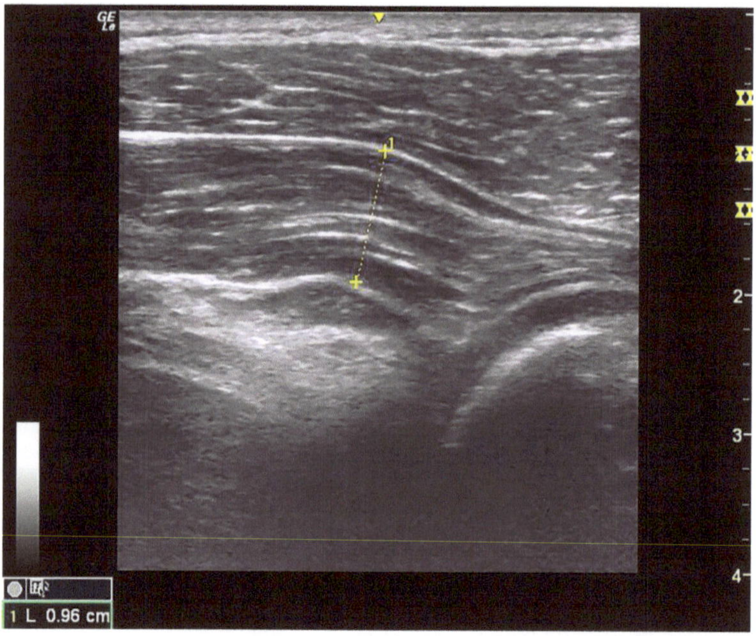

Figure 8-9a

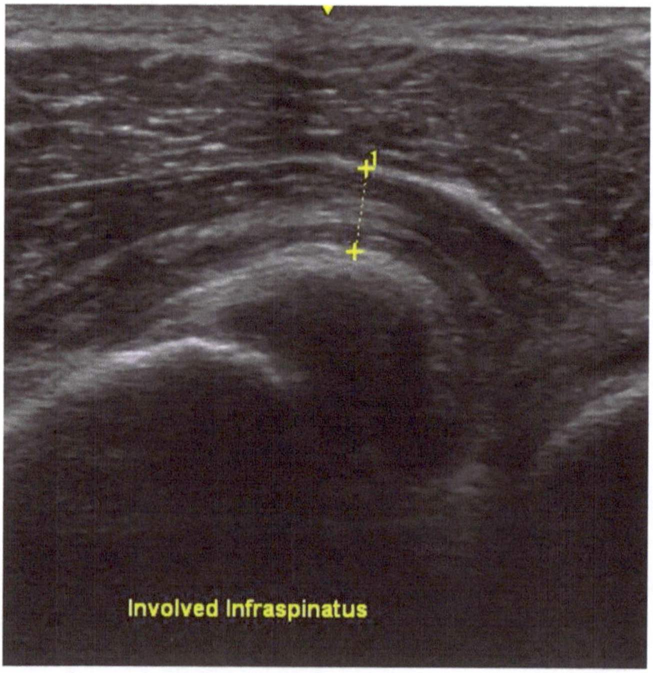

Figure 8-9b

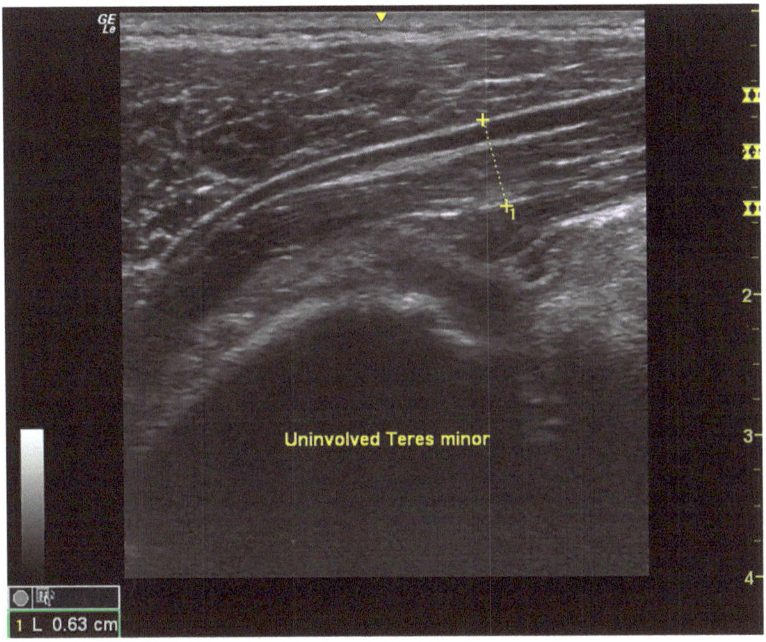

Figure 8-9c

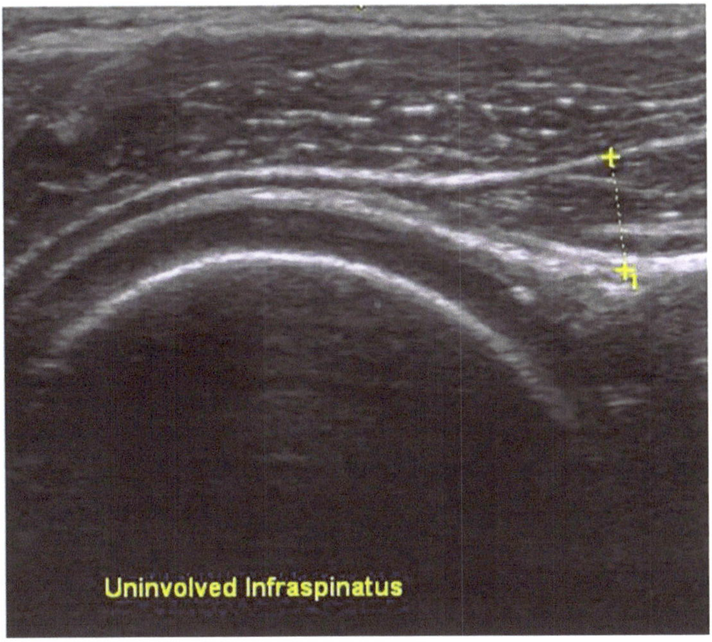

Figure 8-9d

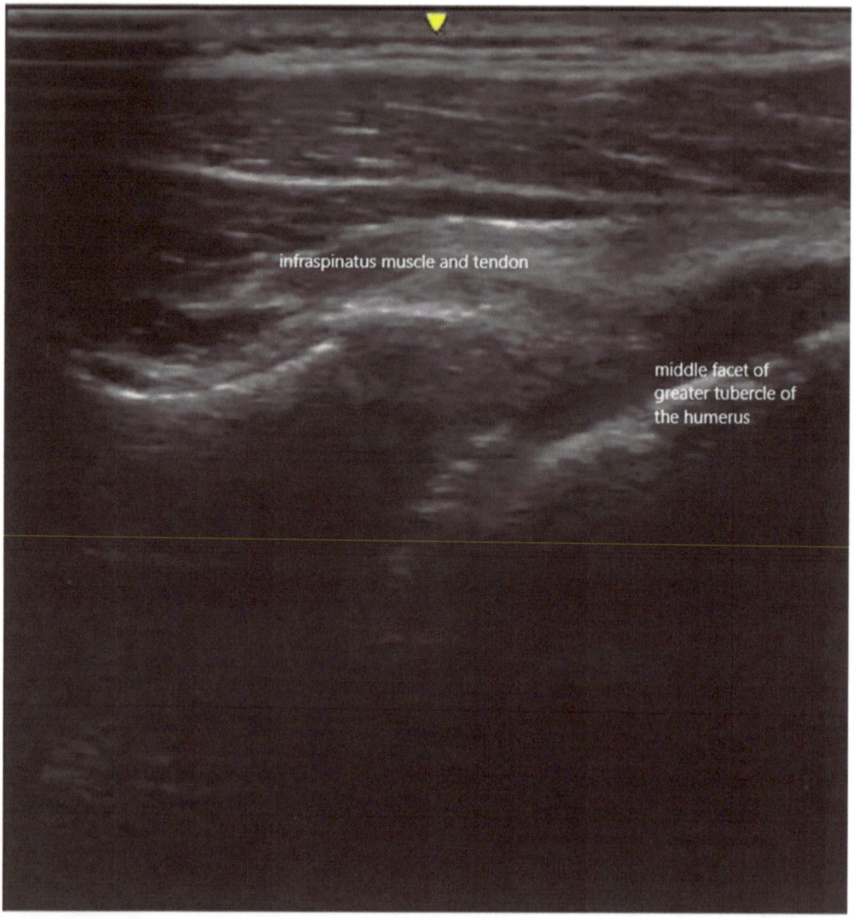

Figure 8-9e

Figure 8-9. This 11-year-old boy with Ehler's Danlos syndrome had chronic dislocations of the shoulder. He experienced one of his many atraumatic dislocations in the orthopaedic office and later underwent a diagnostic arthroscopy. Upon ultrasound imaging, the posterior musculature is less prominent than normal, with the teres minor (a) and infraspinatus (b) being shortened and thickened while in spasm. Comparison views of the opposite shoulder, which did not dislocate, show a thinner and elongated teres minor (c) and infraspinatus (d) not in spasm. (e) shows the infraspinatus insertion onto the cartilaginous middle facet of the greater tubercle of the humerus. *(Courtesy of Christopher Jobe, MD)*

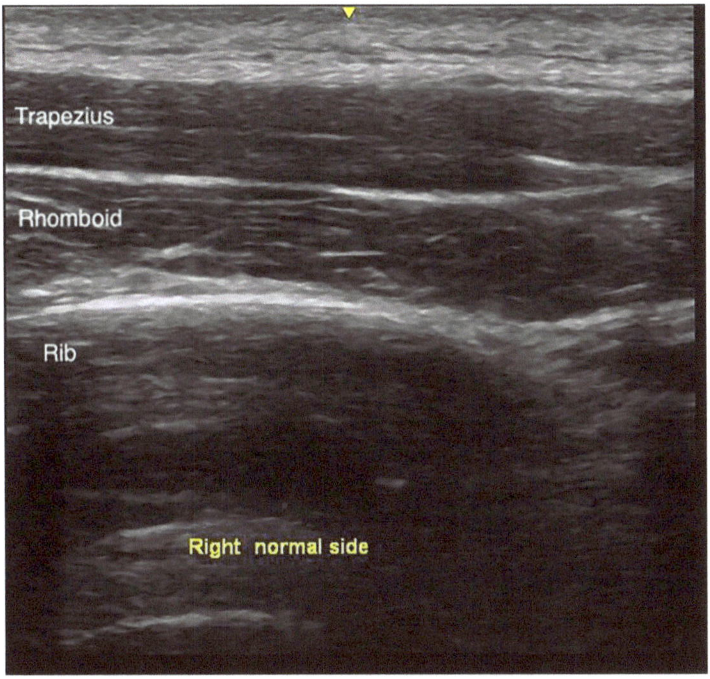

Figure 8-10a

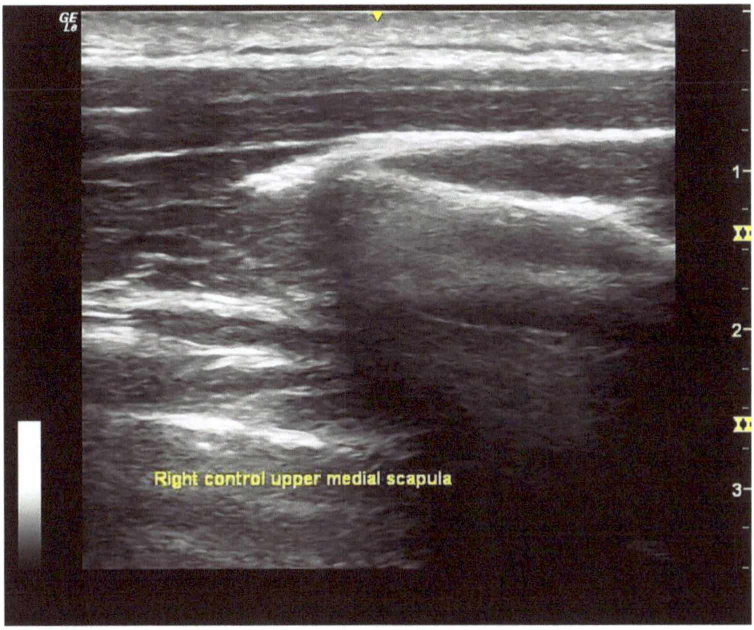

Figure 8-10b

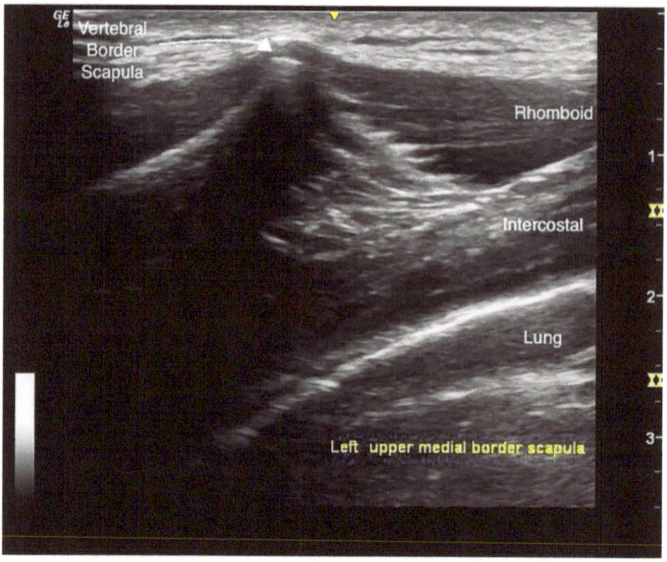

Figure 8-10c

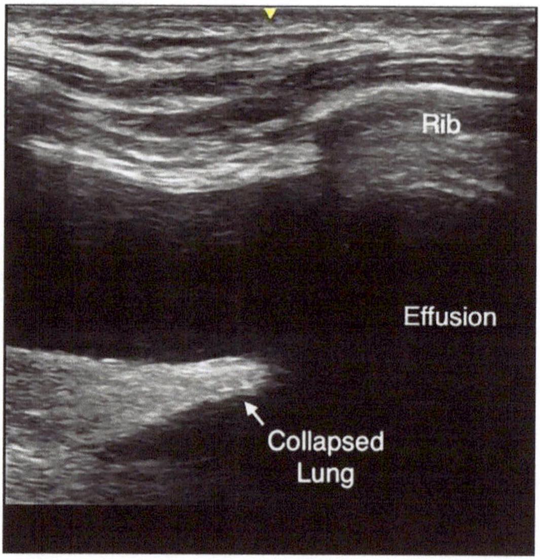

Figure 8-10d

Figure 8-10. Agenesis of trapezius treated with scapulothoracic fusion. A 16-year-old girl referred with what appeared to be Poland's syndrome. Her hand was normal, and the apparent pectoralis agenesis turned out to be secondary to trapezius winging. (a, b) The normal

shoulder showing two layers of muscle lying on rib medial to the scapula. The superficial is the trapezius and the deep is rhomboid. (c) The trapezial agenesis side showed only the rhomboid and the winging of the scapula. The bright line deep is the lung and the parallel muscle is the intercostal muscle at that level. (d) A pleural effusion that occurred two weeks later. As this portion of the lung has no air, its ultrasound appearance is similar to that of the liver, a process the pulmonologists call hepatization. *(Courtesy of Christopher Jobe, MD)*

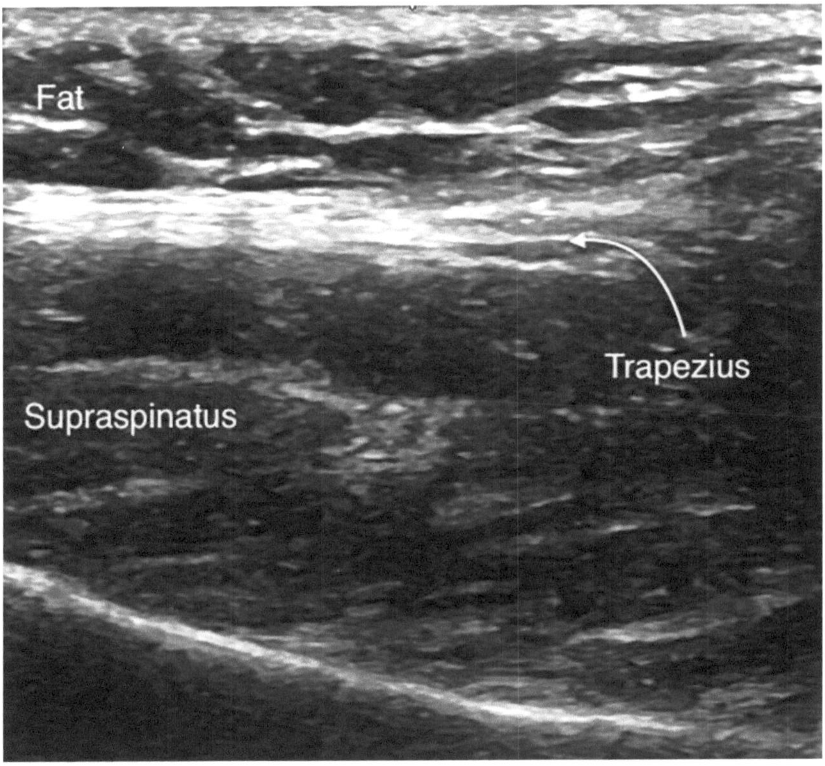

Figure 8-11a

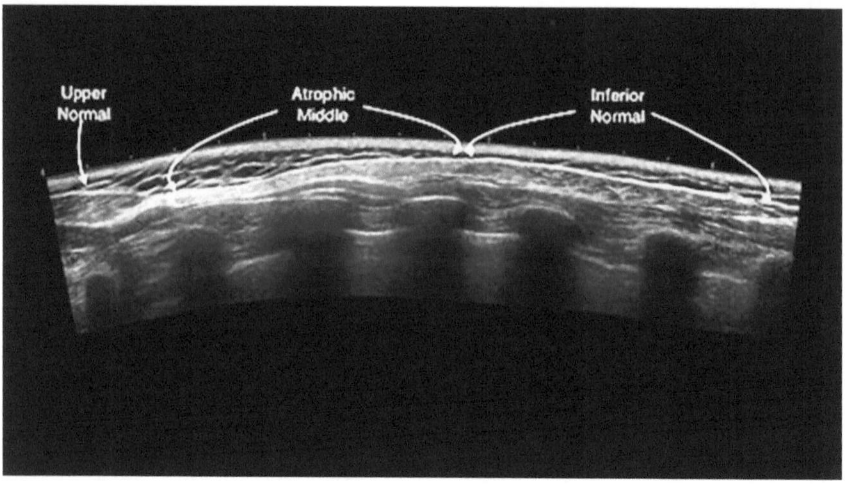

Figure 8-11b

Figure 8-11. This is an adult patient with biceps dislocation, but a full examination picked up an asymptomatic atrophy of the middle trapezius. (a) A long axis view of atrophic trapezius over normal supraspinatus. (b) An extended short axis view of the trapezius over ribs and lung. This illustrates the atrophy and increased echogenicity of the middle trapezius There is middle trapezius atrophy and dislocation of the biceps tendon noted on ultrasound. This was perhaps a result of a mild upper brachial plexus palsy or upper cervical root compression. The missing or atrophic portion of trapezius had no mechanical effect on her arm for many years. Her remaining muscle looks very much like the transfer that Bassem does for trapezius paralysis. This is a good illustration that missing muscle in the shoulder may not have any mechanical effect. *(Courtesy of Christopher Jobe, MD)*

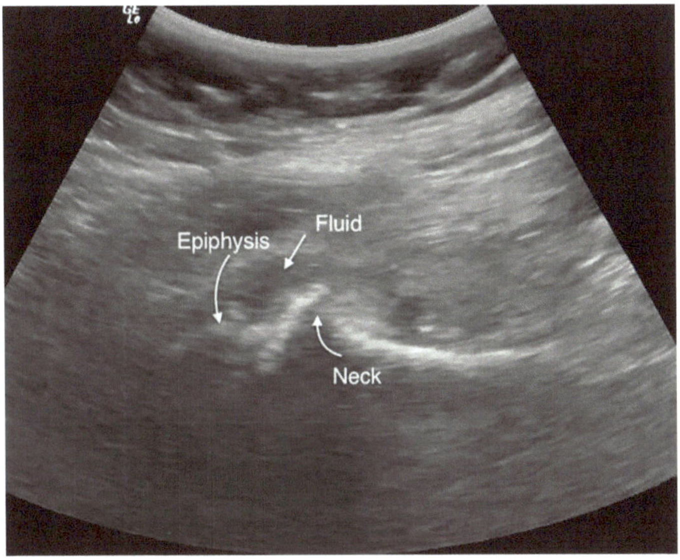

Figure 8-12a

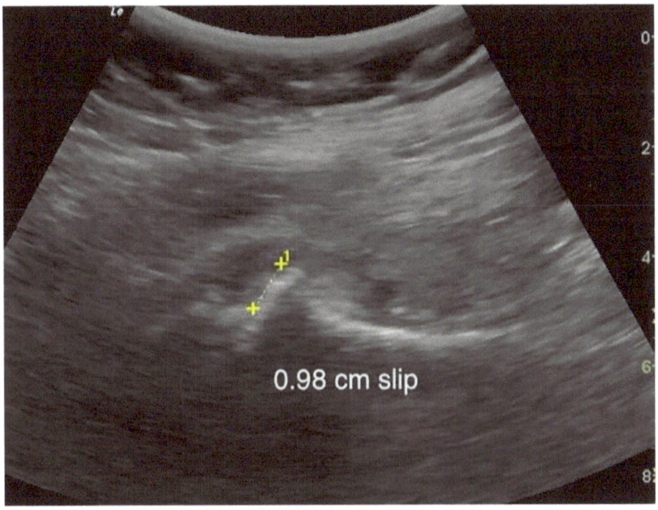

Figure 8-12b

Figure 8-12. (a, b) A child with an acute slipped capital femoral epiphysis was evaluated for hip pain with ultrasound showing a 0.98-cm step-off from a slipped capital femoral epiphysis. The effusion or hemarthrosis, the femoral neck, and the epiphysis can be readily seen on the ultrasound. *(Courtesy of Christopher Jobe, MD)*

Evaluating fracture healing

Authors have shown a high correlation of ultrasonography with X-ray studies in the evaluation of periosteal reactions.[70,71] Maffuli et al. have also proven that ultrasound has a higher effectiveness in imaging of the callus in the early stages of the healing process.[70] Moreover, the use of color or power Doppler allows for evaluation of vascularization of periosteal reactions. Based on the research, it was found that vascular resistance and vessel density in the callus are greatest during the initial healing phase and gradually decrease from 3 to 4 weeks after the fracture. Analysis of the results showed a high value of ultrasonographic evaluation of the vascularity of the callus in predicting normal or delayed healing.[71] Another method for qualitative assessment of periosteal reactions using ultrasonic waves trades on the significant changes in the mineral composition of the callus, comparing it to the healthy bone. Wawrzyk et al. investigated the assessment of changes in the speed of the reflected wave from the callus using transducers, indicating the high efficacy of ultrasound in the evaluation of callus formation after fractures of long bones in children.[72]

Ultrasound of the Spine

Ultrasound of the spine is becoming increasingly accepted as a first-line screening test in neonates with lower spinal cutaneous stigmata and suspected of occult spinal dysraphism. Posterior elements are unossified in newborns, allowing excellent imaging of the intraspinal contents. The advent of new-generation ultrasound machines with high-frequency array transducers and extended field-of-view capability give ultrasound a diagnostic sensitivity equal to that of MRI imaging in young babies. However, advancing age and ossification of the posterior elements limits visualization, and the results are best up to 6 months of age.

High-frequency 7- to 12-MHz linear array transducers are used to obtain spinal ultrasounds with excellent detail and tissue penetration with axial transverse and longitudinal imaging from the craniocervical junction to the tip of the coccyx. Neonates and young infants can be examined over a pillow or blanket roll to exploit opening of the interlaminar and spinous process spaces with slight flexion, while elevating the head and trunk to distend the more dependent thecal sac.[73] On ultrasound, the spinal cord is seen as a hypoechoic tubular structure with an echogenic central canal surrounded by subarachnoid space and dura. The spinal cord is larger and oval in the cervical spine, becomes smaller and round in the thoracic spine, until the round cord enlarges again in the thoracolumbar region above the conus medullaris (Figure 13). At the thoracolumbar region, the spinal cord tapers to form the conus medullaris, which continues as the homogenously, slightly echogenic cord-like filum terminale, which normally measures 1-2 mm in diameter before ending in the distal sacral canal. The conus medullaris is surrounded by echogenic nerve roots. When making a determination of the conus level relative to the vertebrae, radiographic imaging is advisable to confirm the number of rib-bearing vertebrae, which may number from 11 to 13, as ultrasound is not as useful as radiographs in enumerating the vertebrae. This can be important when counting the vertebrae with ultrasound when lateral parasagittal imaging is used to identify the lowest rib and follows this rib medially, to the presumed lowest vertebrae with the rib, usually named T12.

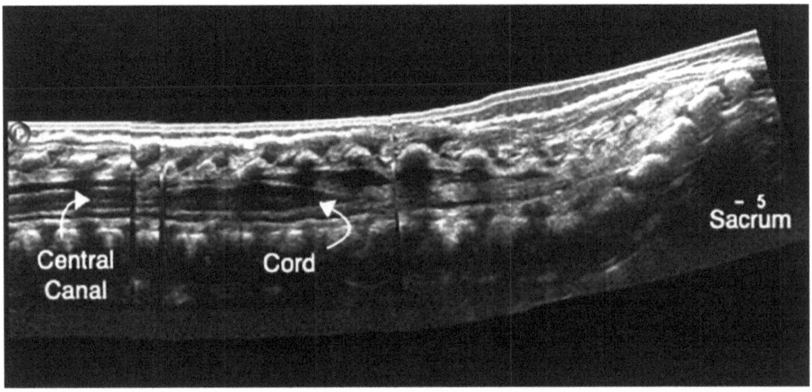

Figure 8-13. An example of a normal ultrasound in a two-week-old neonate with a sacral dimple. Sagittal panoramic sonographic image of the lumbar spine and sacrum obtained with a 12 MHz linear transducer, with the patient in a prone position, shows the normal hypoechoic appearance of the distal cord (arrow indicates distal conus) with an echogenic central canal. The conus medullaris ends normally at the level of the L1-L2 disc space.

The sensitivity of spine ultrasonography in evaluating the neonatal spine is equivalent to MRI in experienced hands and can characterize nearly all spinal anomalies quite well in the early neonatal period. This allows for clinical determination of whether the lesion requires urgent intervention or further radiologic evaluation with studies such as MRI, which might then be delayed until therapeutic intervention is more imminent, or the child is older, larger, and more suitable for advanced imaging with sedation or anesthesia (Figure 14).[74]

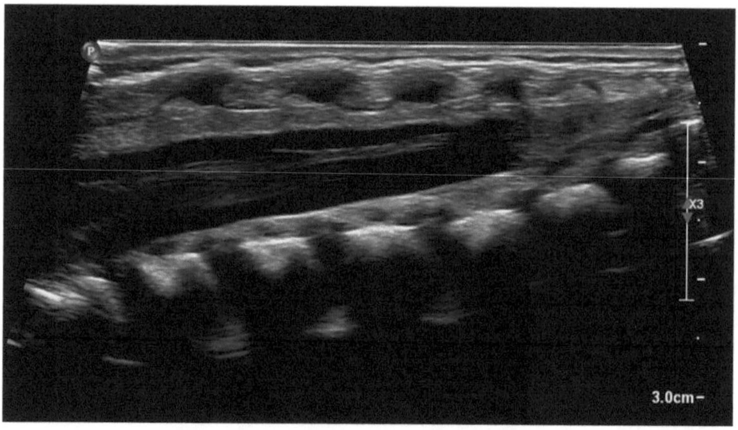

Figure 8-14a

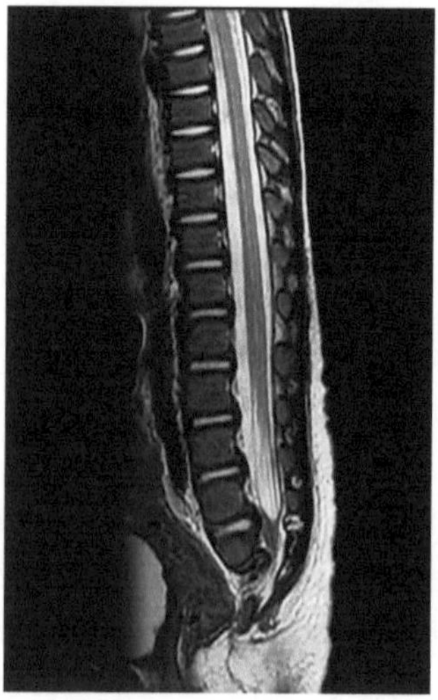

Figure 8-14b

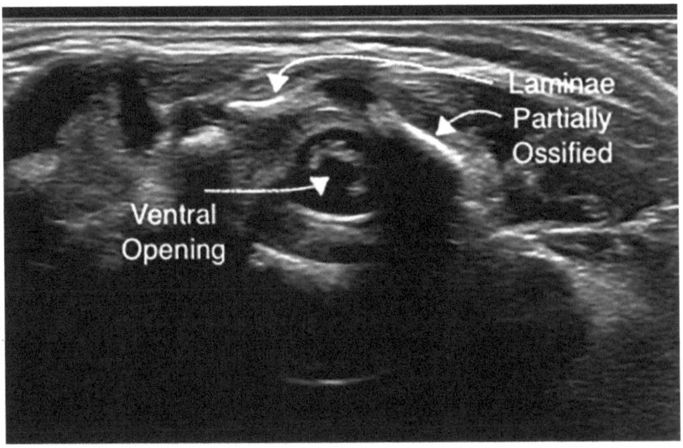

Figure 8-14c

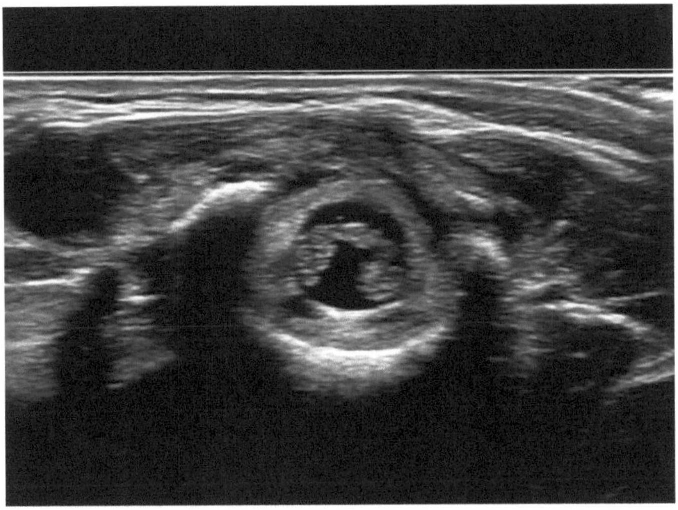

Figure 8-14d

Figure 8-14. A newborn infant with caudal regression syndrome (CRS). At 18 weeks of gestation, compatible data with malformations of the neural tube with sacral agenesis was found, resulting in a CRS diagnosis. During the second trimester of pregnancy, hyperglycemia was detected in the mother, therefore she was placed on insulin treatment. At 40 weeks of gestation, a Caesarian section was performed, obtaining a healthy infant with an Apgar score of 8/9 and a gestational age of 39.6 weeks. (a, Longitudinal ultrasound images

of the 2-day-old newborn showing a low-lying cord at the L4-L5 disc space. B the MRI is shown for comparison, again the low-lying cord is seen ending at about L4(c, d) Axial ultrasound images of a low-lying, distorted conus with a ventral opening. C and also demonstrate how the incomplete ossification of the laminae in the newborn allow ultrasound to visualize the cord.

Spinal cord tethering

The normal conus tip should be seen from the T10-T11 interspace to the superior L3, but most often it is at L1-L2 in neonates. A tethered cord may be suspected if the patient presents with midline dorsal cutaneous abnormalities, including subcutaneous lipomas, hair tufts, skin defects or dimples, skin tags, hemangiomas, and pigmented nevi. The true location of the conus below the level of L2-L3 is considered diagnostic of a tethered cord (Figures 15a-c). In addition, on real-time scanning, there can be a reduction in amplitude or loss of oscillation of the cord and cauda equina due to a tethered spinal cord.[75,76] Normally, brisk oscillations of the cord and cauda equina can be seen in synchrony with the heartbeat, and these may be reduced by tethering in an older infant. The absence of oscillations alone is not clearly pathological in the newborn less than two months of age, but the diagnosis is supported further when thickening of the filum terminale, an intradural lipoma, or a lipomeningocele is also noted.[73]

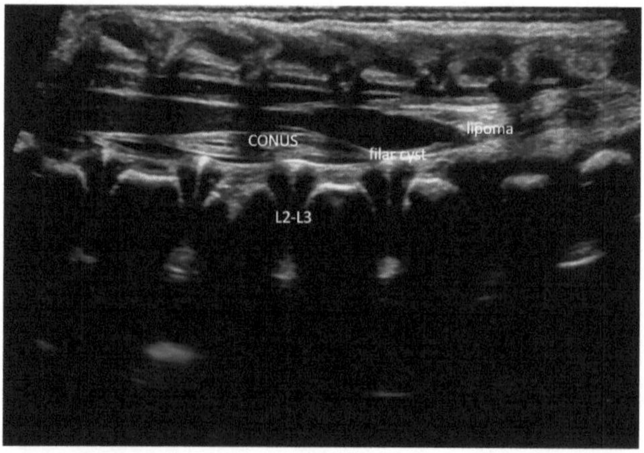

Figure 8-15a

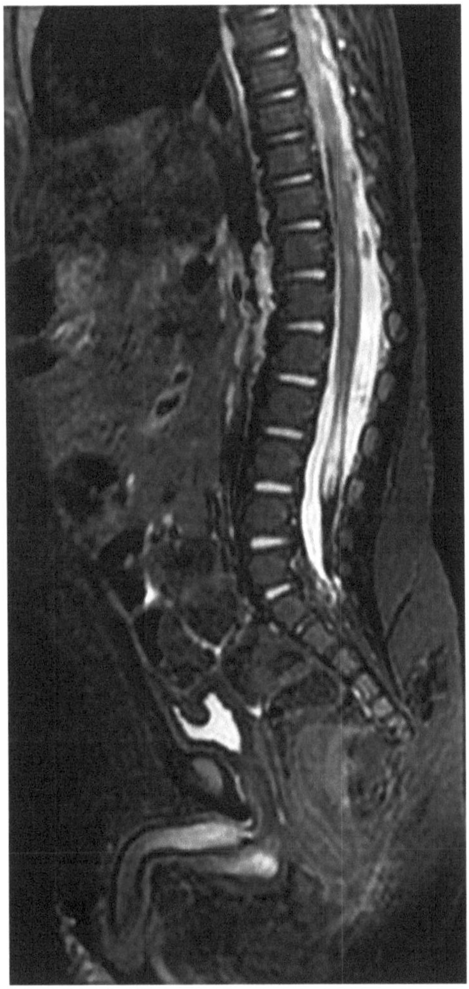

Figure 8-15b

Figures 8-15a and b One-day-old infant with a deep sacral pit. (a) Ultrasound shows the conus medullaris terminating at the L2-L3 disc level. A filar cyst is observed contiguous to the conus While filar cysts alone in newborns are now considered a variant of normal, a normal filum is not identified distally; in its place is a thick echogenic structure compatible with a lipoma (and b). (Short-tau inversion recovery midsagittal magnetic resonance imaging obtained at 4 months confirm the diagnosis of filum terminale lipoma (thick white arrow). The filar cyst is less conspicuous on follow-up.)

Tethering may not be associated with any neurologic abnormalities at birth, but with growth, the cord becomes progressively stretched, and imaging is important to pick up this finding before the mechanical distortion and resulting ischemia cause permanent injury. Torres and DiPietro report that in their 30 years of experience with ultrasound, tethering is identified very reliably, and when the conus is low, and the cord truly tethered, there will be an obvious cause of tethering.[73] The causes include the skin-covered spinal dysraphisms, such as intradural and terminal lipomas, lipomyelocele and lipomyelomeningocele, dorsal dermal sinuses, diastematomyelia, and thickened filum terminale, but if such tethering causes are not identified, perhaps the vertebral counting should be reassessed before concluding that a low-lying conus medullaris is present. Patients with anorectal malformations, such as imperforate anus and anorectal atresia, also have an increased risk for having an occult tethered cord; therefore, these patients should also be screened at birth with ultrasound.

Spinal dysraphism

During the first trimester of pregnancy, the neural tube forms through a primary and secondary neurulation process. The pathophysiology of myelomeningocele is a failed closure of the neural tube during primary neurulation, producing a cystic mass of neuronal elements, including dura, arachnoid, spinal cord, nerve roots, and cerebral spinal fluid within an open bone and skin defect. At the second gestational week, the notochord induces the overlying ectoderm to become neuroectoderm and to form the neural plate, which then folds onto itself and closes bidirectionally to form the neural tube, while simultaneously separating from the overlying ectoderm. Disruption of these processes results in spinal dysraphism.[73] During primary neurulation, the neuroectoderm folds with the last caudal portion, closing approximately on day 27; simultaneously, the mesoderm migrates and forms the posterior vertebral elements, and the ectoderm migrates, forming the skin.

During this first process, the aberrancy *failure of primary disjunction* causes communication and connection of the ectoderm and neuroectoderm, preventing normal mesenchymal migration. This aberrancy results in posterior dysraphic spinal malformations, as seen in myelomeningocele, myelocoele, and dorsal dermal sinuses.[77] Secondary neurulation starts around day 28 and promotes further neural development by forming the caudal spine and filum terminale. During this second process, the aberrancy *premature disjunction* allows perineural mesenchyme to enter the neural groove, which prevents its complete closure, and the neural tube prematurely separates from the overlying ectoderm prior to neural tube closure, producing a closed neural tube defect. The aberrant mesenchymal tissue differentiates into fat, leading to a skin-covered dysraphic spine with associated lipomas, such as lipomeningocele, lipomyelomenigocele, or intradural lipomas.[73,77]

Skin-covered lesions without a subcutaneous mass include caudal mass anomalies, such as a thickened filum terminale, fibrolipoma of filum terminale, caudal regression syndrome, sacrococcygeal teratoma, and anomalies of the cord, such as a split-cord and diastomatomyelia, all of which can be readily seen on ultrasound.[74] Spina bifida aperta, a non-skin-covered open defect, is usually clinically apparent and imaging is limited; in these cases, a cranial ultrasonography study to look for associated defects, like hydrocephalus, is usually performed. Open neural tube defects include myelomeningocele and myelocele; the former accounts for more than 98% of open spinal dysraphisms. The position of the neural plate (placode) establishes the difference between myelomeningocele and myelocele. In the rarer myelocele, the neural placode is flush to the skin, while in the more common myelomeningocele, the unclosed portion of the placode is displaced above the surface skin by the subarachnoid space, with the nerves dropping back from placode through the fluid into the open spinal canal. These severe defects require closure in utero, or typically within 72 hours of birth, to minimize secondary damage. Ultrasound could cause additional trauma or infection and is not done in these open cases, but it can be quite useful in assessment of the uninvolved spine and brainstem. These can be readily assessed for occult malformations in the skin-covered spine and of the ubiquitous Chiari II malformations associated with myelomeningocele in virtually all patients.[73,77]

Although of limited use in the open spinal dysraphisms, neonatal spinal ultrasound is excellent for evaluation of an occult spinal dysraphism, and skin-covered lesions with a subcutaneous mass, like a simple meningocele, lipomyelocele, lipomeningocele, or myelocystocele, are visualized in detail.[73,74,77] On ultrasound, the echogenic intradural lipoma is present within the dural sac, intimately attached to the cord, while filar lipomas are limited to filum terminale (Figure 16).[73] Dimples or shallow pits located less than 2.5 cm above the anus are often associated with spinal dysraphism and should be screened with ultrasound to rule out dermal sinuses or other occult dysraphism.[73,77]

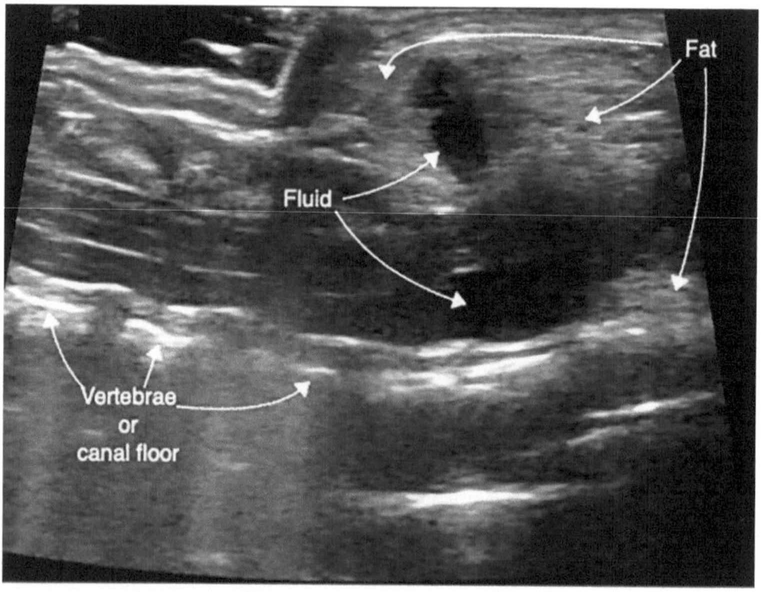

Figure 8-16a

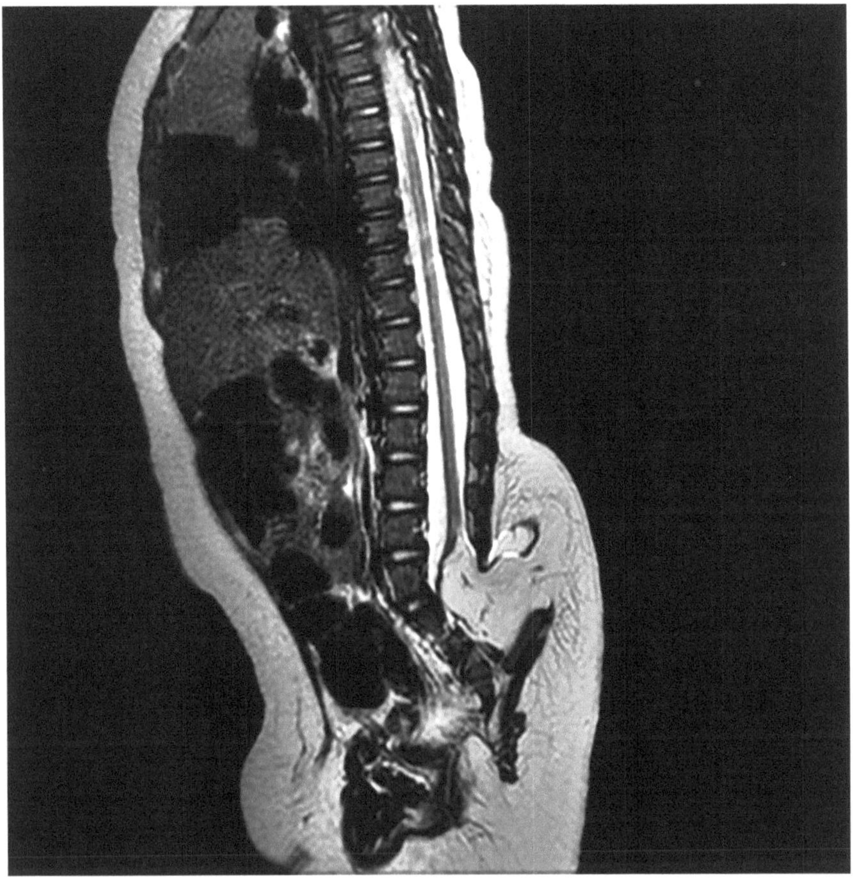

Figure 8-16b

Figure 8-16. Newborn with a lower back mass. (a) Lumbosacral spine ultrasound on the first day of life shows the spinal cord) extending caudally to the level of L4-L5 where it is attached posteriorly to a lipomatous mass that traverses a large posterior sacral bony defect. The mass, which also contains pockets of fluid, corresponds to the clinically palpable abnormality. (b) T2-weighted midsagittal magnetic resonance imaging of the lumbosacral spine obtained at four months of age confirm cord tethering with a lipomyelomeningocele. On , ultrasound fluid is hypoechoic (dark) while on MRI T2- weighted images, it is very bright. On ultrasound, fat has multiple interfaces which render it brighter than muscle but not as bright as bony cortex. On MRI fat is a light gray, not as bright as spinal fluid.

The ultrasonographer must be aware of normal variants readily seen on ultrasound, such as a persistent fetal terminal ventricle in the conus medullaris, due to incomplete regression, causing a ventriculus terminalis, which appears as a hydromyelia confined to the conus, or a filar cyst, which is of uncertain etiology. The latter is now noted to be present on high-resolution ultrasound in most neonates, and is a simple midline cystic structure just caudal to the conus medullaris, displacing the roots.[73]

Other spinal lesions are also readily identifiable by ultrasound. Diastematomyelia is a rare malformation in which the cord is split into two halves, or hemicords, which may reunite distally. These malformations are found 85% of the time between the levels of T9 and L5. Type I diastematomyelias are located within their own separate dural sacs, separated by a bony or fibrous septum, whereas the type II lesions are found within a single sac and may be separated by a fibrous septum. Ultrasonography also helps in the detection of tumors, vascular malformations, and in cases of trauma. Anterior sacral meningoceles may rarely be found and may occur as part of the Currarino triad of presacral mass (dermoid or meningocele), sacrococcygeal osseous defect (crescentic sacrum), and anorectal malformations, such as anal stenosis and anal atresia. These cystic dysraphic lesions may sometimes be confused with a sacrococcygeal teratoma, the most common presacral tumour found in neonates and infants. Fifty to 70% of sacral teratomas are diagnosed at birth because of the obvious bulge, or a prenatal ultrasound diagnosis and a delay in diagnosis may result in large size and surgical complexity, with a higher incidences of malignancy.[73]

Intraoperative spine ultrasound

Ultrasound was first introduced into neurosurgery as far back as 1951, but it failed to get a foothold in the operating theater and was limited to assessment of space-occupying cranial lesions of the brain and differentiating solid from cystic lesions until the 1980s.[78]

Intraoperative ultrasonographic guidance allows the surgeon to correlate the complex anatomy identified on preoperative CT and MRI to the surgical site.[79] In the early 1980s, Masuzawa et al., Dohrmann and Rubin, and Chandler and Knake published on their utilization of ultrasound in the operating room during cranial and spinal surgery.[80-82] By the early 1990s, ultrasound was being used routinely for intramedullary tumor resections, with improved postoperative neurologic function attributed to improved tumor localization, tumor and cyst characterization, placement of myelotomy, and tumor resection monitoring done with ultrasound visualization.[83] Ultrasound identifies pseudoswelling of the spinal cord well, and its real-time nature allows treatment of any CSF-related changes.[84]

Although Reid had first demonstrated use of ultrasound through the flexed-neck interlaminar window in 1978,[5] ultrasound found limited usage in the operating room until Dohrmann and Rubin described their experiences in many operative cases in 1982.[7] The recommended ultrasound setup is with a sterile, 20-mm or smaller transducer probe covered with a disposable plastic bag, with a frequency range of 4 to 10 MHz, placed into the surgical field, where it is bathed in saline to optimize acoustic coupling; there is no need for direct contact with the dura or spinal cord.[78] Early or incidental diagnosis by MRI has shifted the typical tumor case mix from what previously were large, obvious tumors to those with little or no visible changes at the level of the dura, emphasizing the importance of being able to intraoperatively identify tumor location with ultrasound. Doppler techniques have also been shown to be useful in visualizing the feeding arteries. The normal structures can be identified, including the dural-arachnoid, the subarachnoid space, the denticulate ligaments, the dorsal arachnoid septae, the ventral and dorsal roots, and the cauda equina. Components filled with cerebrospinal fluid appear as anechoic areas, and lipomas as hyperechoic. Ultrasound visualizes cystic areas within the spinal cord well, and it also allows for identification and localization of other neural structures and associated lesions such as lipomas, other ectopic tissues such as dermoid and epidermoid cysts, or doubling of the spinal cord and diastematomyelic spurs, bands, and adhesions. In complex intradural cases, ultrasound guidance can protect the patient from inadvertently introduced foreign materials into the thecal sac, such as cotton pledgets or gelfoam. It also can reduce the size of the incision and number of laminectomies necessary to safely identify the lesion, reduces the need for intraoperative radiographs and fluoroscopy, and is quite useful at confirming the adequacy of the decompression or resection without the difficulties associated with intraoperative myelography or MRI (Figure 17).

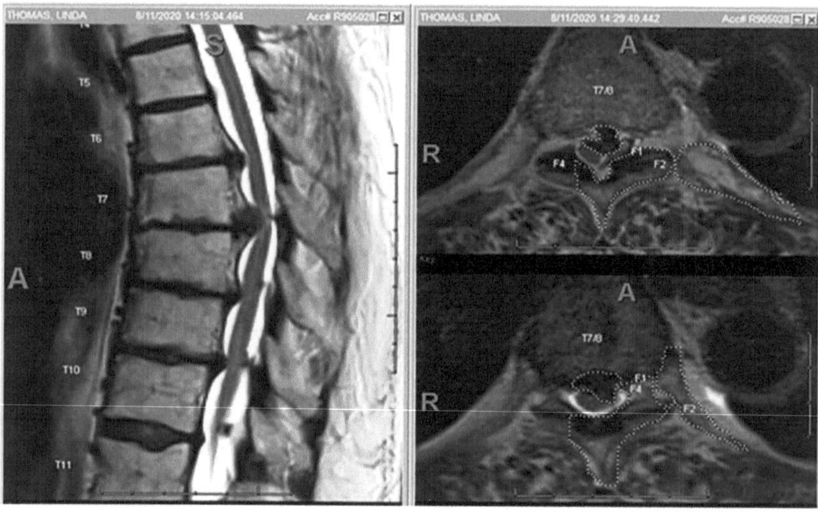

Figure 8-17a

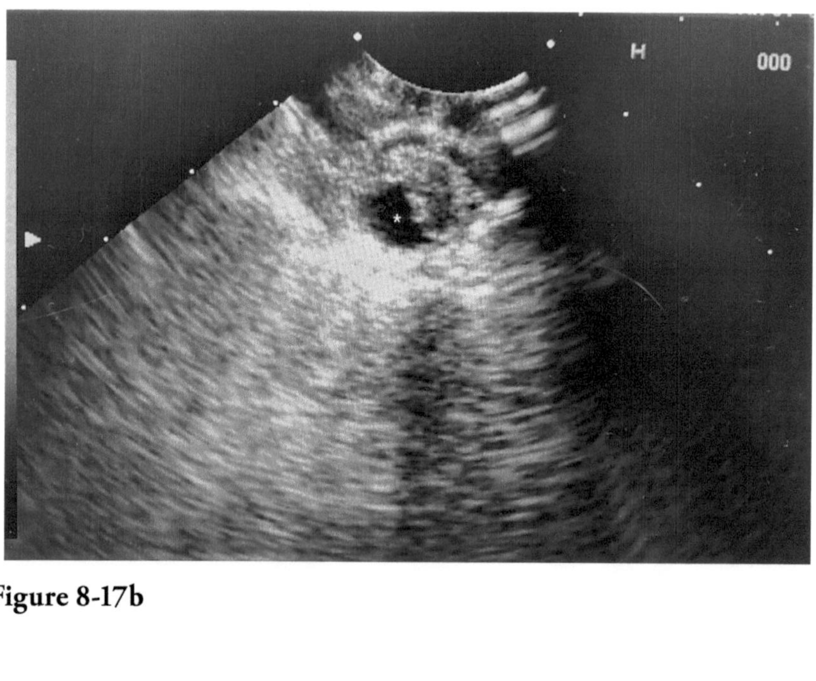

Figure 8-17b

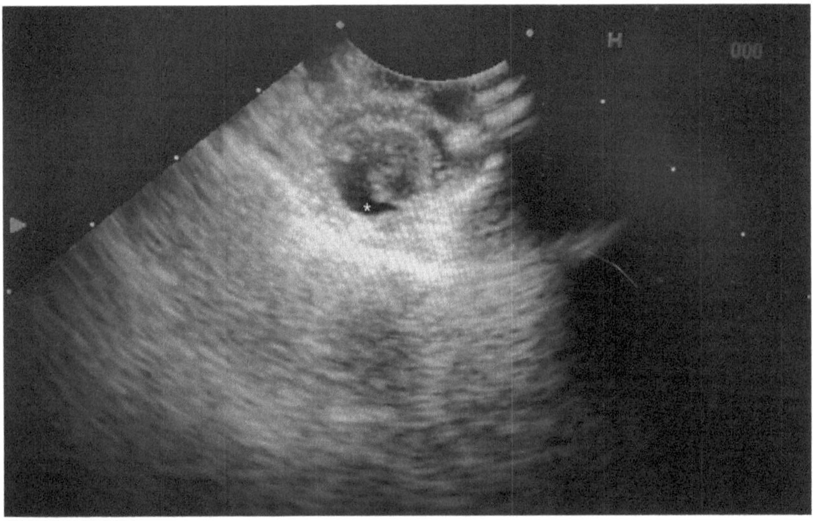

Figure 8-17c

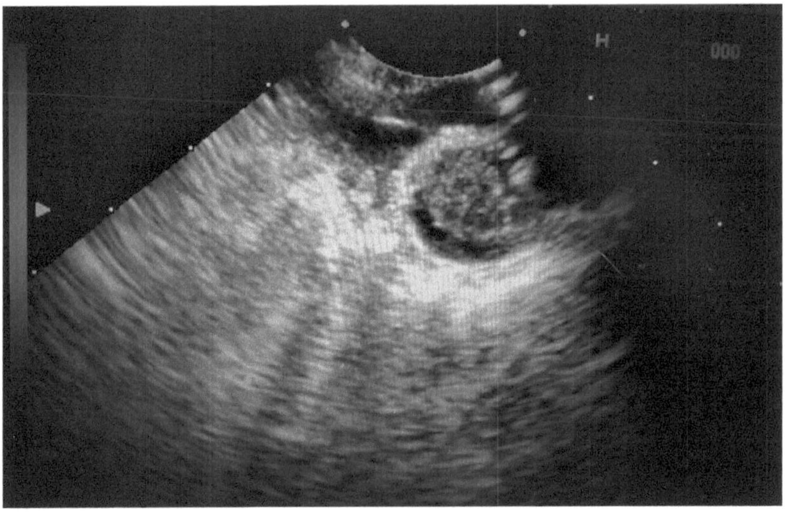

Figure 8-17d

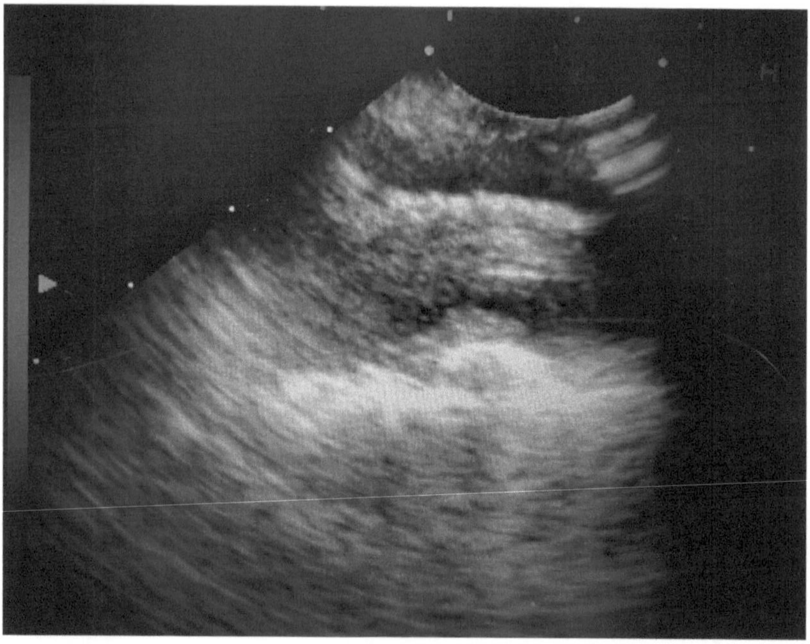

Figure 8-17e

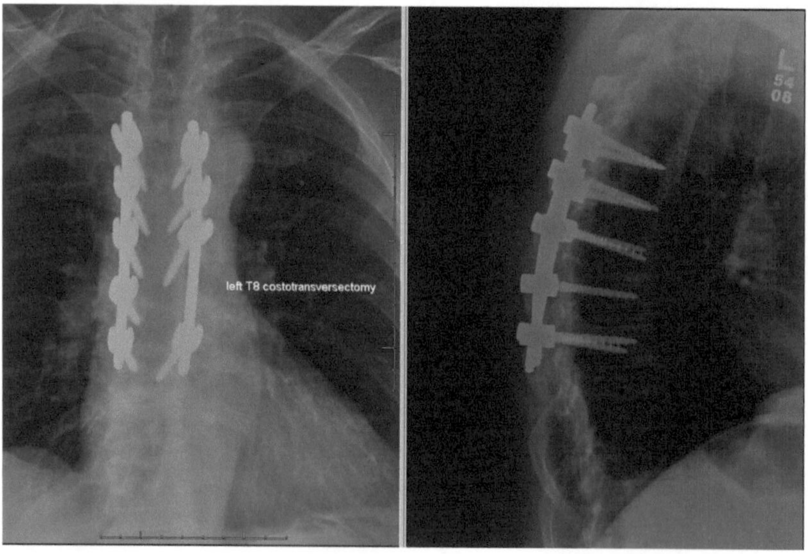

Figure 8-17f

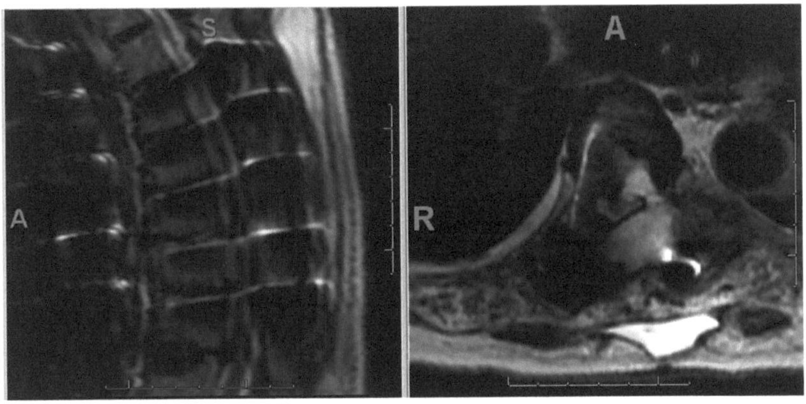

Figure 8-17g

Figure 8-17. A 68-year-old obese woman had undergone multiple prior spine surgeries for low-back degenerative disease at outside hospitals. She presented to us using a wheelchair for ambulation, with severe myelopathic signs and symptoms, which were found to be the result of severe cord compression from a calcified T7/8 disc, among other spine problems that were less urgent. (a) On magnetic resonance imaging and computed tomography, the thoracic disc was displacing the cord to the right and a left-sided T8 costotransversectomy. Anterior cord decompression was necessary, but transthoracic approaches were expected to have much higher complication rates, and we would not see the cord at all while decompressing from the front, a significant risk for further cord injury. All-posterior approaches also allow for simultaneous stabilization and fusion across the wide laminectomies needed to address the pathology. In these cases, intraoperative ultrasound is quite useful to see the cord and compressive lesions during exposure and decompression. Preoperative steroids were given at the start of her surgery, and multimodal monitoring performed throughout surgery. The laminectomies from T5 to T9 were followed by a left T8 costotransversectomy, then a microscopic anterior discectomy and cord decompression. During the final stages of the T7/8 discectomy, the motor-evoked potentials were lost, first in the left, and then in the right lower extremities, followed by a large decrease in the somatosensory evoked potentials; with the motor changes, IV Decadron was administered again, and the blood

pressure elevated to above 85 mmHg. (b) Image taken shortly after cord decompression at the T7/8 disc, showing that the cord was fully decompressed, but there was also a hypoechoic region (*) ventral and lateral, corresponding to what had been the most compressed region of the cord. This is thought to be adjacent to the as-yet unexpanded, deformed spinal cord surrounding a cerebral spinal fluid-filled subdural defect left after the hard calcific disc was resected. (c) Over time, the transverse (axial) ultrasound images showed the cord slowly re-expanding, and there was a smaller hypoechoic, fluid-filled space next to the cord (*). (d) Finally, the cord fully expanded to fill the thecal sac. (e) On sagittal ultrasound imaging, the cord was also seen to have minimal deformity and was adequately decompressed. (f) With final instrumentation of the left rod into the implants, decortication, and bone grafting, the case proceeded to closure as quickly as possible. The motor evoked and somatosensory evoked signals slowly returned, but not to baseline. The patient awoke from surgery at her baseline weakness and was placed into the neuro-spine intensive care unit, where her neurologic changes rapidly improved to above her baseline exam by the morning. The mean arterial pressures were kept above 85 mmHg for 24 hours; by the next day, she was able to ambulate, and reported immediate improvement in pain, sensation and motor strength. (g) Follow-up ultrasound to document the cord status showed that the canal was decompressed on the left completely at the operative level, with minimal residual right-sided effacement.

In our example, it was quite useful to monitor our progress during surgery and guide our spinal cord decompression for an otherwise poorly visualized lesion in the ventral spinal column causing anterior spinal cord compression. We have found that ultrasound particularly facilitates dural exposure in difficult revision surgeries, where the lack of anatomic bony landmarks combined with scarring creates challenges to identifying the dura and associated lesions during the surgical approach. When the distance to the dura through the adherent scar-tissue is reduced to a few millimeters, further dissection can be done under microscope magnification with much greater confidence (Figure 18).

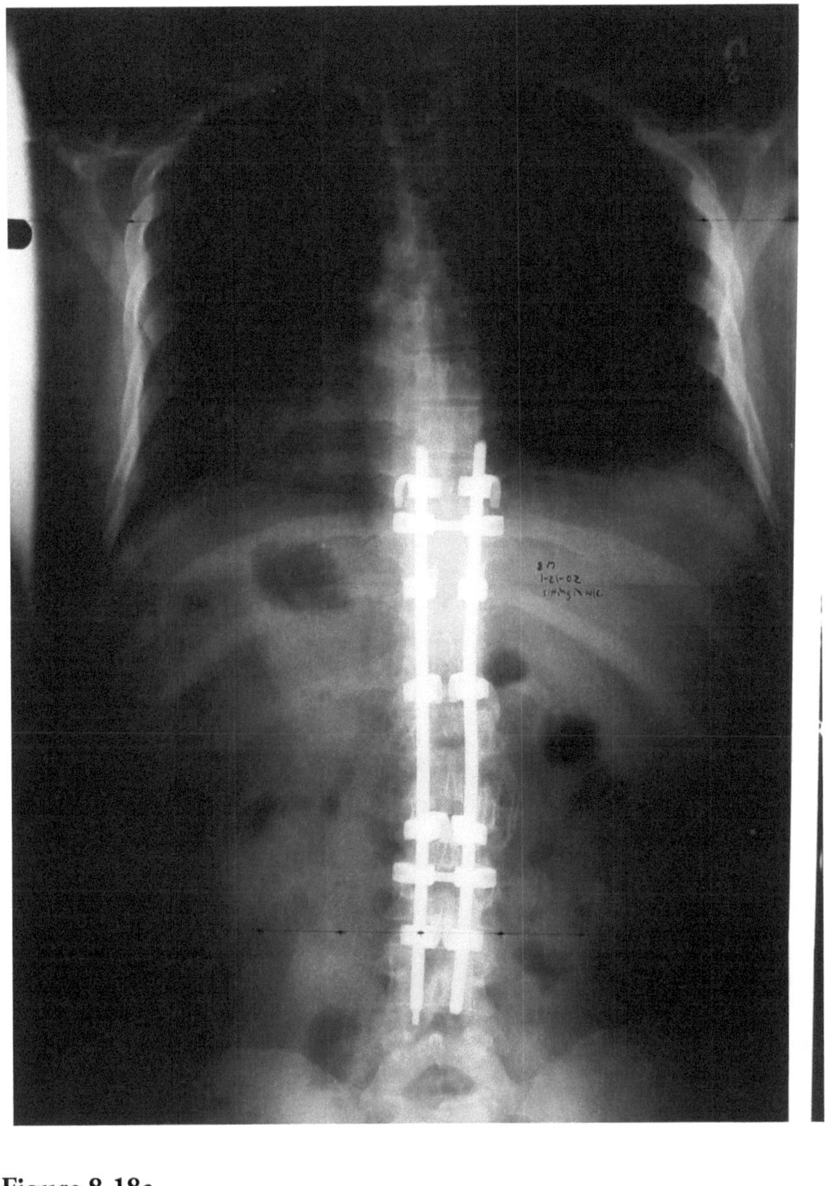

Figure 8-18a

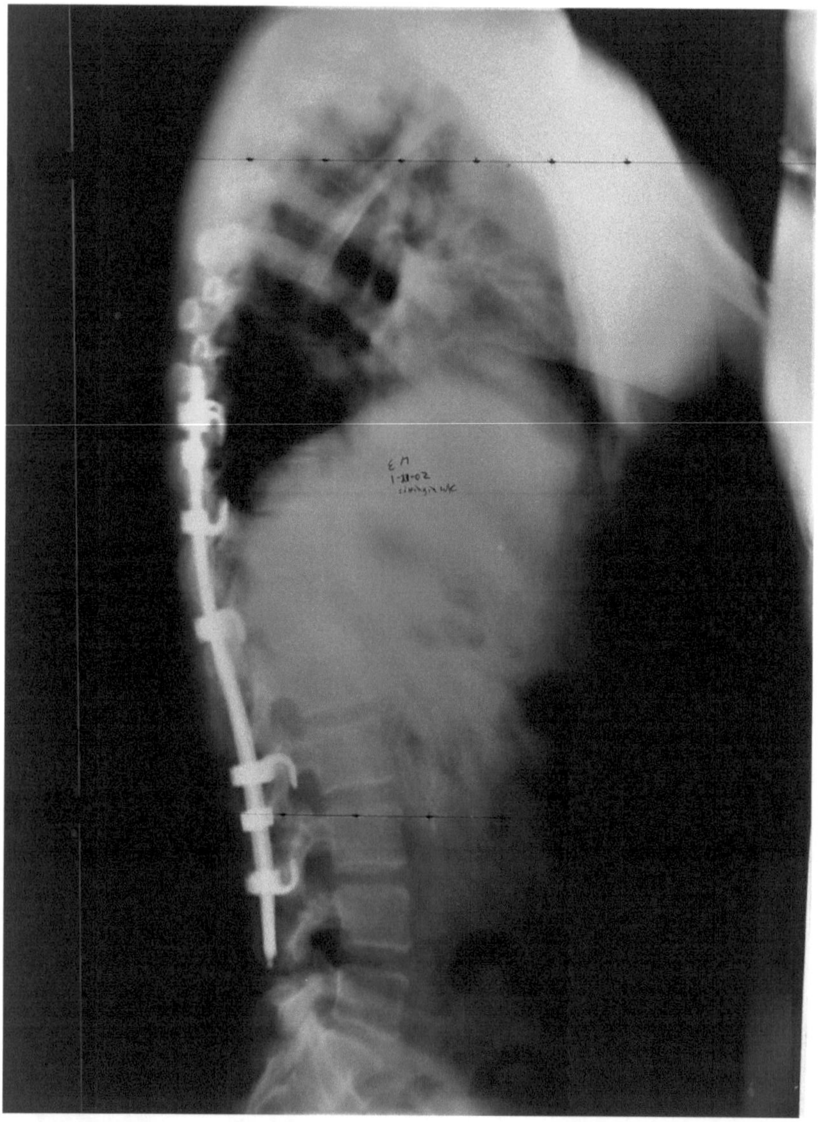

Figure 8-18b

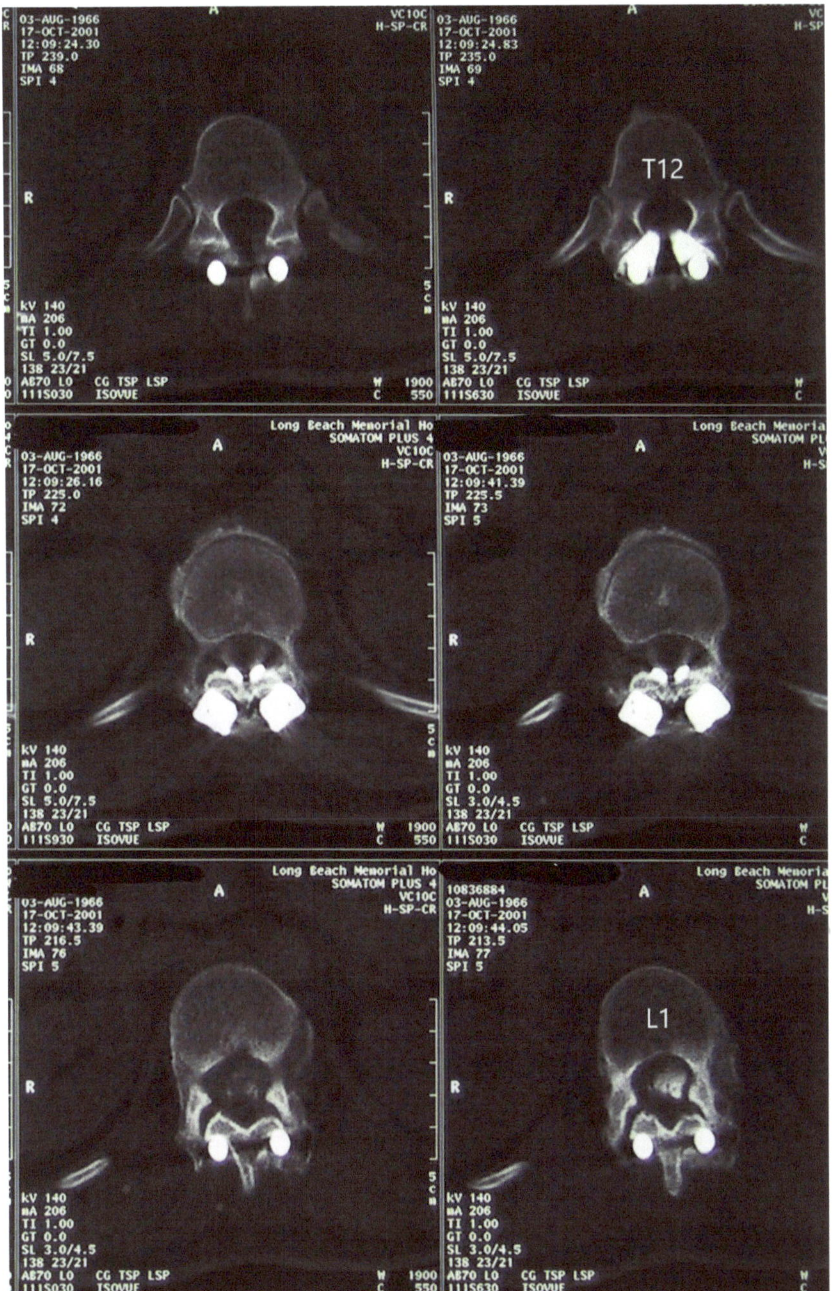

Figure 8-18c

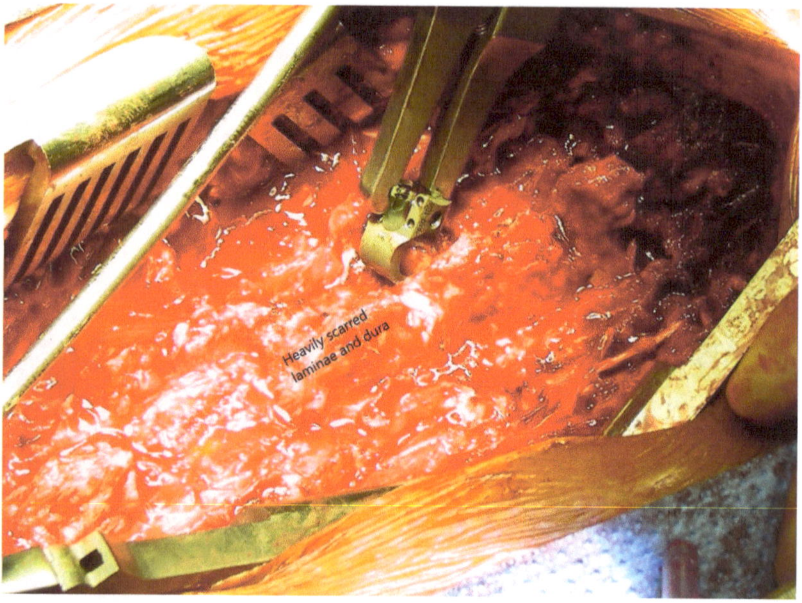

Figure 8-18d

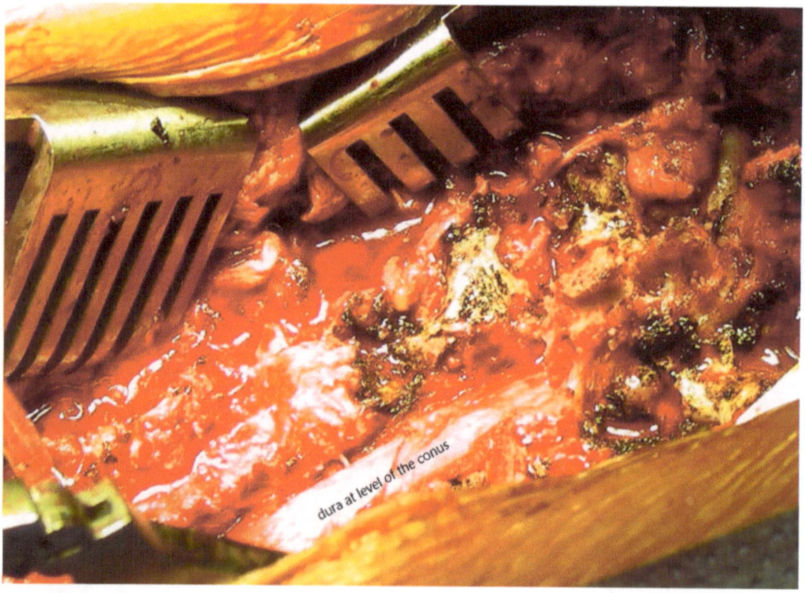

Figure 8-18e

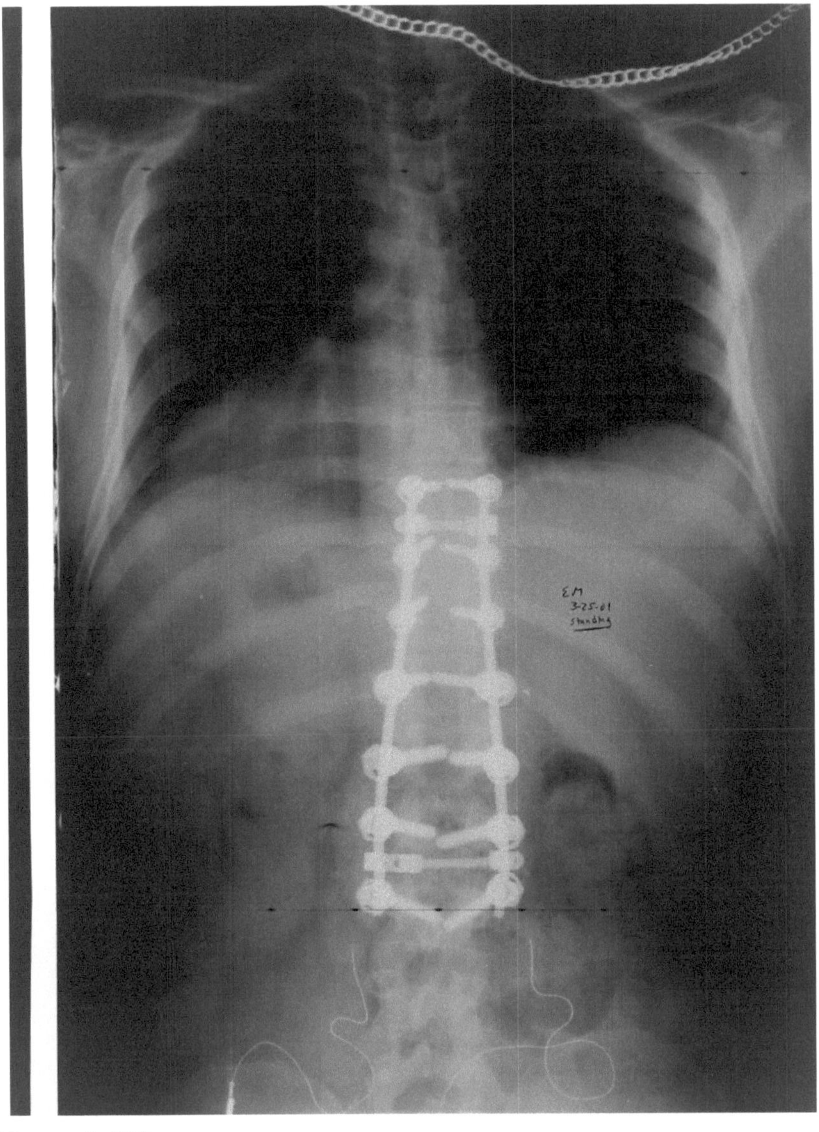

Figure 8-18f

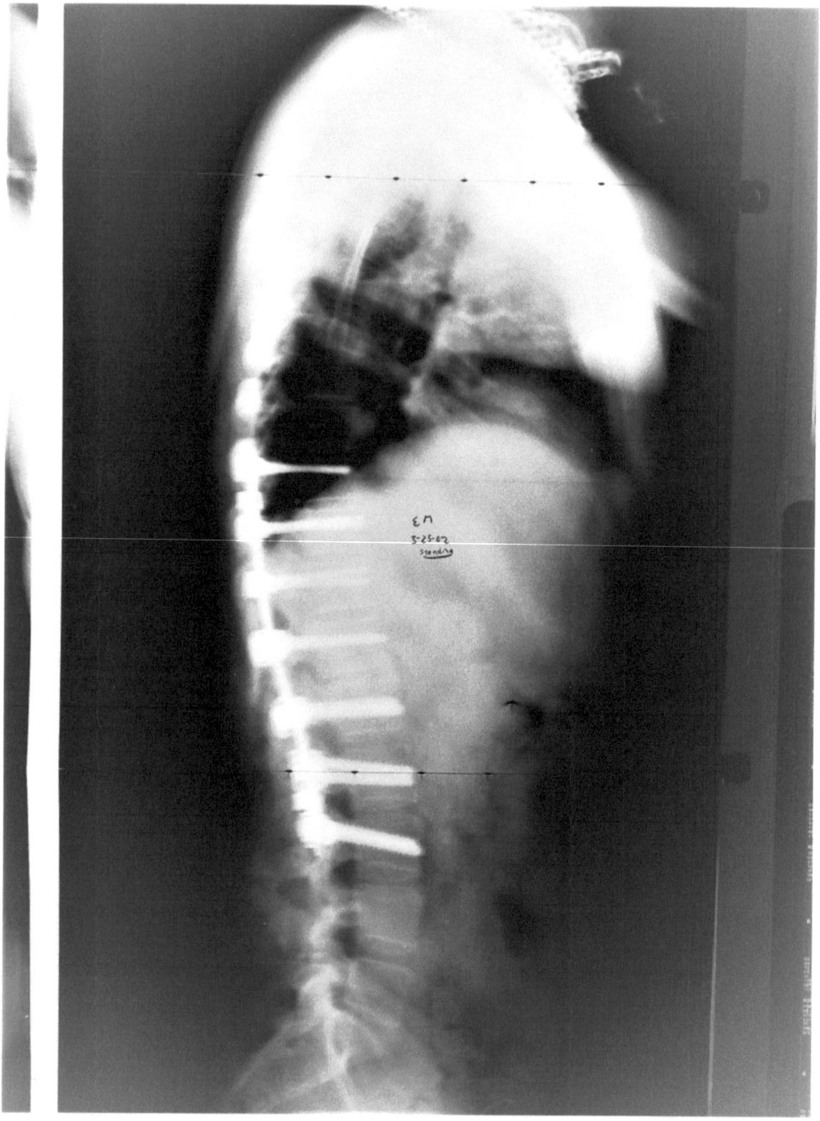

Figure 8-18g

Figure 8-18. Late conus-level spinal cord injury decompression case. (a, b) Sitting whole-spine radiographs of a 35-year-old man two years after an industrial evisceration injury with a T12-L1 fracture dislocation. At the outside trauma center, he was thought initially to have a complete spinal cord injury, and he had had a posterior stabilization T9-L3 with hook and rod instrumentation using indirect

reduction by distraction, but no direct decompression. He had significant residual deficits with a non-ambulatory ASIA B status after this conus-level injury and a painful, multilevel pseudoarthrosis. (c) Selections from a computed tomography myelogram performed due to stainless steel implants preventing MRI, showing residual stenosis with a myelographic block at T12-L1 at the level of the hooks. There is a scarred epidural space with anatomic conus distortion. (d) An intraoperative photograph as the last hook was removed, showing the heavy scarring at the laminae and hooks sites before the decompression. Using ultrasound to guide us through the surgery, we did a revision T11 to L2 laminectomy with spinal cord decompression (e), followed by revision pedicle screw instrumentation and posterolateral fusion T9-L3. Although his bowel bladder dysfunction remained, he had substantial improvement in his lower extremities' strength after surgery, sufficient to regain ambulatory status (ASIA D). (f, g) These are his AP and lateral *standing* whole spine radiographs.

Intraoperative spinal ultrasound is mainly used by neurosurgeons for measurement of cerebrospinal fluid flow in some anomalies like Chiari malformation, or less invasive surgery involving bone decompression without duraplasty.[85] Contrast-enhanced ultrasonography permits assessment of blood flow dynamics, helps define the border between tumor and healthy neural tissue, and can detect residual tumors. Ultrasound has also been used to guide screw placement, and efforts are being used to integrate it into virtual reality surgical navigation.[86-88] Ganau et al. summarized several major papers in the literature on ultrasound application in the spine and brought up ongoing research into the use of microbubbles and nanoparticle contrast agents, which can bypass vascular endothelial cells and accumulate at tissues with ligands.[78] Contrast-enhanced ultrasonography has also been combined with virtual navigation to allow localization of the vessels three-dimensionally during brain surgery and is being developed for use in spine surgery.

The combination of real-time imaging, ease of use, ready accessibility, high sensitivity for most intradural spinal cord lesions, repeatability, low cost, and rapid learning curve make intraoperative ultrasound the imaging modality of choice for spinal cord tumor surgery and a variety of other spinal surgeries, while unfortunately also being an underutilized imaging modality. There is an abundance of literature outlining and demonstrating the utility of ultrasound in pain management and spinal surgery, summarized in Table 2. Less invasive procedures, such spinal injections, can also be more confidently performed with ultrasound guidance in the pediatric age group, especially infants (Figure 19).

Table 2. Research supporting the use of intraoperative ultrasound. Adapted from Ganau M, Syrmos N, Martin AR, Jiang F, Fehlings MG. Intraoperative ultrasound in spine surgery: history, current applications, future developments. *Quant Imaging Med Surg.* 2018 Apr;8(3):261-267. doi: 10.21037/qims.2018.04.02. PMID: 29774179; PMCID: PMC5941206.

Pathology	Experimental and Clinical Evidence
Dysraphism and cerebrospinal fluid disorder	
Chiari malformation; diastematomyelia (split cord); tethered cord; lipomyelomeningoceles and other lipomas; syringomyelia; cystic dilatation ventriculus terminalis	Brock et al. 2017, Fan et al. 2017, Cui et al. 2011 Cokluk et al. 2004, Aschoff et al.1993, Ganau et al. 2012, Zhang et al. 2017
Tumors and other space occupying lesions	
Astrocytomas, ependymomas, meningiomas, schwannomas, cavernomas	Harel et al. 2016, Zhou et al. 2011, Shamov et al. 2013, Nicácio et al. 2009, Friedman et al. 2003
Functional	
Cerebral palsy	Oki et al. 2010, Graham et al. 2018
Trauma	
Acute spinal cord injuries	Hamamoto et al. 2007, Soubeyrand et al. 2014, Huang et al. 2017, Westergren et al. 2001

Vascular	
Dural fistulas, hemangioblastomas and spinal arteriovenous malformations	Prada et al. 2017, Della Pepa et al. 2018
Degenerative	
Rheumatoid arthritis and pseudotumors, synovial cysts, disc herniations, spinal stenosis	Chibbaro et al. 2017, Alaqeel et al. 2015, Ganau et al. 2013, Nishimura et al. 2014
Pedicle screw instrumentation	
Spinal instability	Aly et al. 2011, Kantelhardt et al. 2008, Gueziri et al. 2020

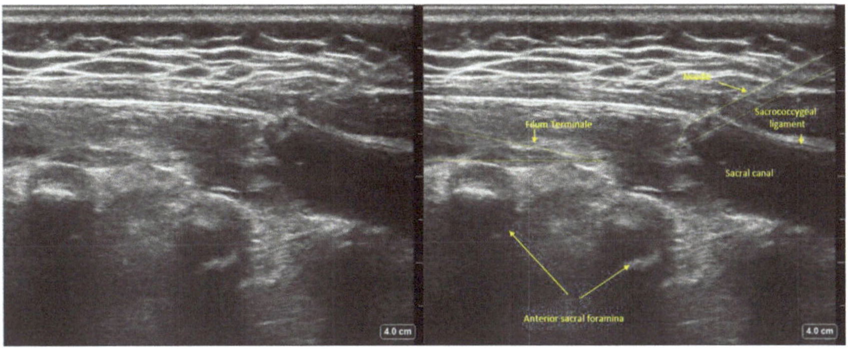

Figure 8-19. Epidural spinal injection through the sacral hiatus and sagittal ultrasound at the sacral hiatus in a newborn. The needle is entering the epidural space via the sacrococcygeal ligament; the filum terminale, the anterior sacral foramina, the sacral canal, the sacrococcygeal ligament, and the needle are labeled in the image to the right. *(Courtesy of Stephanie J. Pan, MD).*

Evaluation and Mapping of Surgical Flap Vascular Anatomy in Plastic Surgery

The development of perforator flaps has popularized minimally invasive free- and pedicled-flap reconstructions for both adult and pediatric patients. Mapping of flaps with ultrasound Doppler or ultra-high frequency ultrasound is a relatively new technique used by plastic surgeons to precisely visualize the perforators piercing the superficial fascia and to follow their course in the hypodermis layer up to, and within, the dermis layer, thus allowing them to precisely mark the superficial fascia perforator vessel location and trace the vascular axiality to optimize the flap design and orientation.[13] For decades surgeons have routinely used handheld Doppler sonography pencil probes operating at 8-10 MHz, with a depth sensitivity of only 20 and 15 mm, respectively, through acoustic coupling gel at the skin-probe interface for identification of vessels (Figure 20). When searching for deep fascial perforators, it has not been useful at depths which are more typical of the flaps desired.[89]

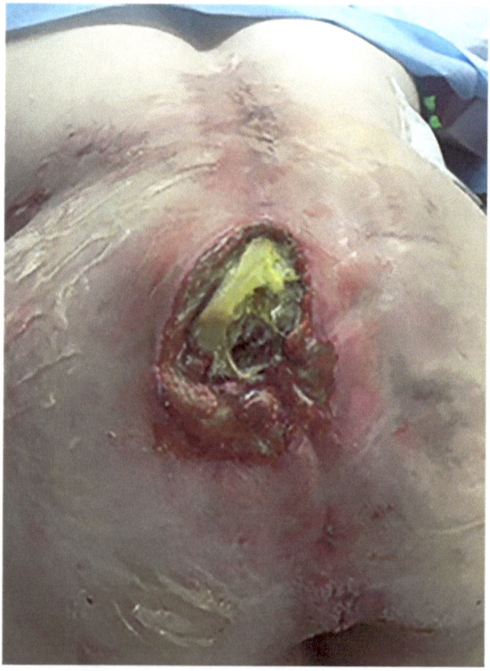

Figure 8-20a

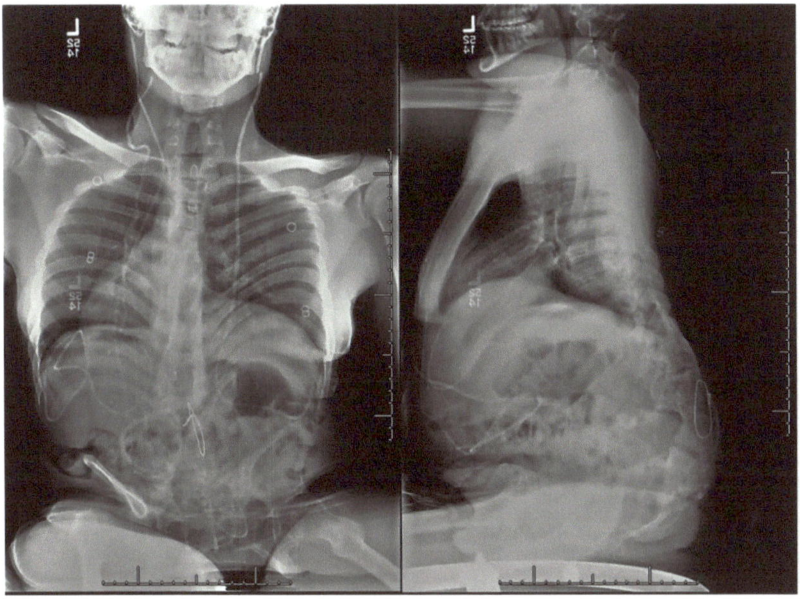

Figure 8-20b

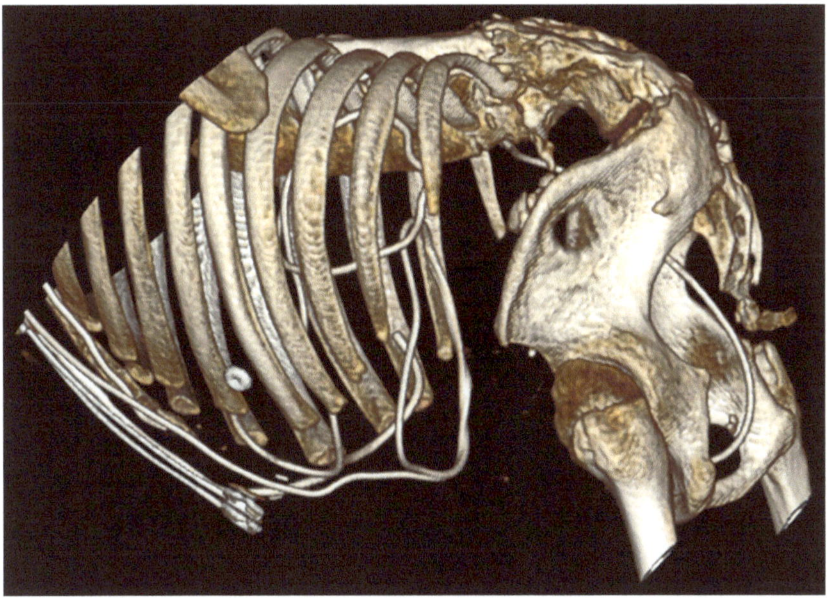

Figure 8-20c

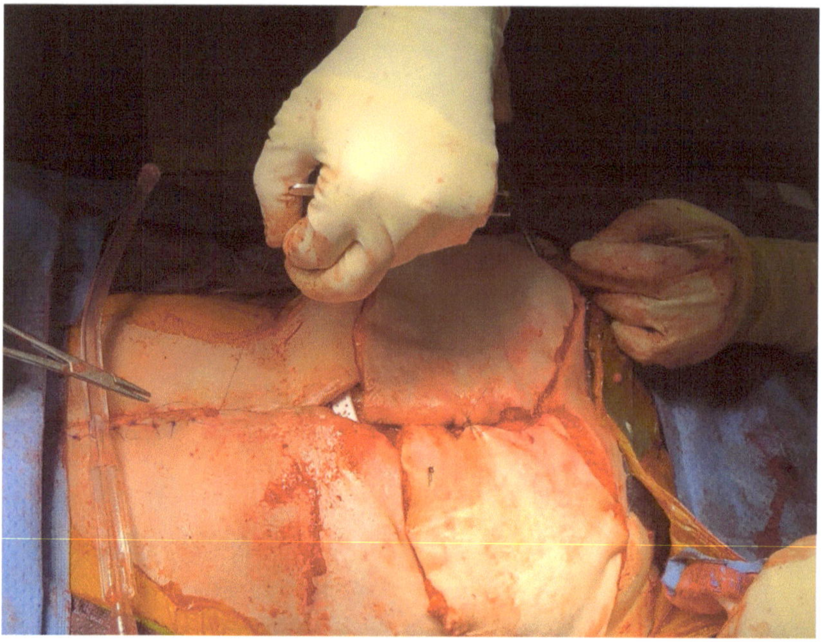

Figure 8-20d

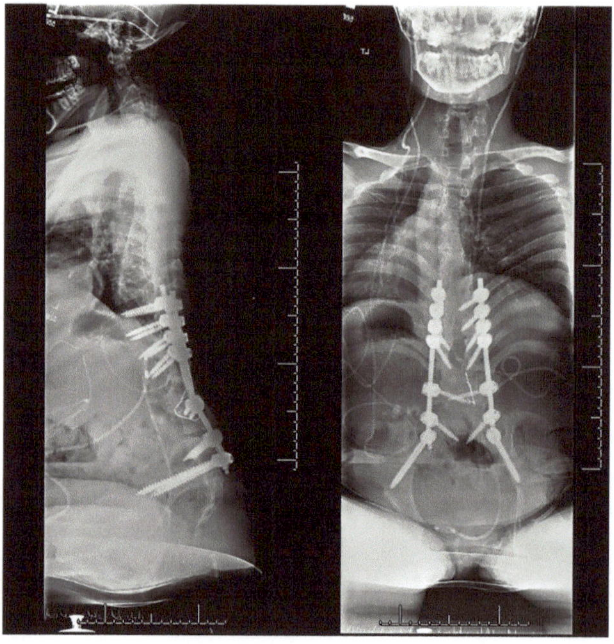

Figure 8-20e

Figure 8-20. Vascular mapping for bilateral advancement gluteal flap creation for a multiply revised infected kyphectomy in a myelomeningocoele patient. The patient had a severe lumbopelvic flexion deformity after a series of prior surgeries in another state, where kyphectomy was performed in infancy and again at 9 years of age. Unfortunately, these attempts were followed by postoperative infections leading to later hardware removal and recurrent deformities which gradually occurred over several years. She then developed a large, chronic sacral decubitus and kyphosis after prior hardware removal and recurrent deformity in the distant past. The patient's decubiti became impossible to control non-operatively and a revision surgery was offered for a third kyphectomy at the apex of the deformity and revision fusion with pedicle screw instrumentation from the thoracic spine to the pelvis. She had multiple office and operative debridements of the decubitus by the plastic surgery service and orthopaedic spine was asked to definitively address the deformity while plastics would provide the definitive soft tissue coverage. (a) This shows the severity of the patient's decubitus ulcer and lumbopelvic kyphosis at the second to the last of her serial incision and debridement surgeries by the plastic surgeons. Ultrasound was used to map out the paths of the superior and inferior gluteal arteries bilaterally on the day of surgery. (b) This shows the preoperative AP and lateral sitting whole spine radiographs of the patient. (c) A three-dimensional reconstruction of the spinal deformity. Bilateral gluteal advancement flaps were used to close the soft tissue defect with full thickness skin flaps over a stable construct (d) These flaps were designed using Doppler mapping of the perforators. (e) These are her 1-year postoperative whole spine sitting radiographs. She is now more than 18 months postoperative and there have been no recurrent decubiti or infections.

Color duplex sonography is based on the same principles as handheld Doppler sonography, but also evaluates the direction of blood flow using the Doppler frequency shift effect and blood flow velocity changes. Color Doppler duplex sonography not only offers information about vessel diameter and course, but can also depict the local three-dimensional footprint of the vascular anatomy. It offers far more information about the anatomy of the vessels and their perforators in reference to the surrounding tissues than a hand-held probe, and it can quantitatively identify the dominant perforators. However, a drawback remains in that it cannot reproduce a two- or three-dimensional image of the complete vascular anatomy to be used by the surgeon during flap design or flap elevation.[89] Direct skin marking and sticky plastic drape overlays with the vascular tree drawn onto the drape have been utilized by plastic surgeons to identify perforator vessels and vascular anatomy during surgery. The newer technique of photoacoustic tomography is an augmented use of ultrasound utilizing near-infrared pulse lasers to excite the red blood cells into releasing ultrasonic waves, which then allows ultrasound imaging to visualize the flow within the vessels.[90]

In-hospital high-definition ultrasound has been used for several years in flap surgery, but is not practical for use in the typical clinic setting. Homsy et al. have explored the use of portable color-flow ultrasound and used it recently in the outpatient setting to facilitate precision flap planning and selection of perforator vessels and reconstructive surgery.[91] After identifying and marking arterial signals using a 5-MHz acoustic Doppler probe, the authors used a tablet computer connected to a linear array L 12-4 ultrasound probe controlled by a software program to obtain high-definition ultrasound images and video recordings. The ultrasound probe was used to identify false positives from the acoustic Doppler, and the true perforators were followed through the subcutaneous tissues to the site of fascial penetration and marked on the skin surface. The largest perforator was selected as the base for the flap design, and the information was correlated to CT angiography images. The thicknesses of the flaps ranged from 2-6 cm, and ultrasound settings were altered to improve vascular clarity. These authors found that the technology allowed in-office vascular mapping and assessments with a short learning time and has substantially reduced the need for CT angiography.[91] The use of high-resolution ultrasound or photoacoustic tomography in planning surgery is now beyond the ability of multidetector CT angiography scanning; it can be used in preoperative and intraoperative planning of traditional perforator flaps used in the coverage of myelomenigocele, sacral ulcers, congenital hand deformities, and traumatic skin defects.[89,91,92]

Conclusion

Ultrasonography is a technique that can be used in the diagnosis of a wide range of conditions, including fractures, hip dysplasia, joint effusions, and spine deformities. Significant research exists that corroborates its value as a diagnostic tool. Adopting ultrasonography as part of the clinical evaluation of pediatric orthopaedic patients provides quick and useful information and can reduce patient exposure to radiation. Ultrasonography is a readily available tool that the pediatric orthopaedic surgeon can master in a short period of time and then broadly apply in practice. Ultrasound, therefore, deserves a wider acceptance and recognition by all orthopaedic surgeons, in particular those caring for younger patients.

References

1. Graf R. Fundamentals of sonographic diagnosis of infant hip dysplasia. *J Pediatr Orthop.* 1984;4(6):735-740. 10.1097/01241398-198411000-00015

2. Harcke HT, Grissom LE. Performing dynamic sonography of the infant hip. *AJR Am J Roentgenol.* 1990;155(4):837-844. 10.2214/ajr.155.4.2119119

3. Adam R, Hendry GM, Moss J, Wild SR, Gillespie I. Arthrosonography of the irritable hip in childhood: a review of 1 year's experience. *Br J Radiol.* 1986;59(699):205-208. 10.1259/0007-1285-59-699-205

4. Wingstrand H, Egund N. Ultrasonography in hip joint effusion. Report of a child with transient synovitis. *Acta Orthop Scand.* 1984;55(4):469-471. 10.3109/17453678408992397

5. Reid MH. Ultrasonic visualization of a cervical cord cystic astrocytoma. *AJR Am J Roentgenol.* 1978;131(5):907-908. 10.2214/ajr.131.5.907

6. Naidich TP, Fernbach SK, McLone DG, Shkolnik A. John Caffey Award. Sonography of the caudal spine and back: congenital anomalies in children. *AJR Am J Roentgenol.* 1984;142(6):1229-1242. 10.2214/ajr.142.6.1229

7. Dohrmann GJ, Rubin JM. Intraoperative ultrasound imaging of the spinal cord: syringomyelia, cysts, and tumors--a preliminary report. *Surg Neurol.* 1982;18(6):395-399. 10.1016/0090-3019(82)90169-0

8. Gerlanc M, Haddad D, Hyatt GW, Langloh JT, St Hilaire P. Ultrasonic study of normal and fractured bone. *Clin Orthop Relat Res.* 1975(111):175-180. 10.1097/00003086-197509000-00025

9. Smeets AJ, Robben SG, Meradji M. Sonographically detected costo-chondral dislocation in an abused child. A new sonographic sign to the radiological spectrum of child abuse. *Pediatr Radiol.* 1990;20(7):566-567. 10.1007/bf02011396

10. Griffith JF, Rainer TH, Ching AS, Law KL, Cocks RA, Metreweli C. Sonography compared with radiography in revealing acute rib fracture. *AJR Am J Roentgenol.* 1999;173(6):1603-1609. 10.2214/ajr.173.6.10584808

11. Verma M, Craig CL, DiPietro MA, Crawford J, VanderHave KL, Farley FA, et al. Serial ultrasound evaluation of pediatric trigger thumb. *J Pediatr Orthop.* 2013;33(3):309-313. 10.1097/BPO.0b013e318287f728

12. Karnik AS, Karnik A, Joshi A. Ultrasound examination of pediatric musculoskeletal diseases and neonatal spine. *Indian J Pediatr.* 2016;83(6):565-577. 10.1007/s12098-015-1957-2

13. Visconti G, Hayashi A, Yoshimatsu H, Bianchi A, Salgarello M. Ultra-high frequency ultrasound in planning capillary perforator flaps: preliminary experience. *J Plast Reconstr Aesthet Surg.* 2018;71(8):1146-1152. 10.1016/j.bjps.2018.05.045

14. Graf R. *Hip sonography: diagnosis and management of infant hip dysplasia.* 2nd ed. New York: Springer Berlin Heidelberg; 2006.

15. Riebel TW, Nasir R, Nazarenko O. The value of sonography in the detection of osteomyelitis. *Pediatr Radiol.* 1996;26(4):291-297. 10.1007/bf01372116

16. Pineda C, Espinosa R, Pena A. Radiographic imaging in osteomyelitis: the role of plain radiography, computed tomography, ultrasonography, magnetic resonance imaging, and scintigraphy. *Semin Plast Surg.* 2009;23(2):80-89. 10.1055/s-0029-1214160

17. Shah NB, Platt SL. ALARA: is there a cause for alarm? Reducing radiation risks from computed tomography scanning in children. *Curr Opin Pediatr.* 2008;20(3):243-247. 10.1097/MOP.0b013e3282ffafd2

18. Montgomery NI, Rosenfeld S. Pediatric osteoarticular infection update. *J Pediatr Orthop.* 2015;35(1):74-81. 10.1097/bpo.0000000000000237

19. Arkader A, Brusalis C, Warner WC, Jr., Conway JH, Noonan K. Update in pediatric musculoskeletal infections: when it is, when it isn't, and what to do. *J Am Acad Orthop Surg.* 2016;24(9):e112-121. 10.5435/jaaos-d-15-00714

20. Krieg AM. A possible cause of joint destruction in septic arthritis. *Arthritis Res.* 1999;1(1):3-4. 10.1186/ar2

21. Agarwal A, Aggarwal AN. Bone and joint infections in children: septic arthritis. *Indian J Pediatr.* 2016;83(8):825-833. 10.1007/s12098-015-1816-1

22. Plumb J, Mallin M, Bolte RG. The role of ultrasound in the emergency department evaluation of the acutely painful pediatric hip. *Pediatr Emerg Care.* 2015;31(1):54-58; quiz 59-61. 10.1097/pec.0000000000000332

23. Gordon JE, Huang M, Dobbs M, Luhmann SJ, Szymanski DA, Schoenecker PL. Causes of false-negative ultrasound scans in the diagnosis of septic arthritis of the hip in children. *J Pediatr Orthop.* 2002;22(3):312-316.

24. Kocher MS, Mandiga R, Zurakowski D, Barnewolt C, Kasser JR. Validation of a clinical prediction rule for the differentiation between septic arthritis and transient synovitis of the hip in children. *J Bone Joint Surg Am.* 2004;86(8):1629-1635. 10.2106/00004623-200408000-00005

25. Caird MS, Flynn JM, Leung YL, Millman JE, D'Italia JG, Dormans JP. Factors distinguishing septic arthritis from transient synovitis of the hip in children. A prospective study. *J Bone Joint Surg Am.* 2006;88(6):1251-1257. 10.2106/jbjs.E.00216

26. Sultan J, Hughes PJ. Septic arthritis or transient synovitis of the hip in children: the value of clinical prediction algorithms. *J Bone Joint Surg Br.* 2010;92(9):1289-1293. 10.1302/0301-620x.92b9.24286

27. Agarwal A, Aggarwal AN. Bone and joint infections in children: acute hematogenous osteomyelitis. *Indian J Pediatr.* 2016;83(8):817-824. 10.1007/s12098-015-1806-3

28. Gilbertson-Dahdal D, Wright JE, Krupinski E, McCurdy WE, Taljanovic MS. Transphyseal involvement of pyogenic osteomyelitis is considerably more common than classically taught. *AJR Am J Roentgenol.* 2014;203(1):190-195. 10.2214/ajr.13.11279

29. Mah ET, LeQuesne GW, Gent RJ, Paterson DC. Ultrasonic signs of pelvic osteomyelitis in children. *Pediatr Radiol.* 1994;24(7):484-487. 10.1007/bf02015005

30. Chau CL, Griffith JF. Musculoskeletal infections: ultrasound appearances. *Clin Radiol.* 2005;60(2):149-159. 10.1016/j.crad.2004.02.005

31. Azam Q, Ahmad I, Abbas M, Syed A, Haque F. Ultrasound and colour Doppler sonography in acute osteomyelitis in children. *Acta Orthop Belg.* 2005;71(5):590-596.

32. Chao HC, Lin SJ, Huang YC, Lin TY. Color Doppler ultrasonographic evaluation of osteomyelitis in children. *J Ultrasound Med.* 1999;18(11):729-734; quiz 735-726. 10.7863/jum.1999.18.11.729

33. Ezzat T, El-Hamid AA, Mostafa M, El-Kady L. Early diagnosis of acute osteomyelitis in children by high-resolution and power Doppler sonography. *The Egyptian Journal of Radiology and Nuclear Medicine.* 2011;42(2):233-242. https://doi.org/10.1016/j.ejrnm.2011.05.002

34. Weber-Chrysochoou C, Corti N, Goetschel P, Altermatt S, Huisman TA, Berger C. Pelvic osteomyelitis: a diagnostic challenge in children. *J Pediatr Surg.* 2007;42(3):553-557. 10.1016/j.jpedsurg.2006.10.048

35. Inusa BP, Oyewo A, Brokke F, Santhikumaran G, Jogeesvaran KH. Dilemma in differentiating between acute osteomyelitis and bone infarction in children with sickle cell disease: the role of ultrasound. *PLoS One.* 2013;8(6):e65001. 10.1371/journal.pone.0065001

36. William RR, Hussein SS, Jeans WD, Wali YA, Lamki ZA. A prospective study of soft-tissue ultrasonography in sickle cell disease patients with suspected osteomyelitis. *Clin Radiol.* 2000;55(4):307-310. 10.1053/crad.1999.0377

37. Bouchoucha S, Benghachame F, Trifa M, Saied W, Douira W, Nessib MN, et al. Deep venous thrombosis associated with acute hematogenous osteomyelitis in children. *Orthop Traumatol Surg Res.* 2010;96(8):890-893. 10.1016/j.otsr.2010.05.006

38. Guillerman RP. Osteomyelitis and beyond. *Pediatr Radiol.* 2013;43 Suppl 1:S193-203. 10.1007/s00247-012-2594-9

39. Trusen A, Beissert M, Schultz G, Chittka B, Darge K. Ultrasound and MRI features of pyomyositis in children. *Eur Radiol.* 2003;13(5):1050-1055. 10.1007/s00330-002-1585-x

40. Royston DD, Cremin BJ. The ultrasonic evaluation of psoas abscess (tropical pyomyositis) in children. *Pediatr Radiol.* 1994;24(7):481-483. 10.1007/bf02015004

41. Breidahl WH, Newman JS, Taljanovic MS, Adler RS. Power Doppler sonography in the assessment of musculoskeletal fluid collections. *AJR Am J Roentgenol.* 1996;166(6):1443-1446. 10.2214/ajr.166.6.8633460

42. Loyer EM, DuBrow RA, David CL, Coan JD, Eftekhari F. Imaging of superficial soft-tissue infections: sonographic findings in cases of cellulitis and abscess. *AJR Am J Roentgenol.* 1996;166(1):149-152. 10.2214/ajr.166.1.8571865

43. Loyer EM, Kaur H, David CL, DuBrow R, Eftekhari FM. Importance of dynamic assessment of the soft tissues in the sonographic diagnosis of echogenic superficial abscesses. *J Ultrasound Med.* 1995;14(9):669-671. 10.7863/jum.1995.14.9.669

44. Chao HC, Lin SJ, Huang YC, Lin TY. Sonographic evaluation of cellulitis in children. *J Ultrasound Med.* 2000;19(11):743-749. 10.7863/jum.2000.19.11.743

45. Chao HC, Kong MS, Lin TY. Diagnosis of necrotizing fasciitis in children. *J Ultrasound Med.* 1999;18(4):277-281. 10.7863/jum.1999.18.4.277

46. Hodgson RJ, O'Connor PJ, Grainger AJ. Tendon and ligament imaging. *Br J Radiol.* 2012;85(1016):1157-1172. 10.1259/bjr/34786470

47. Patel DD, Blumberg SM, Crain EF. The utility of bedside ultrasonography in identifying fractures and guiding fracture reduction in children. *Pediatr Emerg Care.* 2009;25(4):221-225. 10.1097/pec.0b013e31819e34f7

48. Cross KP, Warkentine FH, Kim IK, Gracely E, Paul RI. Bedside ultrasound diagnosis of clavicle fractures in the pediatric emergency department. *Acad Emerg Med.* 2010;17(7):687-693. 10.1111/j.1553-2712.2010.00788.x

49. Tsou PY, Ma YK, Wang YH, Gillon JT, Rafael J, Deanehan JK. Diagnostic accuracy of ultrasound for upper extremity fractures in children: a systematic review and meta-analysis. *Am J Emerg Med.* 2021;44:383-394. 10.1016/j.ajem.2020.04.071

50. Douma-den Hamer D, Blanker MH, Edens MA, Buijteweg LN, Boomsma MF, van Helden SH, et al. Ultrasound for distal forearm fracture: a systematic review and diagnostic meta-analysis. *PLoS One.* 2016;11(5):e0155659. 10.1371/journal.pone.0155659

51. Chen L, Kim Y, Moore CL. Diagnosis and guided reduction of forearm fractures in children using bedside ultrasound. *Pediatr Emerg Care.* 2007;23(8):528-531. 10.1097/PEC.0b013e318128f85d

52. Lee MC, Stone NE, 3rd, Ritting AW, Silverstein EA, Pierz KA, Johnson DA, et al. Mini-C-arm fluoroscopy for emergency-department reduction of pediatric forearm fractures. *J Bone Joint Surg Am.* 2011;93(15):1442-1447. 10.2106/jbjs.J.01052

53. Sumko MJ, Hennrikus W, Slough J, Jensen K, Armstrong D, King S, et al. Measurement of radiation exposure when using the mini C-arm to reduce pediatric upper extremity fractures. *J Pediatr Orthop.* 2016;36(2):122-125. 10.1097/bpo.0000000000000422

54. Litrenta J, Masrouha K, Wasterlain A, Castaneda P. Ultrasound evaluation of pediatric orthopaedic patients. *J Am Acad Orthop Surg.* 2020;28(16):e696-e705. 10.5435/jaaos-d-17-00895

55. Iyer RS, Thapa MM, Khanna PC, Chew FS. Pediatric bone imaging: imaging elbow trauma in children--a review of acute and chronic injuries. *AJR Am J Roentgenol.* 2012;198(5):1053-1068. 10.2214/ajr.10.7314

56. Major NM, Crawford ST. Elbow effusions in trauma in adults and children: is there an occult fracture? *AJR Am J Roentgenol.* 2002;178(2):413-418. 10.2214/ajr.178.2.1780413

57. Skaggs DL, Mirzayan R. The posterior fat pad sign in association with occult fracture of the elbow in children. *J Bone Joint Surg Am.* 1999;81(10):1429-1433. 10.2106/00004623-199910000-00007

58. Blumberg SM, Kunkov S, Crain EF, Goldman HS. The predictive value of a normal radiographic anterior fat pad sign following elbow trauma in children. *Pediatr Emerg Care.* 2011;27(7):596-600. 10.1097/PEC.0b013e318222553b

59. De Maeseneer M, Jacobson JA, Jaovisidha S, Lenchik L, Ryu KN, Trudell DR, et al. Elbow effusions: distribution of joint fluid with flexion and extension and imaging implications. *Invest Radiol.* 1998;33(2):117-125. 10.1097/00004424-199802000-00010

60. Carson S, Woolridge DP, Colletti J, Kilgore K. Pediatric upper extremity injuries. *Pediatr Clin North Am.* 2006;53(1):41-67, v. 10.1016/j.pcl.2005.10.003

61. Broker FH, Burbach T. Ultrasonic diagnosis of separation of the proximal humeral epiphysis in the newborn. *J Bone Joint Surg Am.* 1990;72(2):187-191.

62. Zieger M, Dörr U, Schulz RD. Sonography of slipped humeral epiphysis due to birth injury. *Pediatr Radiol.* 1987;17(5):425-426. 10.1007/bf02396624

63. Ekengren K, Bergdahl S, Ekström G. Birth injuries to the epiphyseal cartilage. *Acta Radiol Diagn (Stockh).* 1978;19(1b):197-204. 10.1177/028418517801901b06

64. Goldfisher R, Amodio J. Separation of the proximal humeral epiphysis in the newborn: rapid diagnosis with ultrasonography. *Case Rep Pediatr.* 2015;2015:825413. 10.1155/2015/825413

65. Lewis D, Logan P. Sonographic diagnosis of toddler's fracture in the emergency department. *J Clin Ultrasound.* 2006;34(4):190-194. 10.1002/jcu.20192

66. Warkentine FH, Horowitz R, Pierce MC. The use of ultrasound to detect occult or unsuspected fractures in child abuse. *Pediatr Emerg Care.* 2014;30(1):43-46. 10.1097/pec.0000000000000064

67. Barata I, Spencer R, Suppiah A, Raio C, Ward MF, Sama A. Emergency ultrasound in the detection of pediatric long-bone fractures. *Pediatr Emerg Care.* 2012;28(11):1154-1157. 10.1097/PEC.0b013e3182716fb7

68. Weinberg ER, Tunik MG, Tsung JW. Accuracy of clinician-performed point-of-care ultrasound for the diagnosis of fractures in children and young adults. *Injury.* 2010;41(8):862-868. 10.1016/j.injury.2010.04.020

69. Lamrani YA, Maâroufi M, Kamaoui I, Ammor H, Houssaini NS, Tizniti S. Neonatal distal femoral epiphyseal dislocation: an ultrasound diagnosis. *J Med Ultrason (2001).* 2011;38(4):221-223. 10.1007/s10396-011-0312-0

70. Maffulli N, Thornton A. Ultrasonographic appearance of external callus in long-bone fractures. *Injury.* 1995;26(1):5-12. 10.1016/0020-1383(95)90544-8

71. Caruso G, Lagalla R, Derchi L, Iovane A, Sanfilippo A. Monitoring of fracture calluses with color Doppler

sonography. *J Clin Ultrasound.* 2000;28(1):20-27. 10.1002/(sici)1097-0096(200001)28:1<20::aid-jcu3>3.0.co;2-w

72. Wawrzyk M, Sokal J, Andrzejewska E, Przewratil P. The role of ultrasound imaging of callus formation in the treatment of long bone fractures in children. *Pol J Radiol.* 2015;80:473-478. 10.12659/pjr.894548

73. Ladino Torres MF, DiPietro MA. Spine ultrasound imaging in the newborn. *Semin Ultrasound CT MR.* 2014;35(6):652-661. 10.1053/j.sult.2014.08.001

74. Lowe LH, Johanek AJ, Moore CW. Sonography of the neonatal spine: part 2, spinal disorders. *AJR Am J Roentgenol.* 2007;188(3):739-744. 10.2214/ajr.05.2160

75. Hill CA, Gibson PJ. Ultrasound determination of the normal location of the conus medullaris in neonates. *AJNR Am J Neuroradiol.* 1995;16(3):469-472.

76. Hoffman HJ, Hendrick EB, Humphreys RP. The tethered spinal cord: its protean manifestations, diagnosis and surgical correction. *Childs Brain.* 1976;2(3):145-155. 10.1159/000119610

77. Iftikhar W, De Jesus O. Spinal dysraphism and myelomeningocele. In. *StatPearls [Internet].* Vol 2021 Jan. Treasure Island, FL: StatPearls Publishing; 2021.

78. Ganau M, Syrmos N, Martin AR, Jiang F, Fehlings MG. Intraoperative ultrasound in spine surgery: history, current applications, future developments. *Quant Imaging Med Surg.* 2018;8(3):261-267. 10.21037/qims.2018.04.02

79. Cokluk C, Jobe KW, Senel A, Iyigun O, Aydin K. Use of intraoperative ultrasonography during the surgical repair of pediatric cystic spinal dysraphism--technical note. *Neurol Med Chir (Tokyo).* 2004;44(9):502-505; discussion 506. 10.2176/nmc.44.502

80. Masuzawa H, Kamitani H, Sato J, Inoya H, Hachiya J, Sakai F. [Intraoperative application of sector scanning electronic ultrasound in neurosurgery (author's transl)]. *Neurol Med Chir (Tokyo).* 1981;21(3):277-285. 10.2176/nmc.21.277

81. Harel R, Knoller N. Intraoperative spine ultrasound: application and benefits. *Eur Spine J.* 2016;25(3):865-869. 10.1007/s00586-015-4222-5

82. Chandler WF, Knake JE. Intraoperative use of ultrasound in neurosurgery. *Clin Neurosurg.* 1983;31:550-563. 10.1093/neurosurgery/31.cn_suppl_1.550

83. Epstein FJ, Farmer JP, Schneider SJ. Intraoperative ultrasonography: an important surgical adjunct for intramedullary tumors. *J Neurosurg.* 1991;74(5):729-733. 10.3171/jns.1991.74.5.0729

84. Ivanov M, Budu A, Sims-Williams H, Poeata I. Using intraoperative ultrasonography for spinal cord tumor surgery. *World Neurosurg.* 2017;97:104-111. 10.1016/j.wneu.2016.09.097

85. Brock RS, Taricco MA, de Oliveira MF, de Lima Oliveira M, Teixeira MJ, Bor-Seng-Shu E. Intraoperative ultrasonography for definition of less invasive surgical technique in patients with Chiari type I malformation. *World Neurosurg.* 2017;101:466-475. 10.1016/j.wneu.2017.02.003

86. Aly AH, Ginsberg HJ, Cobbold RS. On ultrasound imaging for guided screw insertion in spinal fusion surgery. *Ultrasound Med Biol.* 2011;37(4):651-664. 10.1016/j.ultrasmedbio.2011.01.011

87. Kantelhardt SR, Bock CH, Larsen J, Bockermann V, Schillinger W, Rohde V, et al. Intraosseous ultrasound in the placement of pedicle screws in the lumbar spine. *Spine (Phila Pa 1976).* 2009;34(4):400-407. 10.1097/BRS.0b013e31819286ca

88. Gueziri H-E, Yan CXB, Collins DL. Open-source software for ultrasound-based guidance in spinal fusion surgery. *Ultrasound in Medicine & Biology.* 2020;46(12):3353-3368. https://doi.org/10.1016/j.ultrasmedbio.2020.08.005

89. Smit JM, Klein S, Werker PM. An overview of methods for vascular mapping in the planning of free flaps. *J Plast Reconstr Aesthet Surg.* 2010;63(9):e674-682. 10.1016/j.bjps.2010.06.013

90. Tsuge I, Saito S, Yamamoto G, Sekiguchi H, Yoshikawa A, Matsumoto Y, et al. Preoperative vascular mapping for anterolateral thigh flap surgeries: a clinical trial of photoacoustic tomography imaging. *Microsurgery.* 2020;40(3):324-330. 10.1002/micr.30531

91. Homsy C, McCarthy ME, Lim S, Lindsey JT, Jr., Sands TT, Lindsey JT, Sr. Portable color-flow ultrasound facilitates precision flap planning and perforator selection in reconstructive plastic surgery. *Ann Plast Surg.* 2020;84(6S Suppl 5):S424-s430. 10.1097/sap.0000000000002203

92. Kehrer A, Sachanadani NS, da Silva NPB, Lonic D, Heidekrueger P, Taeger CD, et al. Step-by-step guide to ultrasound-based design of alt flaps by the microsurgeon - Basic and advanced applications and device settings. *J Plast Reconstr Aesthet Surg.* 2020;73(6):1081-1090. 10.1016/j.bjps.2019.11.035

Chapter 9 Integrating Ultrasound into your Practice

- Dean W Ziegler, MD
- Spencer H. Moore, MD

As described in the previous chapters, in-office ultrasound provides enhanced evaluation and management of all types of orthopaedic disorders. It is efficient and effective in establishing orthopaedic diagnoses and precisely guiding interventions. It is convenient for both the surgeon and patient while adding educational value for both. Static, dynamic, and functional imaging enhances the understanding of the patient's dysfunction. Along with these areas of increased quality, value is further improved given the relative low cost of diagnostic ultrasound compared to other advanced imaging modalities. The question then is "why is ultrasound not better utilized in the orthopaedic clinic?"

In a survey given to all members of the American Shoulder and Elbow Surgeons, Kruse et al. found the most common excuse for not using in-office ultrasound given by members of the American Shoulder and Elbow Surgeons was a lack of confidence in the ability to determine the reparability of the rotator cuff tear (83.3%)[1]. Other reasons included: not having an ultrasound machine (34%), too busy to use ultrasound in the office for diagnostic purposes (36%), and lack of confidence in diagnosing tears (39%). Only 26.6% of members responded and of those 58% had an ultrasound in their office, 55% used ultrasound for diagnostic purposes in the shoulder and 50% used ultrasound for guided interventions in the shoulder.

Getting Started

The most important concern for many surgeons considering implementing in-office ultrasound is having confidence in obtaining the desired information regarding the structure being imaged. Initially, gaining this confidence starts by getting your hands on any ultrasound machine and beginning to image. As discussed in the introduction, the best person to perform ultrasound imaging is someone who has an excellent three-dimensional anatomic understanding of the structure being imaged. The anatomic understanding is there, given an orthopaedic surgeon's extensive clinical and surgical experience. Competence, as with all skills, comes with practice and use. An orthopaedic surgeon already has enhanced hand eye coordination, especially if they are comfortable with arthroscopy. Obtaining skills in ultrasound is also comparable to obtaining those in arthroscopy. With arthroscopy we start learning diagnostic procedures first, followed by ablative procedures and then finally reconstructive procedures. This will be somewhat similar with ultrasound, although we are not really doing any ultrasonic reconstruction at this point. With ultrasound, diagnostic procedures are somewhat harder to master than injections, given that many injections are already done "blindly" using bony landmarks. Therefore, the educational process tends to proceed with injections, followed by diagnosis, and finally ablation.

As when acquiring any new skill, read whatever you can, including this and other ultrasound texts, watch videos and if possible, attend an instructional lecture either at a meeting, online or at a formal ultrasound course. If you can get your hands on an ultrasound machine that is portable, take it home and start imaging family members, friends or anyone who will sit still long enough to let you. If you are in a training program in which there are faculty that utilize in-office ultrasound, get as much experience with them as possible. After already examining the patient clinically, perform a brief diagnostic ultrasound exam of the anatomic structure in question prior to the attending surgeon performs the diagnostic exam or ultrasound guided intervention. Then compare your findings with those of the attending surgeon, making sure to note how the more experienced surgeon can obtain quality diagnostic images. If you are already in practice, in the same manner, spend time with one of your partners who is already using ultrasound or seek out someone in your community or elsewhere (including one of the authors of this book). Most surgeons experienced in extensively using ultrasound are eager to share knowledge and skills.

Orthopaedic surgeons are comfortable with reading MRI scans and can utilize available MRIs for learning ultrasound skills. Both techniques are used to visualize soft tissues. Comparing your ultrasound images with the MRI is useful in learning, especially if it is a high-quality MRI. As you become more comfortable you will rely on the ultrasound more heavily to examine structures that are near the skin and not obstructed by air or fat. Eventually you will be checking outside MRI images against your ultrasound as you gain more experience, or to check the progress of the disease. Eventually, you will be using ultrasound to gain better information when the MRI is of poor quality, or you value the active, dynamic and functional imaging the ultrasound allows, compared to the static MRI images.

Learning ultrasound involves practice. The learning curve is more like that of a cello rather than a violin: A lot of ultrasound skills can be acquired very quickly. Early on, the learner should work on their own acquiring the basic skills such as turning on the machine, adjusting the focus, adjusting the gain and frequency. Then the learner should attend a course so that they can watch the experts at work. As with acquiring any new talent, you can gain more by watching an expert after you already have some skills.

Once you have access to an ultrasound in clinic, use it to do all the injections you are currently doing with bony references. Perform a brief exam prior to initiating the injection.

As you progress while using ultrasound to help guide injections, becoming comfortable with nonstandard orthogonal planes is important.

When possible, use ultrasound to assess trauma in the emergency room. An example is this shotgun shell piece that was found in the elbow (Figure 1). Ultrasound allows the assessment of the path of entry, the surrounding structures, and the best surgical path for removal.

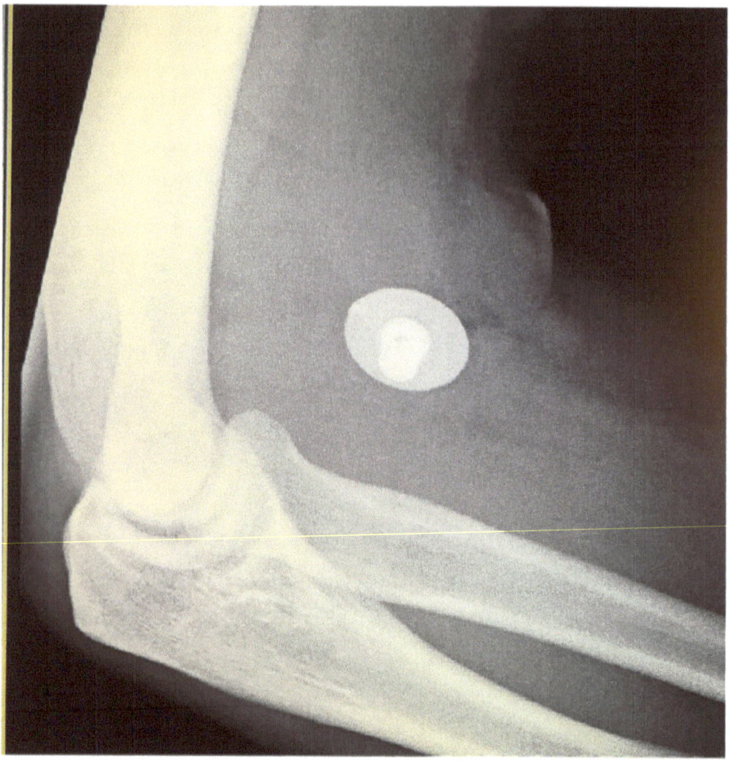

Figure 9-1a: Radiographic image of shotgun casing in elbow.

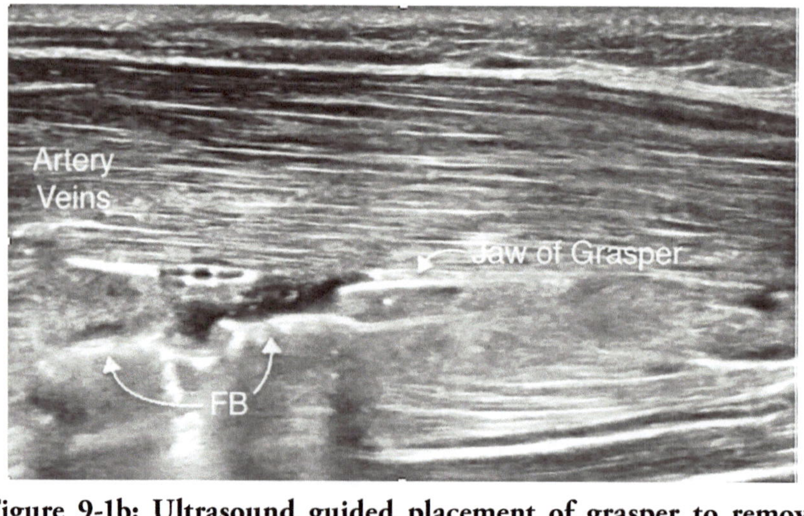

Figure 9-1b: Ultrasound guided placement of grasper to remove shotgun casing foreign body (FB).

Checking your work in the operating room is also beneficial when honing your ultrasound skills. Figure 2 demonstrated an example of a distal tibia fracture screw that is too long and is pushing on the posterior tibial nerve.

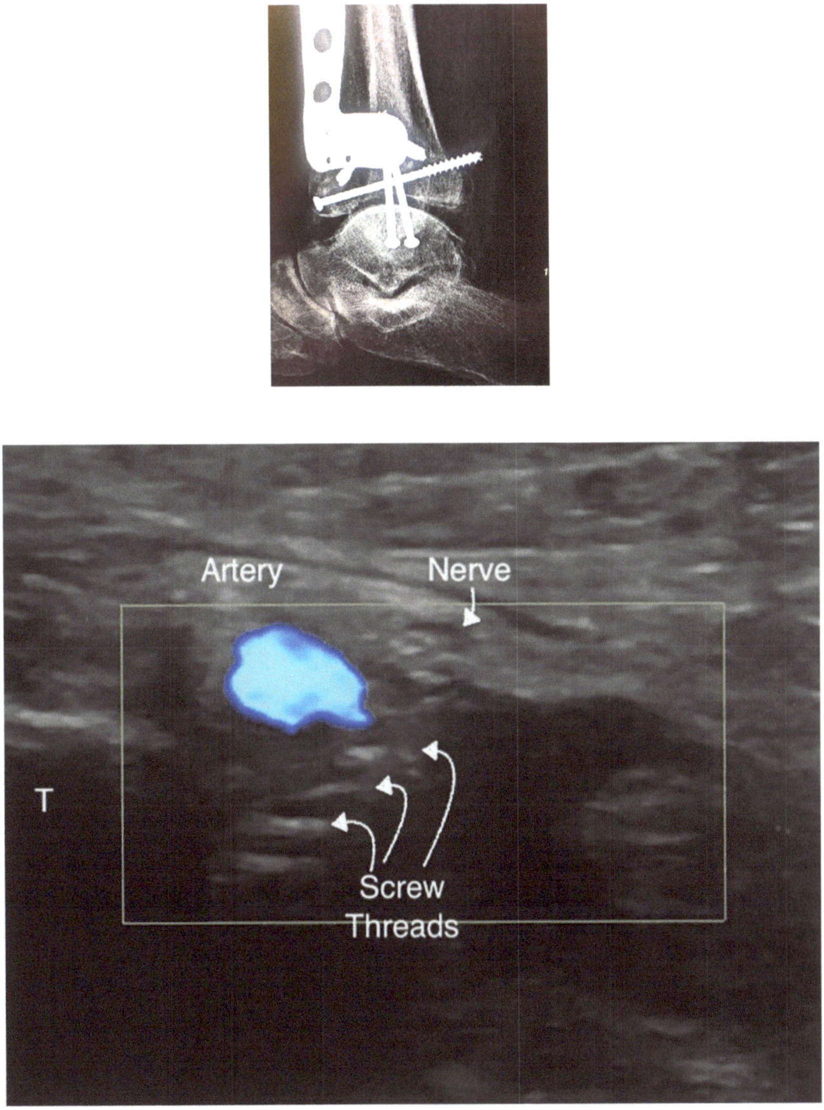

Figure 9-2: Radiograph (a) documenting distal tibia plate screw exiting the posterior tibia with ultrasound confirmation (b) of the screw pushing on the posterior tibial nerve.

In fracture work we like to make sure that our hardware is not pushing on soft tissue in a way that will become a problem later. A prominent radial plate may rub against the FCR. But even more difficult to detect is a screw that is extending beyond the bone on the back side of the radius or on the backside of the distal tibia in a severe ankle fracture. Ultrasound will allow the surgeon to see if it is protruding on an unexposed surface and if it is pushing on important soft tissues.

Utilize ultrasound with other interventional procedures you are comfortable with. These include peripheral nerve blocks. For example, blocking the median and ulnar nerves for in-office fracture reduction. A popliteal block is good for foot and ankle fractures. Nerve block needles are less sharp than our usual injection needles and are less liable to do damage to a nerve. A median nerve block can be done in or out of plane as one would do a hydro dissection for a carpal tunnel release. Ultrasound is also good for draining infections in the office. As usual you will be most comfortable performing interventional ultrasound in those regions of the body where you frequently use the ultrasound for diagnostic purposes.

Obtaining an Ultrasound Machine

When it comes time to buy a machine, the variety of options can be intimidating. It can also be hard to know what you will need when you are first starting out. You do not want to spend more money than necessary, but you also don't want to buy a machine that will need to be upgraded in two years if not two months. It is important to first consider for what applications you will be using the machine. Are you a hand surgeon who is mainly interested in imaging the median nerve and performing small joint injections? If so, a handheld machine may be sufficient, but is probably not going to provide the depth required to perform ultrasound guided hip injections or the quality to do carpal tunnel releases. Also, keep in mind that when your partners recognize your ability to perform diagnostic and interventional ultrasound, they will be sending their patients your way. You may find yourself imaging structures you are not usually evaluating clinically. The following paragraphs will explain the different types of machines, probes, and software features to help you navigate buying your own.

Machine format and size

There are many different system configurations available, which in this book we will divide into four basic categories (listed in order from largest to smallest): console, laptop style, tablet style, and handheld. As you go up in size you get more features, bigger screens, more buttons, and generally better imaging quality, but the tradeoff is reduced mobility and potentially increased cost. Conversely, the smaller machines are highly portable, with some even being able to fit in your pocket but will have far fewer features and the imaging quality will be more limited. However, as with any technology, the quality and features built into the smaller devices continues to improve. Features continue to advance. Designs continuously change.

Console: The console-based machines are the most powerful of the bunch, and the least mobile (Figure 3).

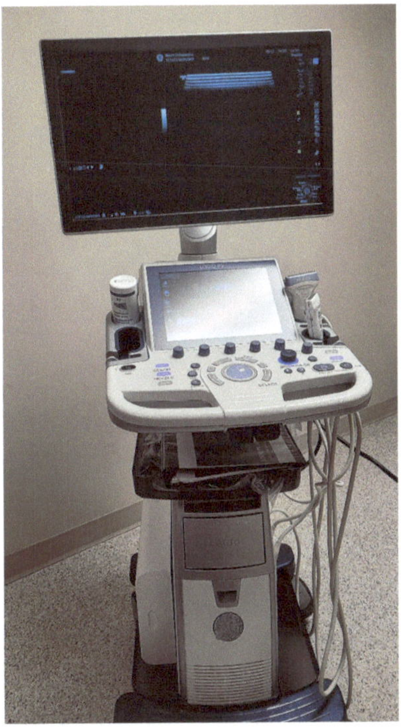

Figure 9-3: Console ultrasound.

These are generally a monitor mounted to a base with a control panel that has lots of buttons. Most of these options are fitted with wheels to allow for movement of the machine around the office, but they are too big to move to multiple locations and perhaps in the bigger machines difficult to move from room to room. These will be your most high powered options and will have every software feature you want, can handle multiple probes at one time, have a big monitor, etc. The console is the gold standard. These also tend to be the most expensive because you are investing in the best image quality and the most features. Consoles can be moved from room to room, and if you plan on doing so, these usually have the best battery life with some options being able to run for hours between charges. These are well-suited to the operating room, and you can share with other surgeons. For example, the machine used by the orthopaedic surgeon for carpal tunnel release can be used by the otolaryngologist to localize parathyroid glands.

Laptop: The laptop-style ultrasound machine is the biggest portable option that still features physical buttons (Figure 4).

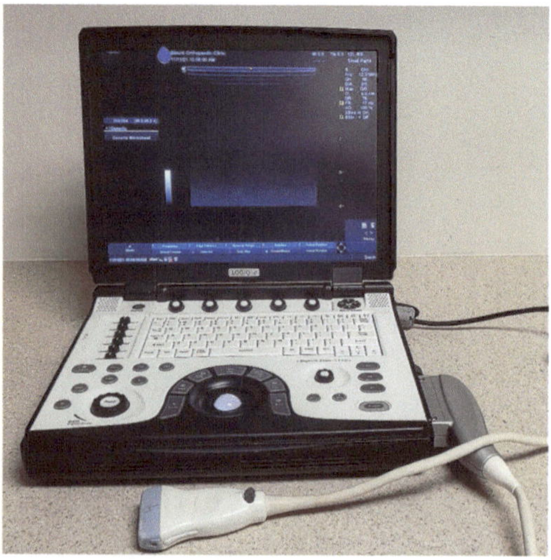

Figure 9-4: Laptop style ultrasound.

These are compact enough that they can be carried with a clinician as they travel to multiple sites. The laptop offers the advantage of physical buttons on the machine itself, a mounted screen, and a good array of software features. Many of these also have the ability to handle different probes, but they typically have to be exchanged out or an adapter may be required to connect more than one probe at a time. These will be slightly more limited in what software options are available than the consoles. Since these will likely be going with the clinician to the point of care, battery life is an important consideration.

Touchscreen: The touchscreen style machine is similar to the laptop in that it is portable and great for use at multiple locations (Figure 5).

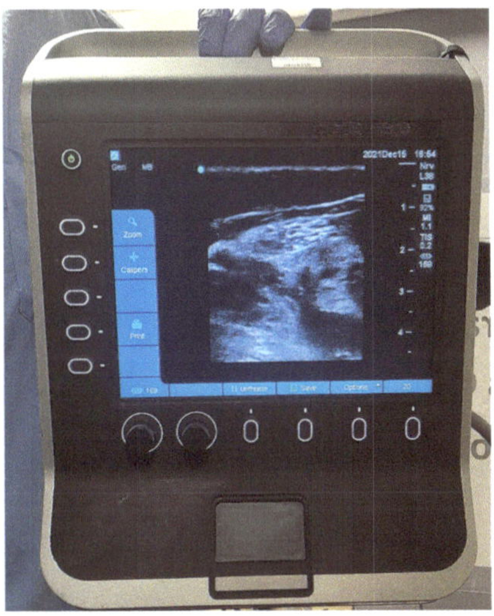

Figure 9-5: Touch screen style ultrasound.

These machines do not have physical buttons and are designed to deliver a more "user friendly" and intuitive interface. In addition, these machines are easier to clean without chemicals leaking between the keys. Because of this, the engineers have hidden or limited certain advanced features in many cases. The intuitive smartphone-like interaction will be welcomed by beginners, however more experienced users can find it frustrating as they will not be able to fine-tune the settings in the same way. Like the laptops, touchscreens generally have smaller screens than the consoles, can handle one probe at a time, and battery life is important to consider.

Handheld: Handheld devices (Figure 6) are those with a smaller setup designed to maximize portability.

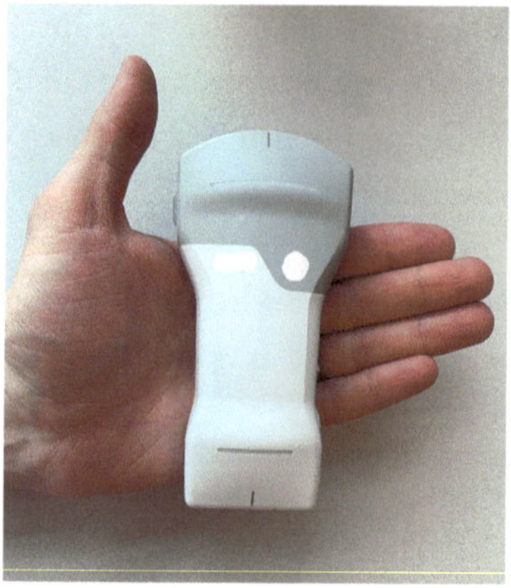

Figure 9-6a

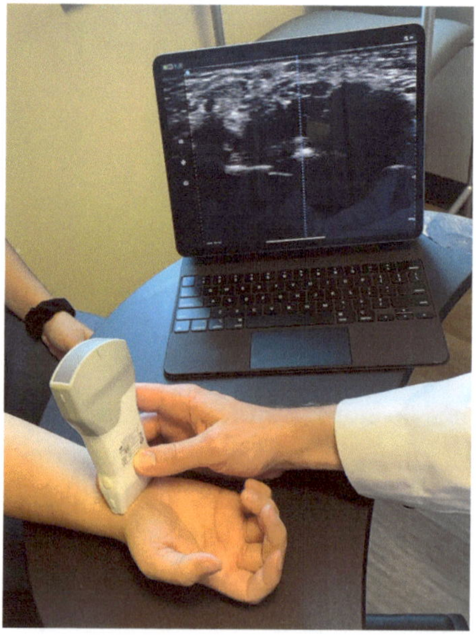

Figure 9-6b

Figure 9-6: Handheld ultrasound probe (a) with wireless connection to surgeon's laptop (b).

These come in numerous different configurations from fixed tablet, probes that can be plugged into any mobile device, and even wireless probes that connect through Bluetooth to your smartphone or tablet. In general, the devices in this category are going to maximize a friendly user interface and portability at the sacrifice of advanced features. Common issues for handheld devices are limited battery life, overheating, limited software features, and limited probe options. These devices will often be cheaper but may frustrate the user as they come to rely on ultrasound more in their practice. Despite these challenges, handhelds have seen a tremendous amount of advancement in their capabilities recently and are growing in popularity.

Probe selection

Perhaps the most important piece of the ultrasound machine is the probe. This is where most of your money is going. Without a high-quality probe, the image quality will suffer. Additionally, it is important to select the right style of probe. The three styles most commonly found are: curvilinear, linear, and hockey-stick. These probes may additionally have buttons, which can be used with the hand on the probe to direct functions on the machine. This can be especially useful when hands are limited and performing ultrasound guided injections, but also can be annoying if you are constantly pushing them accidentally during normal use.

Curvilinear: A curvilinear probe (Figure 7) is a semicircular probe of large size.

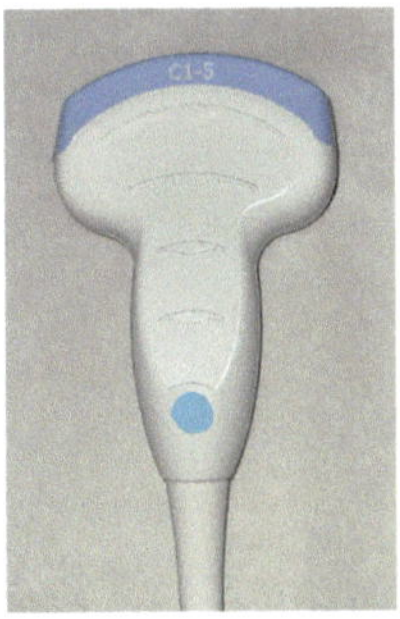

Figure 9-7: Curvilinear probe.

These probes fan out their sound waves so they will image a broader area than a straight linear probe. The thought behind the curvilinear design is to reduce anisotropy by varying the angle of the sound waves produced in the periphery. These are generally restricted to lower frequencies and therefore have better penetration, but worse resolution. MSK applications include imaging the hip and the deep structures of the shoulder in patients with a lot of adipose tissue. Another indication for the curvilinear is for a panorama view of an injection as it offers a longer view of the approach. Therefore, you may diagnose with the linear probe and then inject the same structure with the curvilinear.

Linear: This is the workhorse probe of ultrasound examination. Linear probes (Figures 8a & b) produce a straight soundwave and have a wide range of frequencies. They are slightly more limited in the deep penetration of tissues but have excellent resolution at high frequencies. They are useful for imaging the wrist and hand, foot and ankle, and shoulder.

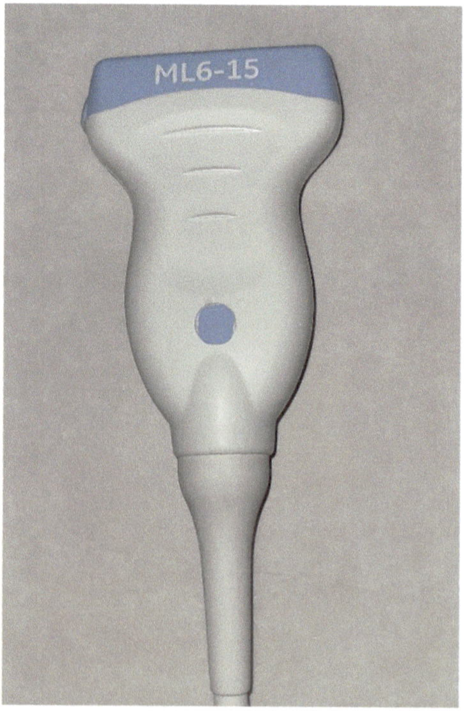

Figure 9-8a: Standard linear probe.

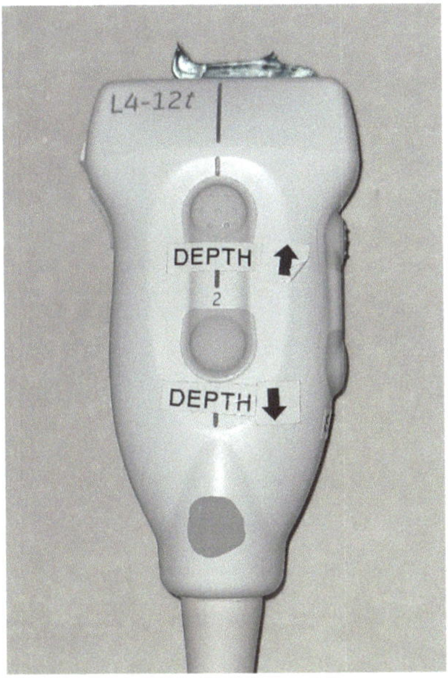

Figure 9-8b: Smaller linear probe including centering lines and remote buttons.

Hockey-stick: These are the smallest probe options, limited to superficial examinations and injections (Figure 9).

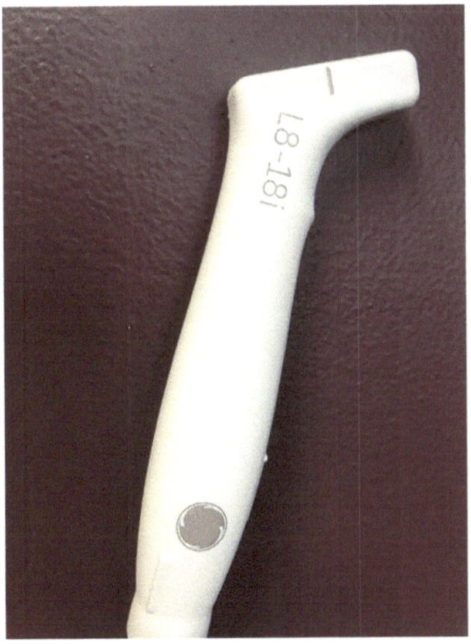

Figure 9-9: Hockey stick probe

They operate at high frequencies so have great resolution but poor penetration. They are smaller so easier to maneuver, but do not image as large of an area as larger probes. Hockey stick probes are great for hand and wrist or superficial structures around the foot and ankle.

Foot pedal

As in arthroscopy, a foot pedal can be used to allow the operator to control imaging while the hands are holding the probe or an instrument.

Software features

The number and variety of software features can make your head spin. To make matters more confusing, certain manufactures advertise proprietary names for features making them hard to compare. For simplicity, common features will be presented here that you will likely encounter when shopping. Some of these are a must, and some are restricted to more experimental applications. In general, you will get more features and greater control over the image quality with consoles, then progressively fewer and more simplified features as the machine becomes more portable.

Recording and saving: You want to make sure that you can record video and stills and have a robust system for saving these for the purposes of future reference and billing. Most machines can export images in the DICOM format, which can be uploaded directly and wirelessly to a PACS system. Other options available include hard drive and cloud storage.

Common measurements: You will almost certainly want to be able to measure from point-to-point and every machine on the market should have the ability to do this (Figure 10).

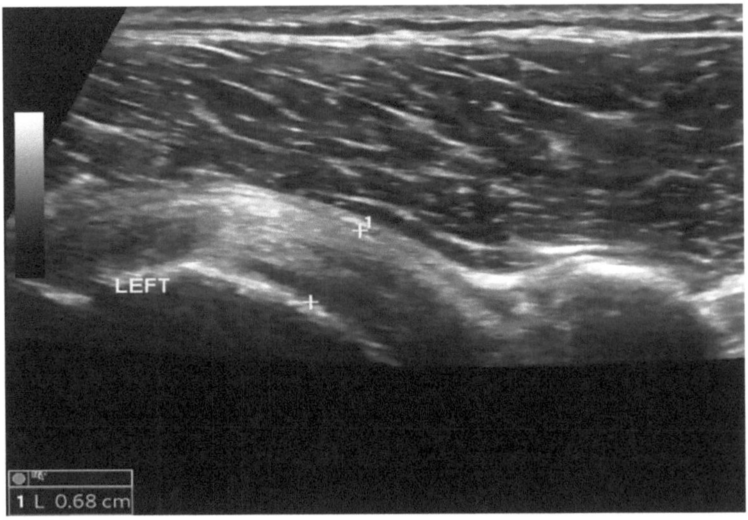

Figure 9-10: Example of linear measurement, in this case the thickness of the subscapularis tendon.

Most machines offer the ability to measure cross-sectional area, though not all the portable options will necessarily have this feature (Figure 11). Consider any other measurements you may need to make and ask regarding the given machine's capabilities.

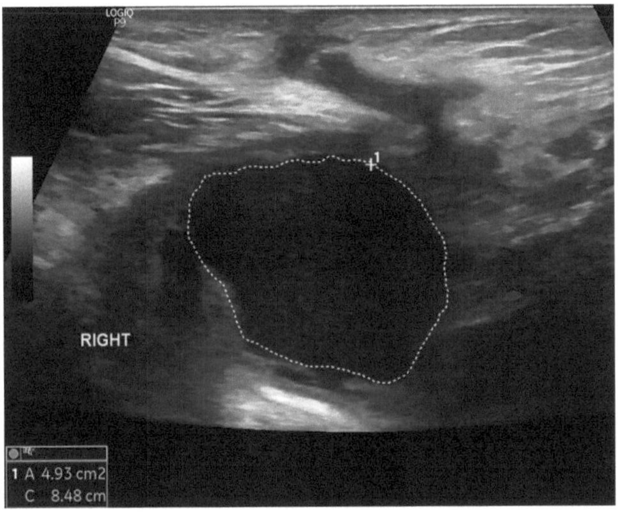

Figure 9-11: Circumference and cross-sectional area measurement of subcutaneous abscess prior to aspiration.

Side-to-side comparison: A useful feature of ultrasound is the ability to perform dynamic and even functional exams. Many machines offer the ability to freeze a frame and continue to examine the patient in a frame next to it for comparison. For example, when imaging the supraspinatus muscle belly, you can compare the size of the muscle in the fossa before and after contraction to help determine the actual functional quality of the muscle (Figure 12).

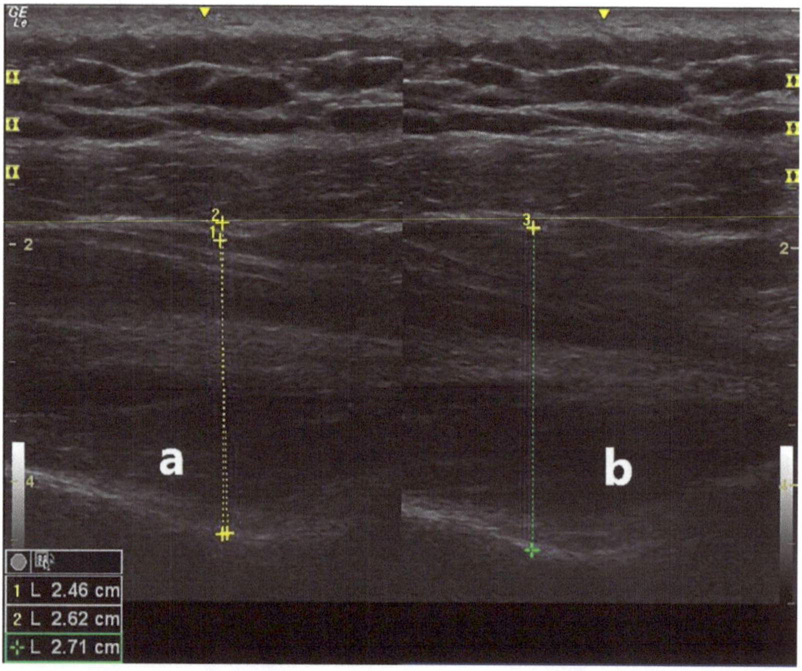

Figure 9-12: Side-to-side comparison on supraspinatus muscle belly. On the left at rest (a) and on the right thickening during isometric contraction (b), including linear measurements in lower left corner.

Doppler: To avoid oversimplifying what can become a complex discussion of ultrasound physics, Doppler allows us to visualize flow within an image. There are two main types of Doppler available that would be useful to know for an orthopaedic surgeon: color and power. Color Doppler provides information about directionality of the flow (usually depicted as blue vs. red) but is less sensitive to lower flow rates. Power Doppler is more sensitive but does not provide information about directionality. Generally, when we are looking at Doppler on ultrasound it is color Doppler. Power Doppler has the useful ability to detect blood flow within a mass of tissue (useful for examining a mass suspected to be tumor or possibly tendon looking for the angiogenesis that forms in response to injury).

Presets: Most devices come with a variety of presets focused on certain applications or anatomic areas. These are a combination of frequency ranges, focal ranges, special features, etc. built in to help deliver good image quality quickly for imaging a certain anatomic area. There are a wide range of preset options, and they are manufacture specific.

Harmonic imaging: This is a more advanced setting that uses the harmonic frequency created by the sound wave going through the tissue to help augment the resolution of the image. Basically, what that means is that this technology helps to improve penetration and image quality. This is not a setting you will likely ever adjust, but a feature that will be advertised and will help to improve overall image quality.

Extended field of view: This feature stitches together multiple images as you translate the probe along a single axis. What this will allow you to do is provide a more complete image of a structure. Possibly helpful to documentation say of the location of a tendon tear since you can provide more context.

Elastography: This is another advanced imaging feature that uses the ultrasound beam to determine the modulus of elasticity within a tissue. Used mainly in Orthopaedic research it currently has limited clinical application. Therefore, at present, it is difficult to justify the increased cost but keep a close eye on this technology.

Spatial compound imaging: In spatial compound imaging the entering sound waves are varied in their direction slightly. This will improve the visualization of structures that are not entirely perpendicular to the probe, for example the ulnar portion of the transverse carpal ligament seen in the short axis of the wrist or the coracoacromial ligament seen in its long axis. This improvement does not carry over when viewed at other angles. The ulnar portion of the TCL can be hypoechogenic if the probe is in the long axis of the wrist.

3D imaging: While this may provide very nice-looking images, it is presently unclear what use it serves in MSK imaging.

Financing your Machine

Getting your practice or hospital system on board with spending money on an expensive machine can be tricky, especially when you are just starting out. However, not only can an ultrasound machine quickly pay for itself, but it is a great practice builder for you and your group. There are a number of billable CPT codes for performing focused or extensive diagnostic exams as well as ultrasound guided injections. To justify the cost of an average price console machine, you would have to do roughly 8 exams a week for 2 years.

You may decide that buying a machine is worth the investment in your own practice. If so, there are leasing options and monthly payment plans offered by many of the larger companies. When purchasing consider the warranty provided and customer service. Also consider asking about any ongoing fees, one well known handheld company requires that you pay for an annual subscription service to be able to save images.

Reimbursement/Coding

Coding for diagnostic and interventional ultrasound, as with all areas of medicine, is constantly changing and evolving. There may be regional variability and variable reimbursement based on insurance carrier. Most insurers base reimbursement on Medicare guidelines and relative value units (RVUs) as with other codes. It is most important to discuss this with your practice administrators and coders.

Most important, you do not need to be a radiologist to perform and bill for musculoskeletal ultrasound. The official statement on ultrasound billing from the American Institute of Ultrasound in Medicine (AIUM) reads: "Any qualified physician who interprets an indicated, appropriately performed, and documented ultrasound examination, should be allowed to bill for imaging services rendered. Representative guidelines for qualifications, performance, and documentation are located at http://www.aium.org/."

All diagnostic ultrasound examinations, including those when ultrasound is used to guide a procedure, require that permanently recorded images be maintained in the patient record. The images can be kept in the patient record or some other archive – they do not necessarily need to be submitted with the claim. Images can be stored as printed images, on a tape or electronic medium. Documentation of the study must be available to the insurer upon request. A written report of all ultrasound studies should be maintained in the patient's record. In the case of ultrasound guidance, the written report may be filed as a separate item in the patient's record, or it may be included within the report of the procedure for which the guidance is utilized.

In the office setting, a physician who owns the equipment and performs the service, may bill the global fee, which is represented by the CPT1 code without any modifiers. If the site of service is the hospital, the -26 modifier, indicating the professional service only was provided, must be added by the physician to the CPT code for the ultrasound service. Payers will not reimburse physicians for the technical component in the hospital setting. If billing for a procedure on the same day as an office visit, add modifier -25 to the office visit code to indicate a "significant, separately identifiable evaluation and management service."

Diagnostic ultrasound is billed as either a complete (76881) or limited exam (76882) with a -50 modifier for bilateral exams. A complete ultrasound for non-vascular extremity needs to be *very* complete, requires *a lot* of imaging and *detailed documentation* for all of it.

The code description for a complete ultrasound is: **76881** Ultrasound of the entire joint (ie, joint space and peri-articular soft tissue structures) real-time with image documentation. This code is describing a complete evaluation of a specific extremity (upper or lower) joint or region (e.g., volar wrist, lateral elbow) and requires examination of the following: the joint space (e.g., effusion); peri-articular soft tissue structures around the joint such as muscles, tendons, or other soft tissue structures); other identifiable abnormalities; and additional evaluations such as dynamic imaging or stress maneuvers as necessary. As with all ultrasounds, permanently recorded images are required along with a written report describing indications of medical necessity for the exam and all the above requirements, or reasons why any could not be captured.

The code description for a limited ultrasound is: **76882** Ultrasound, limited, joint or other nonvascular extremity structure(s) (e.g., joint space, peri-articular tendon[s], muscle[s], nerve[s], other soft tissue structure[s], or soft tissue mass[es]), real-time with image documentation. Orthopaedic surgeons will probably do far more limited exams because orthopaedic surgeons are looking to confirm or deny a particular diagnosis and the limited code (76882) will be used. Code 76882 describes the limited evaluation of a joint (*meaning less than the required elements for a complete exam are imaged*) or imaging of structure(s) within an extremity (non-vascular) other than a joint such as fluid collection, soft tissue masses, nerves, muscles, tendons, etc. As with the complete exam, permanently recorded images are required along with a written report describing indications of medical necessity for the exam.

There are three codes used to report arthrocentesis services with ultrasound guidance. Arthrocentesis, aspiration and/or injection of a small joint or bursa (e.g., fingers, toes), with ultrasound guidance, with permanent recording and reporting uses CPT code 20604. CPT code 20606 is used for an intermediate joint or bursa (e.g., temporomandibular, acromioclavicular, wrist, elbow or ankle, olecranon bursa, and CPT code 20611 for a major joint or bursa (e.g. shoulder, hip, knee joint, subacromial bursa).

To report the use of ultrasound to guide injections or aspirations, the suggested code is 76942 - Ultrasonic guidance for needle placement (e.g., biopsy, aspiration, injection, localization device), imaging supervision and interpretation. Report 76942 in addition to the code for the underlying procedure. Code 76942 is no longer used with joint arthrocentesis/injection (20604, 20606 and 20611), however it is included with CPT code 20526: Injection, therapeutic (e.g., local anesthetic, corticosteroid), carpal tunnel; CPT code 20527 Injection, enzyme (e.g., collagenase) palmar fascial cord (Dupuytren's cord) post enzyme injection; CPT code 20550 Injection(s) single tendon sheath, or ligament, aponeurosis (e.g., Biceps tendon); CPT code 20551 Injection(s) single tendon origin/insertion (e.g., medial/lateral epicondylitis); CPT code 20552 Injection(s), single to multiple trigger point(s) one or two muscle(s); CPT code 20553 Injection(s), single to multiple trigger point(s) three or more muscle(s); CPT code 20612 Aspiration and/or injection of ganglion(s) cyst any location.

Allowable codes for ultrasound guidance may be dependent on diagnostic codes and therefore one or the other or both may need to be modified. Also, the 76942 code is limited to one per patient per day (i.e., patient encounter). However, the bundled joint/bursa codes are not limited to one/day (but 2nd procedure modifier applies). You may not be able to bill the diagnostic code if billing a procedure code in the same region on the same day. As noted above, this should be reviewed with your practice managers and coders.

While it is important to be reimbursed for the work provided, the use of ultrasound adds much more significant value to your practice. It effectively and efficiently (for both you the surgeon and the patient) provides information regarding the specific patient's definitive diagnosis, educates the patient regarding their anatomy and underlying pathology, and further educates you the surgeon regarding musculoskeletal anatomy and pathology. It is extremely convenient and valuable for a patient to leave the clinic with a definitive diagnosis that they have confidence in, not to mention potentially the definitive management with a precisely guided intervention. While all these ultrasound procedures may not be fully reimbursed at a single encounter, the patient satisfaction has great potential for building your practice. Whether you openly promote this or not, primary care physicians, therapists and other front line providers will soon learn the value of sending their patients to you.

Practice Integration

The final barrier for many surgeons considering the use of in-office ultrasound may be how to perform the exams within their already busy clinic day. There may be push back not only from the surgeon, but also administrators, schedulers, and medical assistants. Some may try to bring patients back for diagnostic and interventional ultrasound procedures; however, this takes away from the ultimate efficiency and convenience of ultrasound. Others may have another provider within the group (e.g., non-operative physician or physician's associate) perform the exam or intervention. Again, this takes away from the overall education of the surgeon regarding the patient's specific anatomy and pathology and musculoskeletal anatomy and pathology in general.

No matter how busy you are, integrating ultrasound into your practice can be done. You must get your staff to buy into only it after you have bought into it yourself. Start with injections. While your assistants are getting the patient ready for the intervention see another patient or two. Do a brief exam and educate the patient while giving the injection not only about their pathology but also what to expect with the injection. This will help save time in the long run. For diagnostic exams, see several patients while your staff is getting the patient set up for the exam. While performing the exam discuss management options including risks and benefits of potential interventional procedures. That way, by the time the exam is completed, the patient can make an educated decision regarding which direction they would like to proceed. Since, this may include an ultrasound-guided injection, your staff will learn to anticipate it and be ready to seamlessly add it on to the end of the exam if desired.

It will only take a short time before you, your staff and your patients will actively seek the use of in-office ultrasound, making all of you question how you practiced so long without it.

References:

1. Kruse KK, Dilisio MF, Wang WL, Schmidt CC. Do we really need to order magnetic resonance imaging? Shoulder surgeon ultrasound practice patterns and beliefs. *JSES Open Access.* 2019;3(2):93-98. Published 2019 Apr 26. doi:10.1016/j.jses.2019.01.004

Subject Index

Volume 1

Volume 2